CO-BZC-237

NEUROPOISONS
THEIR PATHOPHYSIOLOGICAL ACTIONS

Volume 2–Poisons of Plant Origin

CONTRIBUTORS

Margaret Anderson	*Department of Biological Sciences, Smith College, Northampton, Massachusetts, U.S.A.*
P. B. Bradley	*Medical Research Council Neuropharmacology Unit, The Medical School, University of Birmingham, Birmingham, England*
I. Briggs	*Medical Research Council Neuropharmacology Unit, The Medical School, University of Birmingham, Birmingham, England*
D. R. Curtis	*Department of Pharmacology, Australian National University, Canberra, Australia*
Jose del Castillo	*Laboratory of Neurobiology and Department of Pharmacology, University of Puerto Rico, San Juan, Puerto Rico, U.S.A.*
Graham A. R. Johnston	*Department of Pharmacology, Australian National University, Canberra, Australia*
R. D. O'Brien	*Section of Neurobiology and Behavior, Cornell University, Ithaca, New York, U.S.A.*
Ronald W. Ryall	*Department of Pharmacology, University of Cambridge, Hills Road, Cambridge, England*
Theodore A. Slotkin	*Department of Physiology and Pharmacology, Duke University, Durham, North Carolina, U.S.A.*

NEUROPOISONS
THEIR PATHOPHYSIOLOGICAL ACTIONS

Volume 2–Poisons of Plant Origin

Edited by
L. L. Simpson
Departments of Pharmacology and Psychiatry
College of Physicians and Surgeons
Columbia University
New York, New York

and

D. R. Curtis
Department of Pharmacology
Australian National University
Canberra, Australia

PLENUM PRESS · NEW YORK AND LONDON

Library of Congress Cataloging in Publication Data

Simpson, Lance L.
Neuropoisons; their pathophysiological actions.

Vol. 2 edited by L.L. Simpson and D.R. Curtis.
Includes bibliographies.
CONTENTS: v. 1. Poisons of animal origin.—v. 2. Poisons of plant origin.
1. Poisons—Physiological effect. 2. Nervous system—Diseases. 3. Neuropharmacology. I. Curtis, David R., joint author. II. Title. [DNLM: 1. Animals, Poisonous. 2. Nervous System Diseases—Chemically induced. 3. Nervous System Diseases—Drug therapy. WD400 S613n]
RA1211.S55 615.9 76-128511
ISBN 0-306-37122-7

A Division of Plenum Publishing Corporation
227 West 17th Street, New York, N.Y. 10011

United Kingdom edition published by Plenum Press, London
A Division of Plenum Publishing Company, Ltd.
4a Lower John Street, London W1R 3PD, England

Printed in the United States of America

Contents of Volume 1

Preface

In Volume 1 of this series, attention was focused on neuropoisons of animal origin. In the present volume, attention has been shifted to poisons of plant origin. In both cases, we have attempted to identify those poisons for which there is a large measure of clinical or research interest.

Our efforts in compiling the series have been aided by three groups of individuals. First, we are grateful to the investigators who contributed chapters. Their labors are the substance of this two-volume work. Second, we are pleased to acknowledge the support of Mr. Seymour Weingarten and Plenum Press in our project. And third, we have been immeasurably aided by our assistants, Mrs. Ruby Hough in New York City and Mrs. Helena Walsh in Canberra. To all these persons, we are indebted.

Dr. Lance L. Simpson
New York City

Dr. David R. Curtis
Canberra

Contents

Chapter 4
Atropine **157**
by R. D. O'Brien

Chapter 5
Neurotoxic Amino Acids **179**
by Graham A. R. Johnston

Chapter 6
Convulsant Alkaloids **207**
by D. R. Curtis and G. A. R. Johnston

Chapter 7
Ergot Alkaloids and Related Substances **249**
by P. B. Bradley and I. Briggs

Chapter 1

Reserpine

Theodore A. Slotkin

Department of Physiology and Pharmacology
Duke University Medical Center
Durham, North Carolina, U.S.A.

I. INTRODUCTION

Reserpine, an alkaloid obtained from the roots of *Rauwolfia serpentina* (Fig. 1) and related species, is one of the drugs of antiquity. Primitive doctors have used *Rauwolfia* to treat a wide variety of diseases (Raymond-Hamet, 1939), and at least two of these actions have found a place in modern therapeutics, namely the antihypertensive and tranquilizing properties. In this respect, it is interesting to note that one of the common ancient names of *Rauwolfia* translates as "madman's medicine" (Saxton, 1960). References to the actions of *Rauwolfia* in the European literature date back to the sixteenth century (Rieppel, 1955), and the genus was named a century later in honor of Leonhard Rauwolf (*d.* 1596), an Augsburg physician who probably was not even acquainted with the plants (Rieppel, 1955). The first detailed description of the medicinal uses of *Rauwolfia* appeared in Rumpf's *Herbarii Amboinensis Auctuarium* (1755).

Despite the early interest in *Rauwolfia*, the attention of Western researchers was not revived until the 1930s, when the antihypertensive and antipsychotic actions of *R. serpentina* were again described (Sen and Bose, 1931); subsequently, detailed studies by Bhatia (1942) in India and by Vakil (1949) in Britain confirmed these reports. Further impetus was provided by the isolation of reserpine from *R. serpentina* by Müller *et al.* in 1952. Since then, thousands of articles have been published on all aspects of the chemistry and pharmacology of reserpine. This chapter reviews some of the

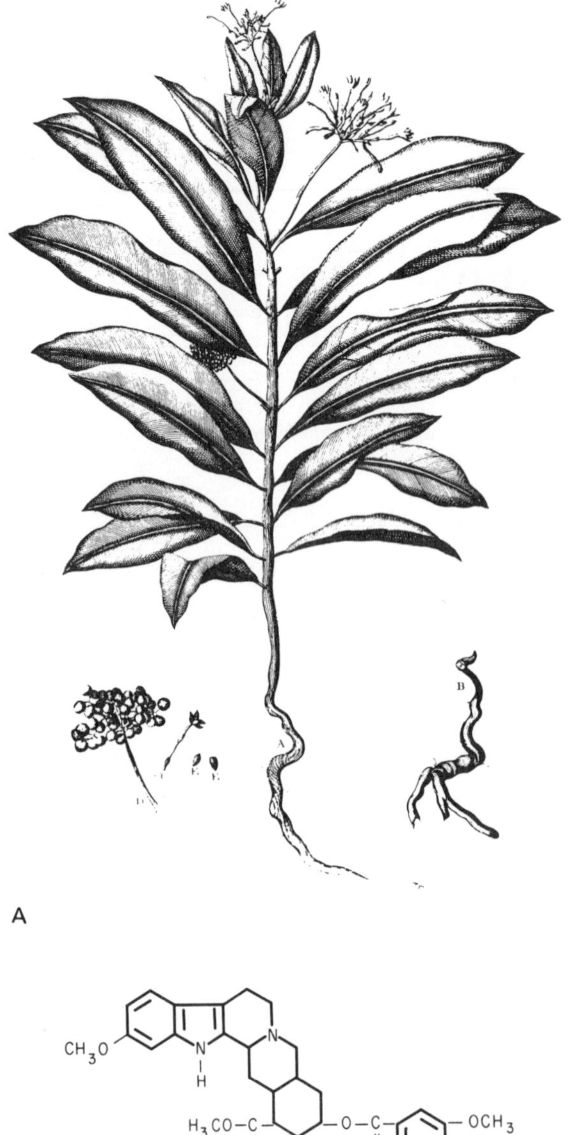

Fig. 1. (A) *Rauwolfia serpentina.* Reproduction of original engraving from Rumpf's *Herbarii Amboinensis Auctuarium* (1755). (B) Chemical structure of reserpine.

general aspects of the actions of reserpine, with particular attention to effects on nervous tissue.

II. BOTANY, PHARMACOGNOSY, AND CHEMISTRY

There are in excess of 100 recorded species of *Rauwolfia* (dogbane family, Apocynaceae), and these contain more than 50 different alkaloids (Lucas, 1963). The various species are found in tropical and subtropical regions of Central and South America, Africa, India, and Southeast Asia. *R. serpentina,* medicinally the most important species, is a woody shrub, generally less than a meter in height, bearing white blossoms, and is found primarily in India and portions of Southeast Asia and Indonesia (Saxton, 1960; Woodson *et al.,* 1957). The content of alkaloids in *R. serpentina* is about 1% by weight (Woodson *et al.,* 1957).

Reserpine is found in nearly all the species of *Rauwolfia*, and *R. serpentia* contains in addition about 20 related alkaloids (Lucas, 1963). These include ajmalicine, ajmaline, chandrine, corynanthrine, rauwolfinine, rescinnamine, reserpiline, serpentine, and yohimbine; only reserpine and rescinnamine have been found clinically useful, along with deserpidine (found primarily in *Rauwolfia* species other than *R. serpentina*) and syrosingopine (semisynthetic) (Schlittler and Plummer, 1964).

The first total synthesis of reserpine was achieved by Woodward *et al.* (1956*a,b*) and was later modified to permit more economical synthesis as well as chemical modification of the final product (Schlittler and Plummer, 1964). Subsequent X-ray crystallographic studies (Pepinsky *et al.*, 1957) and structural work (Woodson *et al.*, 1957) demonstrated that the absolute configuration of reserpine is 11,17α-dimethoxy-16β-carbomethoxy-18β-(3′,4′,5′-trimethoxybenzoyloxy)-3β,20α-yohimbane. While several stereoisomers of reserpine have been prepared synthetically (MacPhillamy *et al.*, 1955; Robinson *et al.*, 1961; Rosen and O'Connor, 1961), none of these retains pharmacological activity (Schlitter and Plummer, 1964).

Reserpine base (pK_b = 6.6) is a colorless powder nearly insoluble in water or solutions containing mineral salts but freely soluble in glacial acetic acid or chloroform. It is also soluble in aqueous solutions of organic acids or in mixed solvents such as citric acid, benzyl alcohol, polyethylene glycol, and water (Carlsson, 1965). The phosphate salt is readily soluble in water in concentrations up to about 0.01 M. Since reserpine is somewhat light sensitive, it is best stored in a dark bottle.

Detailed reviews of the botany, pharmacognosy, and chemistry of *Rauwolfia* species can be found in Woodson *et al.* (1957), Saxton (1960), Lucas (1963), and Schlittler and Plummer (1964).

III. DISTRIBUTION, BINDING, METABOLISM, AND EXCRETION OF RESERPINE

Reserpine falls into the class of drugs typified by thiopental (Brodie, 1964) and harmine (Slotkin *et al.*, 1970), which have a high degree of lipid solubility and consequently disappear from the bloodstream very rapidly (Hess *et al.*, 1956; DeFelice, 1957; Maass *et al.*, 1969). Due to the lipid solubility, reserpine levels decline slowly in adipose tissue, but rapidly (3–5 hr) in other tissues (Plummer *et al.*, 1957). In view of reserpine's actions on neural tissue, special consideration has been given to measurement of brain levels of the drug. In 1956, Hess *et al.* reported that the reserpine-induced depletion of brain serotonin persisted long after the drug was no longer detectable (2 hr), and this led to the suggestion that reserpine was a "hit-and-run" drug, one whose actions persisted after the drug itself had disappeared. However, subsequent studies utilizing radioactively labeled reserpine have demonstrated that a small amount of reserpine is persistently bound to brain tissue (Sheppard *et al.*, 1958; Manara and Garattini, 1967). Thus after a dose of 0.1 mg/kg in guinea pigs, a maximum brain level of reserpine of 12 ng/g is reached in 30 min; this declines to 7 ng/g in 2 hr but then remains steady for 48 hr (Plummer *et al.*, 1957). Similarly, traces of reserpine can be found in brains of treated mice as late as 120 hr after administration (Maggiolo and Haley, 1964), and traces of a pulse dose of radiolabeled reserpine are detectable in the feces of chronically reserpinized humans even after 10 days (Numerof *et al.*, 1958).

In peripheral nervous tissue, experiments on the binding of reserpine to subcellular components indicate that the long-term persistence of the drug may reflect binding to the putative site of action, namely catecholamine storage vesicles:

1. When isolated adrenal medullary storage vesicles are incubated with reserpine and then washed several times, the inhibition of amine uptake persists (Kirshner, 1962, Carlsson *et al.*, 1962, 1963), suggesting an irreversible action.
2. The degree of depletion of cardiac norepinephrine is directly proportional to the concentration of persistently bound reserpine (Alpers and Shore, 1969), which indicates that the bound reserpine is pharmacologically active.
3. Prior administration of unlabeled reserpine decreases the amount of subsequently administered ^{3}H-reserpine which is persistently bound to the storage vesicle (microsomal) fraction of mouse heart (Wagner and Stitzel, 1972), suggesting that the number of binding sites is fixed and that saturation can occur.

4. Eighteen hours after ^{3}H-reserpine administration, about half of the radioactivity associated with adrenergically innervated tissues can be removed by administration of unlabeled reserpine but at 30 hr none is removed (Norn and Shore, 1971*a*), indicating that the fraction of total drug persistently bound increases with time.
5. Stimulation of the neuron does not result in loss of bound ^{3}H-reserpine (Norn and Shore, 1971*b*); since vesicle membranes remain behind after secretion while the soluble contents of the vesicles are released (see Kirshner and Viveros, 1972), this suggests that the persistent binding is to the membrane of the storage vesicle.

Similar long-term binding occurs in the central nervous system; the subcellular distribution of reserpine in brain homogenates indicates that retention occurs in the microsomal fraction (Fig. 2) (Manara *et al.*, 1972). One hour after the *in vivo* administration of labeled reserpine to rats, the distribution of label was identical to the distribution when reserpine was added *in vitro* to brain homogenates of untreated rats, suggesting that physical and chemical factors determined the initial distribution of drug. Twenty-four hours after the *in vivo* administration of labeled reserpine, the distribution was quite different, with a marked increase in the percentage

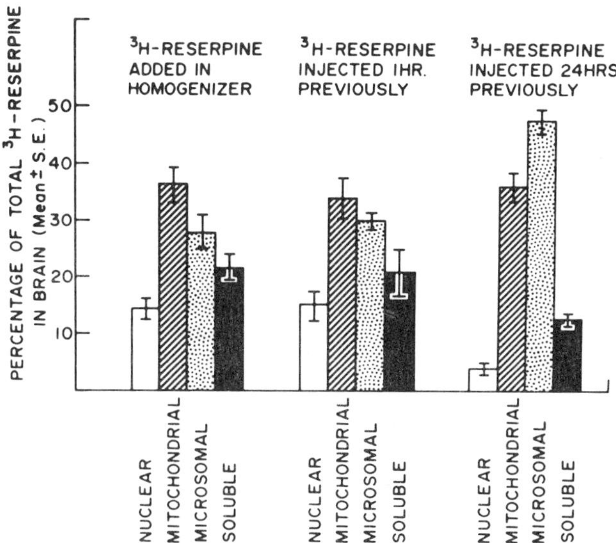

Fig. 2. Subcellular distribution of ^{3}H-reserpine in rat brain. Total dpm/g of brain tissue: 110,000 dpm/g added to homogenizers containing brains of untreated animals, 74,000 dpm/g at 1 hr, 7900 dpm/g at 24 hr. From Manara *et al.* (1972).

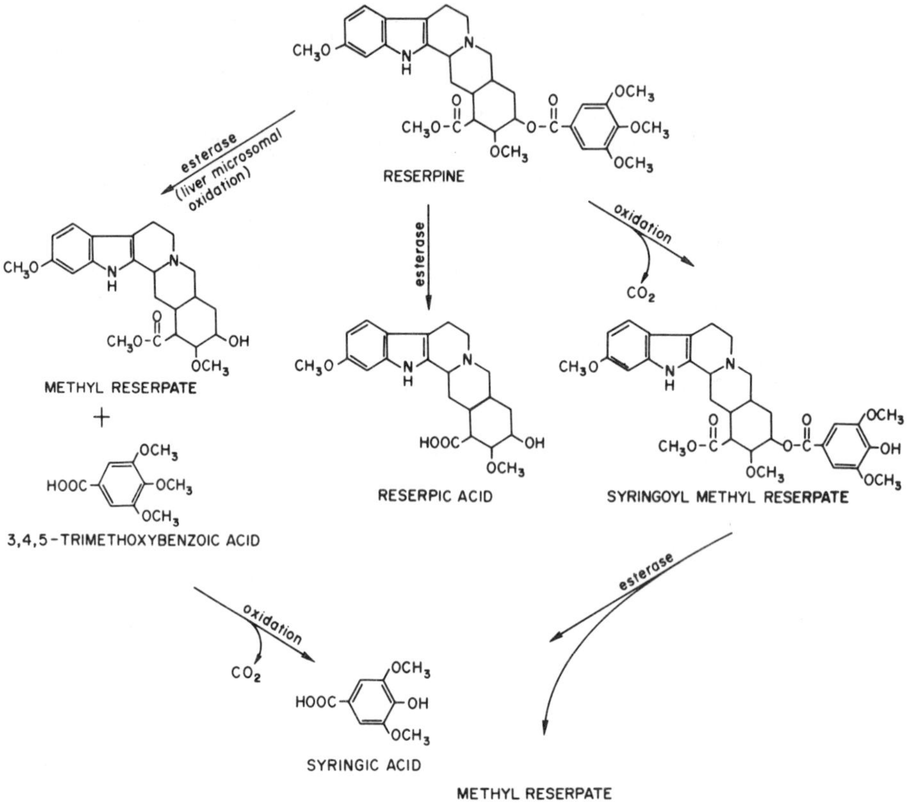

Fig. 3. Scheme of the metabolism of reserpine.

found in the storage vesicle–containing (microsomal) fraction (Fig. 2). Thus persistent binding occurs in brain as well as peripheral nervous tissue; the bound reserpine is not concentrated in any particular region, but rather is distributed throughout the brain (Enna and Shore, 1971).

Reserpine is a diester (positions 16 and 18), and hydrolysis occurs both *in vivo* and *in vitro* to give the metabolic products reserpic acid, methyl reserpate, and trimethoxybenzoic acid (Fig. 3) (Dhar *et al.*, 1955; Glazko *et al.*, 1956; Sheppard *et al.*, 1955; Plummer *et al.*, 1957), all of which are either inactive or less active than reserpine (Shore *et al.*, 1957). Recent studies suggest that the hydrolysis of the ester at the 18-position occurs mainly in the liver and that hydrolysis occurs secondarily to the action of a microsomal mixed-function oxidase (Stitzel *et al.*, 1972). Thus the metabolism of reserpine can be inhibited by hexobarbital, aniline, or SKF 525-

A, compounds which do not interfere with liver esterases but which do affect the liver microsomal oxidation system (Stitzel *et al.*, 1972). As a consequence of metabolism of reserpine by the liver, intraperitoneal administration produces a diminished effect compared to the subcutaneous route, since the drug must pass through the portal circulation after absorption from the peritoneal space (Rosecrans, 1967).

Most of administered reserpine is metabolized within several hours of drug administration (Numerof *et al.*, 1955), and very little is excreted unchanged (DeFelice, 1957; Plummer *et al.*, 1957). Some hydrolysis of the ester groups occurs in the intestine, and species differences in intestinal esterase activity may be in part responsible for differences in sensitivity to orally administered reserpine. In humans, fecal excretion of reserpine consists mostly of unchanged drug, suggesting that intestinal hydrolysis is unimportant (Maass *et al.*, 1969) and that most of the methyl reserpate found in the urine is the result of hydrolysis by the liver. Consequently, man, like the dog and monkey, is more sensitive to oral reserpine than the rat, whose intestinal esterase activity is high (Sheppard *et al.*, 1955; Glazko *et al.*, 1956; Plummer *et al.*, 1957).

In addition to hydrolysis of ester linkages, the 4-methoxy carbon on the trimethoxybenzoic acid moiety can be removed to form syringoyl methyl reserpate or syringic acid, and carbon dioxide (Fig. 3) (Sheppard *et al.*, 1957).

IV. EFFECTS ON BIOGENIC AMINES

Following the elucidation of much of the general pharmacology of reserpine in the early 1950s, Shore *et al.* (1955) and Pletscher *et al.* (1955) discovered that reserpine produced a marked depletion of brain serotonin accompanied by a rise in excretion of serotonin breakdown products. More importantly, in subsequent studies it was shown that reserpine also depleted catecholamines, resulting in adrenergic blockade (Carlsson and Hillarp, 1956; Bertler *et al.*, 1956). Finally, several years later, independent reports by Kirshner (1962) and Carlsson *et al.* (1962, 1963) demonstrated conclusively that the reserpine-induced depletion of catecholamines resulted from blockade of a magnesium-ATP-activated uptake system at the level of the adrenergic storage vesicle.

Because of the complex interplay of factors regulating synthesis, storage, release, and degradation of catecholamines and serotonin, it is important to review several of the salient points concerning these processes in order fully to understand the effects of reserpine on them. The current presentation is not intended as a definitive review of all aspects of the dynamics of neuronal amines, but rather represents a useful model based on numerous studies (primarily of peripheral adrenergic neurons and the adrenal medulla) published in the last two decades. For recent reviews, see Kopin (1968), Axelrod (1971), and Trendelenburg (1972).

A. General Aspects of Adrenergic and Serotonergic Transmission

A schematic representation of an adrenergic neuron varicosity appears in Fig. 4. The precursor of catecholamines, tyrosine, is in plentiful supply in the bloodstream (5×10^{-5} M) and may be actively accumulated by the neuron (step 1). In the cytoplasm, tyrosine is hydroxylated to form 3,4-dihydroxyphenylalanine (DOPA) (step 2) by the highly specific enzyme, tyrosine hydroxylase. Tyrosine hydroxylase is a mixed-function oxidase containing Fe^{2+} and requiring molecular oxygen and a pteridine cofactor (probably tetrahydrobiopterin) (Fig. 5); it is generally acknowledged that the activity of this enzyme is rate limiting in norepinephrine synthesis, since there is a comparative excess of the enzymes for the subsequent steps. There exist at least two mechanisms by which tyrosine hydroxylase activity (and therefore catecholamine synthesis) is regulated: first, there is end-product feedback inhibition of cytoplasmic norepinephrine on tyrosine hydroxylase activity, presumably through competition of norepinephrine with the pteridine cofactor. Additionally, the activity of tyrosine hydroxylase is increased by neural stimulation; this second process is apparently an enzyme induction and therefore requires *de novo* synthesis of the enzyme. Inhibitors of tyrosine hydroxylase include α-methyl-*p*-tyrosine (competitive with tyrosine) and various catechols (competitive with the pteridine cofactor).

The DOPA that is formed by hydroxylation of tyrosine is then decarboxylated in the cytoplasm to form dopamine (Fig. 4, step 3; Fig. 5). In contrast to tyrosine hydroxylase, DOPA decarboxylase is nonspecific and is also called "L-aromatic amino acid decarboxylase." It requires pyridoxal phosphate; its activity toward DOPA is inhibited competitively by α-methyl DOPA, which is also decarboxylated to α-methyldopamine.

Dopamine can be deaminated and inactivated by monoamine oxidase within the neuron (Fig. 4, step 4), a process which is inhibited by monoamine oxidase inhibitors, such as tranylcypromine, harmine, pargyline, and iproniazid; in addition, dopamine is accumulated by the storage vesicles (step 5) by an ATP-Mg^{2+}-stimulated mechanism. It is this uptake mechanism which is inhibited by reserpine, and most of the pharmacological and biochemical effects produced by reserpine result from changes in the disposition of amines caused by the inhibition.

Once dopamine is within the storage vesicle, it is acted on by dopamine β-hydroxylase (step 6), an enzyme which is associated partly with vesicle membranes and partly with soluble proteins within the vesicle. Dopamine β-hydroxylase, like tyrosine hydroxylase, is a mixed-function oxidase which, in the presence of copper, molecular oxygen, and a reducing agent (probably ascorbate), converts dopamine to norepinephrine (Fig. 5);

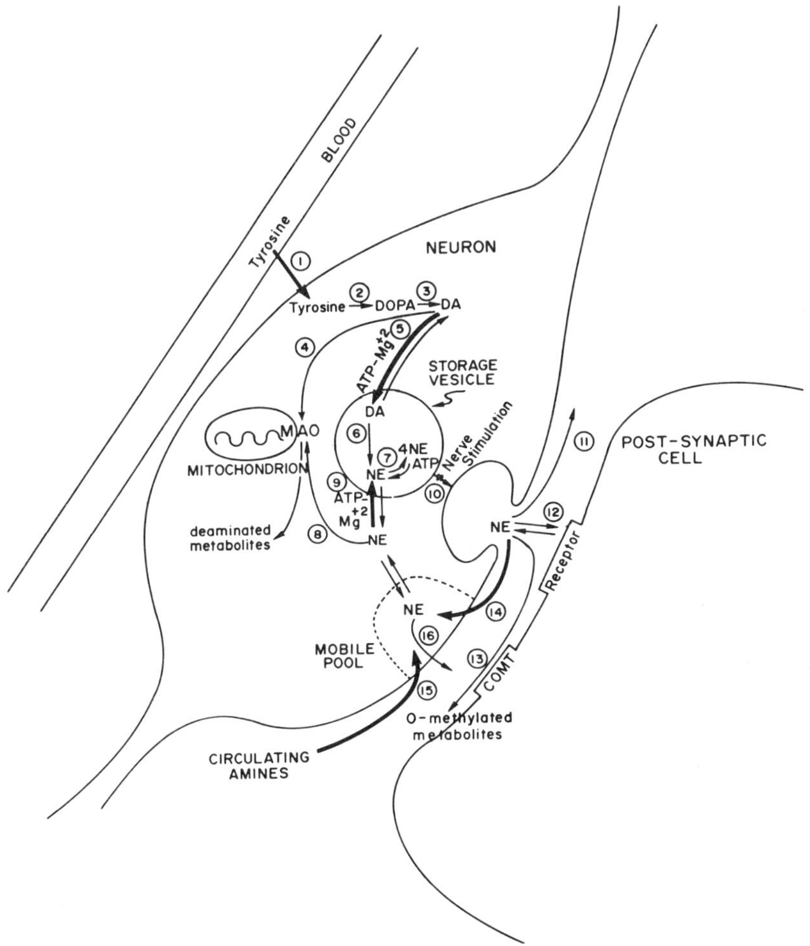

Fig. 4. Schematic representation of the adrenergic neuron. Heavy arrows denote active (energy-requiring) processes. Numbered steps are discussed in text. Abbreviations: DOPA, 3, 4-dihydroxyphenylalanine; DA, dopamine; NE, norepinephrine; MAO, monoamine oxidase; COMT, catechol-*O*-methyltransferase.

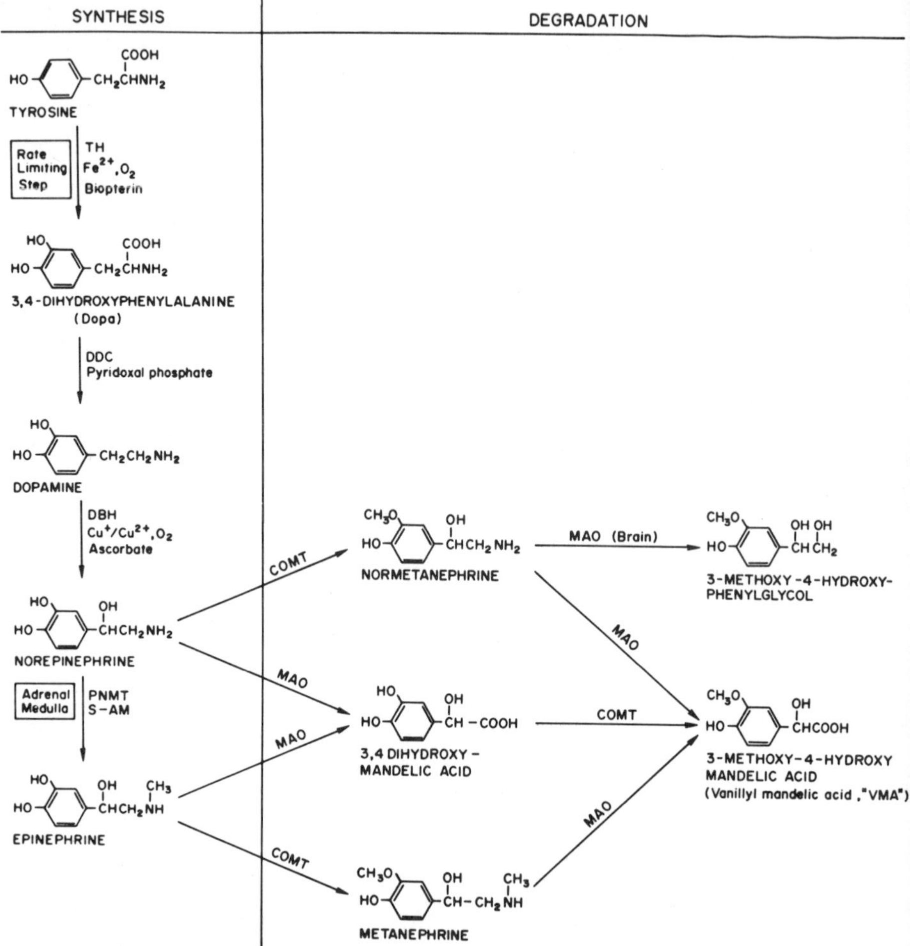

Fig. 5. Synthesis and degradation of catecholamines. Abbreviations: TH, tyrosine hydroxylase; DDC, DOPA decarboxylase; DBH, dopamine β-hydroxylase; PNMT, phenylethanolamine *N*-methyltransferase; S-AM, *S*-adenosylmethionine; MAO, monoamine oxidase; COMT, catechol-*O*-methyltransferase.

it is inhibited by disulfiram and copper-chelating agents (cyanide, for example). The enzyme also resembles tyrosine hydroxylase in that its levels are increased by neural stimulation. The norepinephrine formed in the vesicle can combine with ATP in the molar ratio of 4:1 to form a storage complex (possibly involving participation of proteins such as chromogranin A, and divalent cations) which is osmotically inactive (Fig. 4, step 7); in addition to blocking vesicular uptake, reserpine may have an effect on the formation of the complex.

The vesicle pool represents the major source of catecholamine storage, and the uptake and storage of catecholamines in the vesicles are crucial to the maintenance of the stores, since norepinephrine in the cytoplasm will be inactivated by monoamine oxidase (step 8). The dynamic equilibrium between cytoplasmic and vesicular norepinephrine favors storage, since the same active uptake which accumulates dopamine in the vesicles also takes up norepinephrine (step 9); the vesicular uptake of norepinephrine is potently inhibited by reserpine, which then shifts the storage equilibria toward dissociation of the complex and consequent washout into the cytoplasm.

On stimulation of the nerve, the membrane is depolarized, and there are sodium and calcium influx and potassium efflux; with the participation of the Ca^{2+}, the storage vesicles fuse temporarily with the cell membrane and the soluble contents of the vesicles are extruded into the synapse (step 10) while the vesicle membranes then detach from the interior of the cell membrane and remain behind (exocytosis); the release of catecholamines may also require the prior release of acetylcholine ("Burn–Rand hypothesis"). Secretion is prevented by adrenergic neuron–blocking agents (guanethidine and bretylium).

Once norepinephrine appears in the synapse, several events can occur. It can diffuse away from the synapse (step 11). It can combine with its receptor on the postsynaptic cell and thereby elicit a physiological response (step 12); this can be antagonized by adrenergic α- and β-blocking agents (phentolamine and propranolol). Also associated with the postsynaptic cell is the enzyme catechol-*O*-methyltransferase, which can inactivate norepinephrine (step 13); the enzyme is inhibited by tropolone derivatives.

By far the major pathway for removal of norepinephrine from the synapse is reuptake across the neuronal membrane (step 14) by an active pump which utilizes a Na^+-K^+-activated ATPase. It is inhibited by ouabain, cocaine, and tricyclic antidepressants, but not by reserpine. The pump, which also removes circulating amines (step 15), can be utilized by compounds related to norepinephrine but less active pharmacologically (false transmitters); these substances, such as metaraminol, amphetamine, octopamine, and α-methylnorepinephrine, then displace norepinephrine from a so-called mobile pool (step 16) and the displaced norepinephrine appears in the synapse. Ultimately, displacement of norepinephrine by false transmitters occurs in the storage vesicles, at which point adrenergic transmission is blocked or reduced because nerve stimulation now releases a less active amine than norepinephrine.

In the adrenal medulla, similar processes occur in the synthesis, storage, and release of catecholamines, but there are several important differences:

1. There is an additional synthetic step. Norepinephrine is *N*-methylated to form epinephrine by the enzyme phenylethanolamine *N*-methyltransferase, with *S*-adenosylmethionine serving as the methyl donor (Fig. 5). Since the enzyme is cytoplasmic, norepinephrine must first diffuse out of the vesicles and the epinephrine formed is then taken back up into the vesicles by the ATP-Mg^{2+}-stimulated (reserpine-inhibited) system.
2. The storage vesicles are much larger (1000–3000 A) than in adrenergic neurons (500–800 A).
3. Release is elicited by exposure to acetylcholine secreted by the splanchnic nerve.
4. Release of amines occurs into the general circulation rather then into a synapse.
5. There is no reuptake system in the cell membrane.

The degradation of catecholamines by monoamine oxidase and catechol-*O*-methytransferase is shown in Fig. 5. The metabolism of dopamine, although not shown, proceeds similarly. Because of the differences in localization of the enzymes, the relative amounts of each metabolite have been used to indicate whether amines have been functionally released: norepinephrine released into the synapse will be metabolized primarily by *O*-methylation to form normetanephrine, while intraneuronal norepinephrine will be preferentially deaminated to form 3,4-dihydroxymandelic acid (Fig. 5). Such inferences from metabolite formation have been vital in establishing the modes of action of reserpine and other drugs affecting adrenergic function. In human brain, the major degradation product of norepinephrine is 3-methoxy-4-hydroxyphenylglycol (Fig. 5); this observation provides an additional tool with which to evaluate alterations in brain catecholamines.

Serotonin is synthesized in a two-step process (Fig. 6). Tryptophan is converted by tryptophan hydroxylase to 5-hydroxytryptophan, which is then decarboxylated to form serotonin. In the pineal gland only, two additional steps convert serotonin to melatonin (Fig. 6). Serotonin is degraded primarily by monoamine oxidase to form 5-hydroxyindoleacetic acid (HIAA); it has been suggested that direct sulfate conjugation or *N*-methylation of serotonin may also occur.

Studies on the uptake, storage, and release of serotonin have been hampered by the lack of a peripheral model (such as sympathetic neurons or the adrenal medulla for catecholamines), but it is generally accepted that serotonergic neurons carry on the same basic functions that adrenergic neurons do: storage in vesicles, vesicular uptake of serotonin, active neuronal uptake from the synapse, etc. However, there are notable differences between serotonergic and adrenergic neurons; there is no intravesicular synthetic step, the neuronal uptake of serotonin is not ouabain sensitive, and also serotonin depletion is less marked than catecholamine depletion after reserpine and more marked after *p*-chlorophenylalanine. Reserpine is postulated to act in the same way in serotonergic and adrenergic neurons, namely by inhibition of the storage vesicle uptake system, and while most mechanistic inferences have been drawn primarily from effects on catecholamines, similar effects seem to hold true for serotonin. For a more detailed discussion of serotonin synthesis, uptake, storage, and release, see Barchas *et al*. (1972).

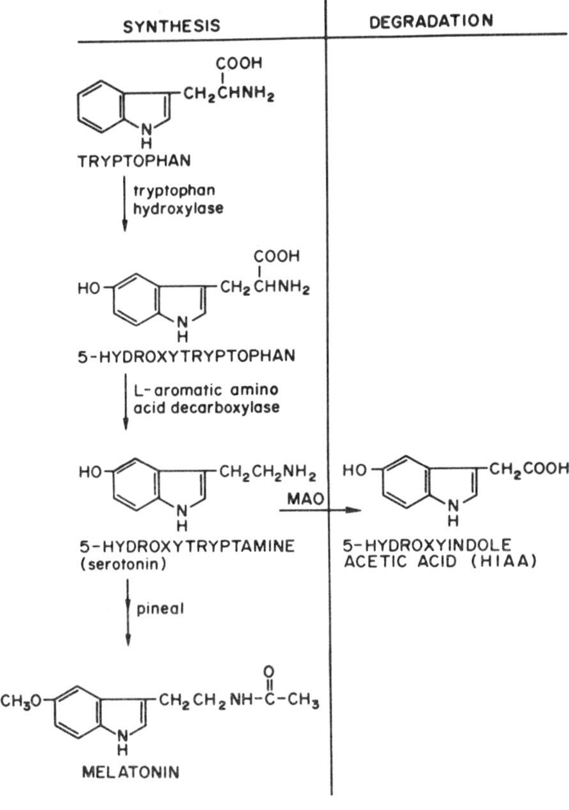

Fig. 6. Synthesis and degradation of serotonin.

From the foregoing processes occurring in adrenergic and serotonergic neurons, it is evident that reserpine-induced blockade of vesicular uptake and the consequent depletion of amines will have a wide variety of effects on the dynamics of neurotransmitter disposition. The rest of this section is devoted to a discussion of these changes and the mechanistic inferences which can be made from them.

B. Effects on Biogenic Amine Levels

A vast literature exists on the effects of reserpine on biogenic amine levels. Only a small number of these reports are reviewed in this chapter; for further information, see the reviews by Carlsson (1965), Stjärne (1972), and von Euler (1972).

In every tissue examined which contains catecholamines, reserpine produces a marked depletion. In rabbits given 5 mg/kg of reserpine intravenously, Carlsson *et al.* (1957*a*) observed a rapid decrease in brain catecholamines, a somewhat slower decrease in the heart, and a much slower decrease in the adrenals (Fig. 7), the last requiring 5 hr for maximal depletion. Recovery took 10 days in the peripheral tissues and a period of several weeks in the brain. Similarly, Bertler (1961) has observed depletion of rabbit brain norepinephrine and dopamine after 1 mg/kg of reserpine, and Berkowitz *et al.* (1971) reported reserpine-induced depletion of catecholamines from all sympathetically innervated tissues in the cardiovascular system.

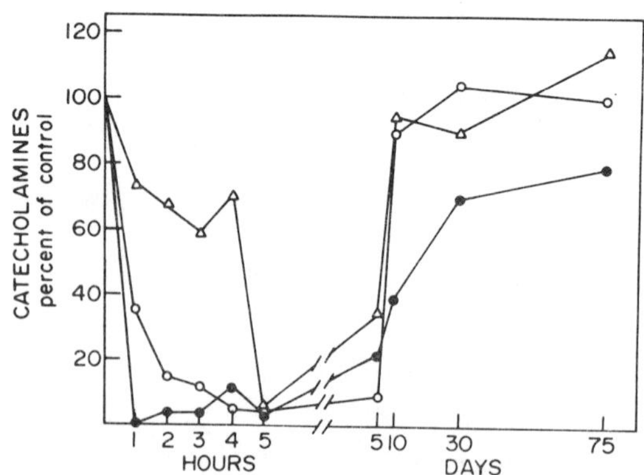

Fig. 7. Depletion and recovery of catecholamines from rabbit adrenal (Δ), heart (O), and brain (●) after 5 mg/kg of reserpine intravenously. From Carlsson *et al.* (1957*a*).

In general, the rate at which depletion occurs in a given tissue is determined by the rate at which the adrenergic neurons in that tissue (or, in the case of the adrenal medulla, the splanchnic nerve) are being stimulated (Bertler, 1961; Carlsson, 1965). Thus the rapid turnover of catecholamines in the brain makes that tissue most susceptible to depletion, while the slow turnover in the adrenal medulla results in a slower rate of loss. Since reserpine causes reflex sympathetic stimulation, this provides an additional mode of amine depletion: amines are lost via secretion, and the increased turnover accelerates the onset of functional blockade of adrenergic transmission. Thus prior administration of a ganglionic blocking agent (which reduces the rate of stimulation of the postganglionic neurons) reduces the rate of catecholamine depletion in sympathetically innervated tissues, particularly in the adrenal medulla (Viveros *et al.*, 1969*a*).

The depletion of neuronal scrotonin after reserpine administration proceeds in much the same manner as does depletion of catecholamines, although in general serotonergic neurons are less sensitive than adrenergic neurons (Barchas *et al.*, 1972). Decreases in serotonin are also seen in blood, platelets, intestine, and lung (Carlsson, 1965). In addition to differences in depletion of each amine, there are considerable differences in the susceptibility of various species; rats are considerably more resistant to reserpine-induced depletion than are guinea pigs or rabbits (Carlsson, 1965).

Of all the pharmacological and biochemical effects of reserpine, the most important is the depletion of catecholamines and serotonin which results from blockade of vesicular uptake. The immediate consequence of depletion is interference with adrenergic ("chemical sympathectomy") and serotonergic neurotransmission with consequent changes in cardiovascular and temperature regulation, endocrine function, mood, etc.; the alterations which result from depletion are the subject of Sections V, VI, and VII.

C. Effects on Biogenic Amine Synthesis and Metabolism

The actions of reserpine on catecholamine synthesis are complex, consisting of at least three distinct actions:

1. Inhibition of hydroxylation of dopamine via
   a. interference with vesicular uptake.
   b. loss of vesicle integrity due to secretion from reflex stimulation.
2. Initial increase in end-product feedback inhibition of tyrosine hydroxylase, followed by later removal of inhibition.
3. Transsynaptic induction of tyrosine hydroxylase and dopamine β-hydroxylase.

Since dopamine β-hydroxylase is localized solely within the storage vesicles, it is to be expected that blockade of dopamine uptake into the vesicles will result in a functional inhibition of the enzyme (Kirshner, 1962). In splenic nerve and in nerve trunk particles, Stjärne and Lishajko (1966) and Roth and Stone (1968) observed decreased conversion of dopamine to norepinephrine. Similar results were obtained in brain by Glowinski *et al.* (1966) and in heart by Jonsson and Sachs (1970); although some synthesis of ^{3}H-norepinephrine from ^{3}H-dopamine occurs after reserpine administration, in general the incorporation is far below control levels. In perfused rabbit heart, Rutledge and Weiner (1967) demonstrated reserpine-induced reductions in synthesis of dopamine and norepinephrine from labeled tyrosine. When a monoamine oxidase inhibitor was given prior to reserpine, the decreased synthesis of dopamine was markedly reversed, indicating that reserpine inhibited apparent dopamine synthesis indirectly: by preventing entry of dopamine into the storage vesicles, reserpine made the dopamine accessible to deaminative metabolism. On the other hand, monoamine oxidase inhibition produced only a small reversal of the decrease in norepinephrine synthesis, indicating that, unlike dopamine, the synthesis of norepinephrine was dependent on vesicular uptake and that inhibition of uptake by reserpine denied the dopamine access to dopamine β-hydroxylase.

It is interesting to note that the small degree of reversal of reserpine inhibition of norepinephrine synthesis seen after monoamine oxidase inhibitors can be further enhanced in the adrenal medulla by the administration of large amounts of DOPA (Bertler *et al.*, 1961). These data suggest that the reversal is due to an increase in intracellular dopamine which then competes with reserpine for uptake sites; in addition, the higher dopamine concentrations would shift the type of vesicular uptake toward a reserpine-insensitive mechanism (see Sections IVE,G).

In the adrenal medulla, there is also a loss of vesicle integrity after reserpine as a result of the high degree of reflex stimulation-induced secretion. After vesicles have released their contents, they are no longer capable of taking up amines; in addition, there is a loss of the soluble dopamine β-hydroxylase, which is secreted along with the other soluble vesicle proteins, catecholamines, and nucleotides (Viveros *et al.*, 1969*b*). The secretion is prevented by pretreatment with ganglionic blocking agents (Viveros *et al.*, 1969*b*; Slotkin and Edwards, 1973). Since there is a vast excess of dopamine β-hydroxylase compared to tyrosine hydroxylase, the loss of the former enzyme probably does not contribute to reduced catecholamine synthesis.

Because of the efficient neuronal reuptake of catecholamines released into the synapse, blockade of vesicular uptake by reserpine should result in an initial *increase* in cytoplasmic norepinephrine after neural stimulation. Thus one would expect to see a decrease in tyrosine hydroxylase activity as a result of increased feedback inhibition by cytoplasmic norepinephrine; as depletion of catecholamines occurs, the feedback inhibition would subside. Weiner *et al.* (1972) administered 2 mg/kg of reserpine to mice and measured tyrosine hydroxylase activities in vasa deferentia at several time periods after drug administration (Fig. 8). Reserpine produced an initial decrease in activity, but the activity returned to normal by 26 hr; in contrast, administration of the injection vehicle alone produced an increase in tyrosine hydroxylase activity (presumably stress related). These data show that reserpine does indeed produce a transient decrease in the activity of the rate-limiting enzyme in norepinephrine synthesis. However, Boadle-Biber and Roth (1972) have suggested that reserpine may inhibit tyrosine hydroxylase directly.

Agents which lower blood pressure, such as reserpine and phenoxybenzamine, evoke a reflex increase in stimulation of the sympathetic nervous system and the adrenal medulla, which in turn causes an

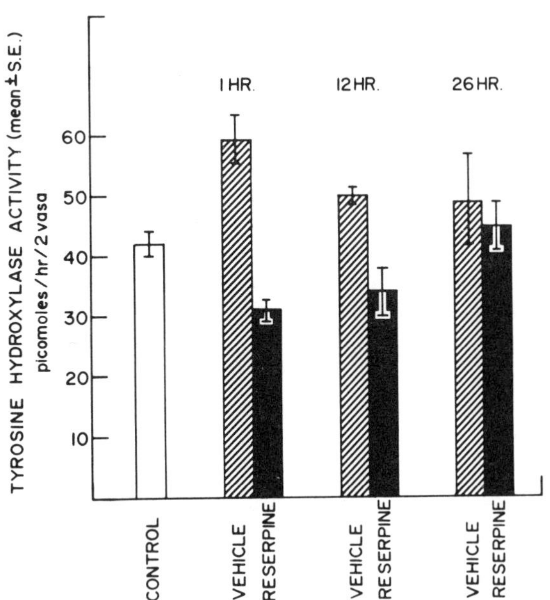

Fig. 8. Tyrosine hydroxylase activity in mouse vasa deferentia after administration of reserpine, 2 mg/kg intraperitoneally in 5% ascorbate, or of ascorbate vehicle. Vehicle-treated mice show stress-related increases in activity, while reserpine treatment produces a short-term (less than 1 day) decrease. From Weiner *et al.* (1972).

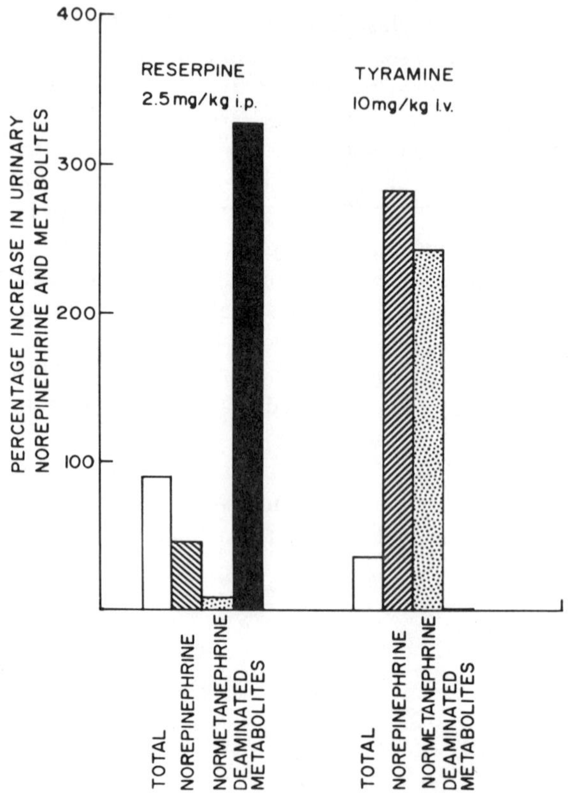

Fig. 9. Urinary excretion of ^{3}H-norepinephrine and its metabolites in rats after reserpine or tyramine administration. Animals were given 100 μCi of ^{3}H-norepinephrine intravenously followed by reserpine or tyramine 10 hr later, and urine was collected over the subsequent 4-hr period. From Kopin and Gordon (1963).

increase in the levels of tyrosine hydroxylase and dopamine β-hydroxylase ("transsynaptic induction") (Viveros *et al.*, 1969*b*, 1971; Axelrod *et al.*, 1970; Axelrod, 1971, Patrick and Kirshner, 1971; Bhagat *et al.*, 1971). The increases can be prevented by prior decentralization and subsequently restored in the adrenal medulla by exposure to the neurotransmitter, acetylcholine (Patrick and Kirshner, 1971), indicating that the induction is a consequence of stimulation rather than catecholamine depletion *per se*. The increases in both enzymes are functional increases: the resynthesis of catecholamines is probably rate limiting in the recovery from depletion (Slotkin and Kirshner, 1973*a*; Slotkin and Edwards, 1973), and an increase in the rate-limiting enzyme would accelerate reestablishment of the stores.

In addition, the persistent effect of reserpine probably necessitates in part the resynthesis of storage vesicles to permit recovery after reserpine, and the increased dopamine β-hydroxylase reflects accelerated resynthesis of vesicles.

Thus the effects of reserpine on catecholamine synthesis can be divided into two phases: initially, there is a decrease in catecholamine synthesis resulting from blockage of dopamine uptake into storage vesicles along with direct and feedback inhibition of tyrosine hydroxylase. Later, the rate of synthesis is increased, due in part to removal of feedback inhibition and also to transsynaptic induction of tyrosine hydroxylase and dopamine β-hydroxylase.

The effects of reserpine on the degradation of biogenic amines are considerably less complex than effects on synthesis. Because monoamine oxidase is localized intraneuronally, while catechol-*O*-methyltransferase is associated with the postsynaptic cell, blockade of vesicular uptake, which results in the intraneuronal release of amines, will cause an increase in deaminated vs. *O*-methylated metabolites. After administration of 2.5 mg/kg of reserpine to rats, Kopin and Gordon (1963) found a large increase in urinary excretion of deaminated metabolites but only a small change in normetanephrine (Fig. 9); on the other hand, tyramine, which releases norepinephrine from the mobile pool into the synapse, produced an increase in norepinephrine and normetanephrine excretion but not of deaminated metabolites. When ^{3}H-norepinephrine is administered intraventricularly, identical effects of reserpine on the metabolism of brain catecholamines can be observed (Sulser *et al.*, 1969). Similarly, reserpine causes a rise in brain levels of deaminated dopamine metabolites, 3,4-dihydroxyphenylacetic acid and homovanillic acid (3-methoxy-4-hydroxyphenylacetic acid), and the rise in the former metabolite precedes the latter, indicating that metabolism by monoamine oxidase occurs first (Andén *et al.*, 1963, 1964); serotonin metabolism is also affected by reserpine administration, with marked increases in urinary excretion of 5-hydroxyindoleacetic acid (Shore *et al.*, 1955; Carlsson, 1965) and elevations in brain levels of the metabolite (Andén *et al.*, 1963).

D. Effects on Biogenic Amine Uptake, Retention, and Release

The uptake and storage of biogenic amines in neuronal tissue play vital roles in the maintenance of normal levels of the amines and consequently affect neurotransmission. Numerous studies have been carried out on catecholamine uptake and storage systems in virtually all adrenergically innervated tissues as well as in the central nervous system and the

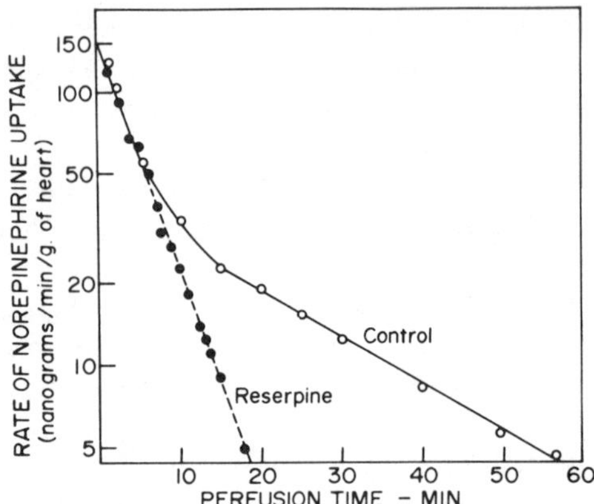

Fig. 10. Rate of uptake of ^{3}H-norepinephrine in isolated perfused hearts from control and reserpine-pretreated rats; medium contained 200 ng/ml ^{3}H-norepinephrine. From Iversen *et al.* (1965).

adrenal medulla (see review by Kirshner *et al.*, 1971); the general characteristics of uptake into intact tissues and the effects of reserpine from one such study are shown in Fig. 10 (Iversen *et al.*, 1965). The rate of uptake of norepinephrine in isolated perfused rat heart exhibits a biphasic character, with an initially high rate of uptake and a subsequently slower rate. Pretreatment of the animals with reserpine results in an elimination of the slow phase of uptake. In addition, the subcellular locus of the incorporated norepinephrine is altered by reserpine, with a marked decrease in the amount of label in the microsomal (storage vesicle–containing) fraction but no decrease in the soluble or mitochondrial fractions (Iversen *et al.*, 1965). Thus reserpine administered *in vivo* appears to block incorporation into the storage vesicles but does not affect the uptake across the neuronal membrane; neuronal uptake represents the rapid initial rate of incorporation and vesicular uptake the slower, subsequent rate. In addition, studies utilizing fluorescence histochemistry (Hillarp and Malmfors, 1964; Hamberger *et al.*, 1964) demonstrate that reserpine depletes catecholamines from sympathetic nerves but that subsequent administration of norepinephrine along with a monoamine oxidase inhibitor results in a reappearance of histofluorescence. The histofluorescence does not have a typical "beaded" appearance of untreated nerves but rather shows a uniform distribution throughout the neuron. In the absence of a monoamine oxidase inhibitor, no fluorescence is detected. These data indicate that uptake into the neuron proceeds normally after reserpine but that incorporation into vesicles does not occur.

The specific site of action of reserpine has been identified in studies utilizing isolated adrenal storage vesicles (Kirshner, 1962; Carlsson *et al.*, 1962, 1963) and neuronal vesicles from many sources (see reviews by von Euler, 1972; Shore, 1972; Stjärne, 1972). These studies indicate that:

1. There is an ATP-Mg^{2+}-stimulated uptake mechanism in the storage vesicles.
2. The major effect of reserpine is the inhibition of this uptake.

Thus, when isolated bovine adrenal vesicles are incubated with epinephrine, the degree of uptake is markedly increased by the addition of ATP and Mg^{2+}, but the increase is eliminated by reserpine (Fig. 11). However, when vesicles are incubated *in vitro*, no actual *net* accumulation of amines occurs, even in the presence of ATP and Mg^{2+}, because there is also a spontaneous efflux of endogenous amines which occurs simultaneously with the uptake of exogenous amines; thus in the absence of ATP and Mg^{2+} there is a net loss of amines, while in the presence of ATP and Mg^{2+} the uptake balances the efflux. In vesicles partially depleted of their contents, net accumulation of catecholamines does occur in the presence of ATP and Mg^{2+}, and is blocked by reserpine (Lishajko, 1971). These studies indicate the significance of the blockade of ATP-Mg^{2+}-stimulated uptake by reserpine: since the major fraction of neuronal amines is stored in the vesicles, uptake of norepinephrine *in vivo* is generally inhibited more than 90% by reserpine administration (Muscholl, 1960; Hertting *et al.*, 1961). Serotonin uptake into various tissues is similarly affected

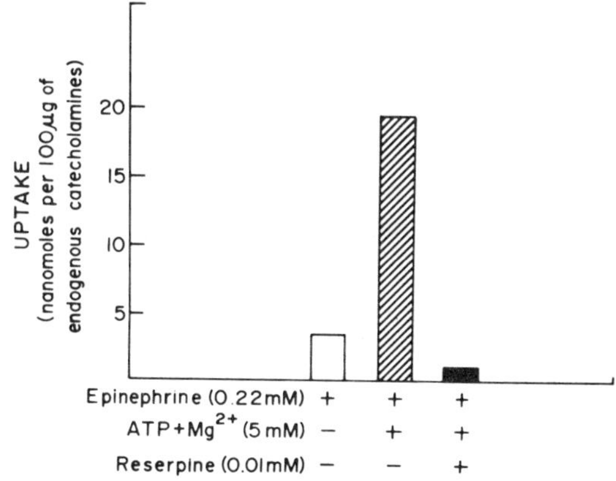

Fig. 11. Uptake of ¹⁴C-epinephrine by isolated bovine adrenal medullary vesicles. Vesicles were incubated for 20 min at 30°C in isotonic sucrose. From Slotkin *et al.* (1971).

(Carlsson, 1965; Barchas *et al.*, 1972). As a result, administration of reserpine leads to the depletion of catecholamines and serotonin.

A detailed discussion of the mechanism of reserpine inhibition of vesicular uptake appears in Section IVG.

The catecholamine–ATP storage complex may represent an additional site of action of reserpine. The complex itself is inherently stable, since adrenal vesicles in isotonic media and in the absence of amines or energy utilization maintain their stores for several days at 0°C (Falck *et al.*, 1956) despite the fact that the membrane is permeable to catecholamines and ATP at this temperature (Hillarp, 1959; Kirshner *et al.*, 1966). The latter observation also indicates that the complex is nondiffusible; it is also osmotically inactive, since the intravesicular amine and ATP concentrations are 0.6 and 0.15 M, respectively. The complex may contain, in addition to amines and ATP, proteins (perhaps chromogranins), divalent cations, or RNA, and may exist in a gel form or in high molecular weight aggregates (Hillarp, 1958; Holtz and Palm, 1966; Phillipu and Schümann, 1966; Smith, 1968; Berneis *et al.*, 1969). Recent studies have demonstrated that mixtures of catecholamines, ATP, and divalent cations form a multimolecular complex *in vitro* and that reserpine alters the phase separation of the complex in aqueous solutions (Berneis *et al.*, 1970). Similar observations have been made with serotonin–ATP mixtures (Pletscher *et al.*, 1971). The obvious implication is that reserpine may have an effect on the storage process that is distinct from uptake. However, several factors militate against this interpretation:

1. The aggregates do not form at physiological temperatures.
2. Reserpine appears to be bound to the storage vesicle membranes rather than inside the vesicle (see Section III).
3. In conditions under which amines leak from isolated adrenal vesicles at a rate dependent on stability of the storage complex (isotonic sucrose, no ATP or Mg^{2+}, 30–37°C), reserpine does not affect the rate of efflux (Slotkin *et al.*, 1971).

Thus the evidence that reserpine disrupts the storage complex is not conclusive.

When adrenal storage vesicles are incubated in chloride-containing isotonic salt medium (rather than sucrose), a spontaneous release of catecholamines (as well as ATP and proteins) occurs which is also stimulated by ATP and Mg^{2+} (Oka *et al.*, 1966; Poisner and Trifaró, 1967; Ferris *et al.*, 1970; Lishajko, 1971). Interestingly, the release is blocked by *N*-ethylmaleimide, which blocks the vesicle membrane ATPase and ATP-Mg^{2+}-stimulated amine uptake; however, reserpine has little or no effect on the release process except at high concentrations (0.05–0.1 mM), where enhanced release is observed (Ferris *et al.*, 1970). In neuronal vesicles incubated in isotonic sucrose, reserpine reduces the spontaneous efflux of amines, thus reducing the exchangeability of the amine store (Klein and Lagercrantz, 1971; Lagercrantz, 1971); however, since the effect on the uptake of amines is fiftyfold greater than the effect on release, the significance of the latter observation remains to be assessed.

In conclusion, the depletion of catecholamines and serotonin by reserpine, and the consequent interruption of neurotransmission, is most likely due to blockade of ATP-Mg^{2+}-stimulated catecholamine uptake into the storage vesicles rather than effects on the storage complex or on release.

E. Adrenergic False Transmitters and Reserpine-Resistant Amine Pools

When norepinephrine is infused in fully reserpinized animals, the actions of some pharmacological agents on adrenergic function are restored for a short period of time (Burn and Rand, 1958, 1960, 1962); for example, the catecholamine-releasing effect of drugs which utilize the neuronal uptake system reappears after the norepinephrine infusion (Nasmyth, 1962; Smith, 1963; Lundborg and Waldeck, 1971). What is occurring, obviously, is the replenishment of the mobile pool of norepinephrine. Since reserpine does not affect neuronal uptake, norepinephrine is removed from the synapse and enters the mobile pool, from which it is eventually inactivated by monoamine oxidase, thus accounting for the transient nature of the recovery. During this period in which appreciable unchanged norepinephrine is present, catecholamine releasers such as tyramine, metaraminol, octopamine, α-methylnorepinephrine, and amphetamine (Fig. 12) would be able to produce their typical sympathomimetic effects. However, since physiological release of catecholamines from stimulated nerves probably involves release from the storage vesicles, one would not expect the infusion of norepinephrine to restore the response to stimulation; DeSchaepdryver *et al.* (1963) and Gaffney *et al.* (1963) have demonstrated this lack of physiological recovery in dogs. Replenishment of the mobile pool and displacement of norepinephrine by other amines are preventable by administration of blockers of uptake at the neuronal membrane (see Section IVG). These studies indicate that the cytoplasmic mobile pool of norepinephrine represents a pharmacologically important reserpine-resistant pool.

Many of the drugs which displace norepinephrine from the mobile pool also have the ability to replace norepinephrine in the storage vesicles; these compounds are generally called "false transmitters" because nerve

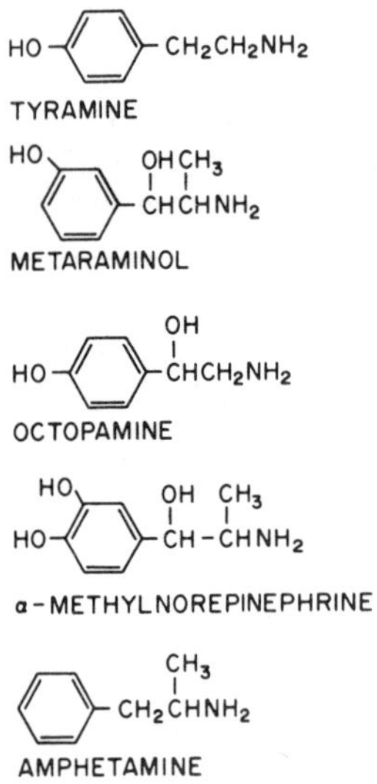

TYRAMINE

METARAMINOL

OCTOPAMINE

α-METHYLNOREPINEPHRINE

AMPHETAMINE

Fig. 12. Structures of drugs which displace catecholamines from the mobile pool and/or storage vesicles.

stimulation subsequent to administration of one of these drugs leads to the release of the pharmacologically less active compound along with norepinephrine. Consequently, most false transmitters have both sympathomimetic and sympatholytic effects: the initial administration leads to displacement of norepinephrine from the mobile pool into the synapse, producing actions similar to nerve stimulation. Once norepinephrine is replaced in the vesicle by the false transmitter, nerve stimulation results in a below-normal adrenergic effect. In this section, the interactions of reserpine with the two most widely studied false transmitters, α-methylnorepinephrine and metaraminol, are discussed; for a recent review of false transmitters, see Muscholl (1972).

When α-methylnorepinephrine is incorporated into storage vesicles, it is less readily depleted by reserpine than is norepinephrine (Lindmar and Muscholl, 1965; Schümann *et al.*, 1965; Muscholl and Sprenger, 1966; Carlsson and Waldeck, 1968). Since the α-methyl group confers resistance to monoamine oxidase, the increased ratio of cytoplasmic to vesicular amines after reserpine will result in the preferential destruction of norepinephrine. In addition, the α-methyl group increases the affinity of the amine for the vesicular uptake system (Slotkin and Kirshner, 1971), although it decreases the stability of storage (Lundborg and Stitzel, 1967*a*; Slotkin and Kirshner, 1971). Since the primary effect of reserpine is competitive blockade of vesicular uptake, the incorporation of norepinephrine will be inhibited to a greater extent than that of α-methylnorepinephrine at low concentrations of reserpine, but at concentrations of reserpine which produce total blockade of uptake, both amines will be depleted (Lindmar and Muscholl, 1965; Muscholl and Sprenger, 1966).

In addition to resistance to deamination and higher affinity for uptake into vesicles, α-methylnorepinephrine and, to a greater extent, metaraminol utilize a second vesicular uptake system which is not stimulated by ATP and Mg^{2+} and is not blocked by reserpine (Carlsson *et al.*, 1967; Lundborg and Stitzel, 1967*a,b*; Slotkin *et al.*, 1971; Slotkin and Kirshner, 1971). The differences between the two uptake mechanisms can be characterized as follows:

1. Specificity: Catecholamines utilize the reserpine-sensitive system; metaraminol utilizes the reserpine-insensitive system (Fig. 13A).
2. Stimulation: There is a marked increase in catecholamine uptake with ATP and Mg^{2+}, but only a small increase in metaraminol uptake (Fig. 13B).
3. Concentration: The uptake of catecholamines by the stimulated mechanism occurs at low concentrations; higher concentrations are required for the nonstimulated mechanism (Fig. 13B). Consequently, reserpine blockade is overcome by higher catecholamine concentrations (Fig. 13C) by at least two mechanisms—increased

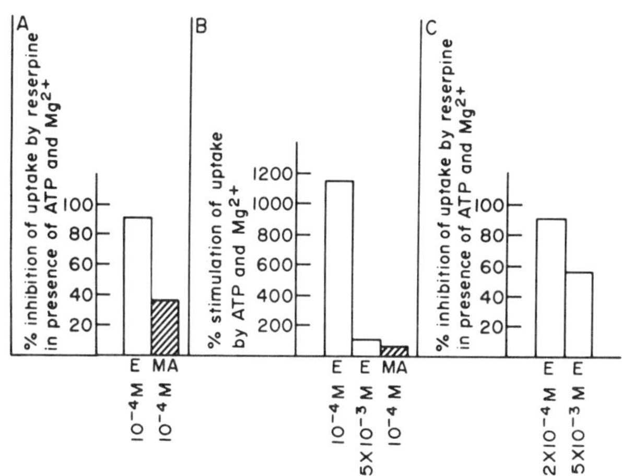

Fig. 13. Differences between the two uptake mechanisms in isolated bovine adrenal medullary vesicles. (A) Specificity of inhibition by reserpine. (B) Stimulation by ATP plus Mg^{2+} and effect of epinephrine concentration. (C) Overcoming of reserpine blockade at high epinephrine concentrations. Abbreviations: E, epinephrine; MA, metaraminol. From Slotkin *et al.* (1971) and Slotkin and Kirshner (1971).

competition with reserpine for stimulated uptake sites and changeover to the second (unstimulated, reserpine-resistant) uptake mechanism.

4. Temperature: Both mechanisms are temperature dependent.

These studies indicate that there is a reserpine-resistant uptake of amines in storage vesicles and that in general false transmitters have a higher affinity for the reserpine-resistant mechanism than do catecholamines. Farnebo (1971) has recently demonstrated that the reserpine-resistant vesicular pool is functional *in vivo*: ^{3}H-metaraminol, but not ^{3}H-norepinephrine, is incorporated into neuronal storage vesicles of reserpinized rat iris, and the ^{3}H-metaraminol is released on neural stimulation.

F. Interactions with Other Agents

Many drugs other than reserpine alter biogenic amine levels and the effects of biogenic amines, and, not surprisingly, these drugs can potentiate, antagonize, or otherwise interact with reserpine. The preceding section dealt with one class of such drugs, false transmitters; in this section, the effects on reserpine action by benzoquinolizines and the antagonism produced by catecholamine precursors, monoamine oxidase inhibitors, and tricyclic antidepressants are discussed, along with the influence of several other drugs.

1. Tetrabenazine

Certain derivatives of benzoquinolizine, notably tetrabenazine (Fig.14), have the ability, like reserpine, to deplete catecholamines and serotonin and to produce blockade of vesicular amine uptake mechanisms (Carlsson *et al.*, 1963). However, tetrabenazine has a considerably shorter duration of action than reserpine, with depletion rarely lasting more than 24 hr (Pletscher *et al.*, 1958), which suggests a more readily reversible action on the vesicles. Since both tetrabenazine and reserpine presumably compete for the same site in the membrane, pretreatment of animals with tetrabenazine protects them from the long-lasting amine depletion and pharmacological effects of reserpine (Quinn *et al.*, 1959; Carlsson, 1965). This interaction of tetrabenazine and reserpine has important mechanistic implications:

a. The protective effect of tetrabenazine indicates that the long-lasting nature of the inhibition by reserpine depends on binding to a

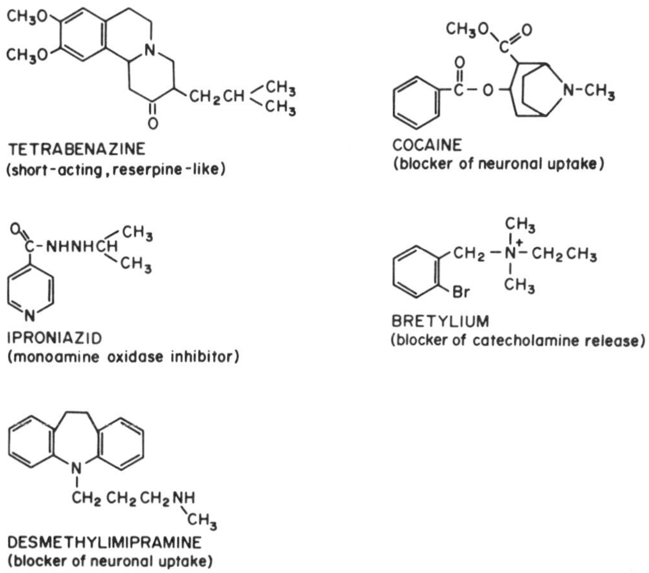

TETRABENAZINE
(short-acting, reserpine-like)

COCAINE
(blocker of neuronal uptake)

IPRONIAZID
(monoamine oxidase inhibitor)

BRETYLIUM
(blocker of catecholamine release)

DESMETHYLIMIPRAMINE
(blocker of neuronal uptake)

Fig. 14. Structures of some drugs which antagonize the effects of reserpine.

specific site in the vesicle rather than on physicochemical factors such as lipid solubility (which would be unaffected by tetrabenazine pretreatment).

b. The short-acting characteristic of tetrabenazine indicates that this molecule lacks that part of the structure of reserpine responsible for long-term binding, presumably the D-E-F ring system and additional substituent groups (see Fig. 16 and Section IVG).

2. *Catecholamine Precursors*

In view of the existence of the reserpine-resistant "mobile pool" as well as reserpine-resistant vesicular uptake at high concentrations of amines, it is to be expected that the administration of large amounts of precursors of catecholamines and serotonin will result in a partial, short-acting reversal of the pharmacological effects of reserpine. Thus after treatment of reserpinized animals with 5-hydroxytryptophan or DOPA, serotonin and dopamine are synthesized in the neurons (Udenfriend *et al.*, 1957; Carlsson *et al.*, 1957*b*) and the visible effects of reserpine are markedly alleviated (Everett and Toman, 1959; Blaschko and Chruściel, 1960; Degkwitz *et al.*, 1960; Smith and Dews, 1962; Seiden and Carlsson, 1963,

1964). It is interesting to note that some of the dopamine formed is converted to norepinephrine despite the continued blockade of vesicular uptake, especially when a monoamine oxidase inhibitor is administered (Carlsson, 1965). How can this conversion take place? First, if sufficient precursor is administered, the concentration of dopamine might become high enough (especially after monoamine oxidase inhibition) to overcome the blockade of uptake or to utilize the reserpine-resistant uptake mechanism; second, emptied vesicle membranes in the neuronal cytoplasm would be in above-normal abundance because of secretion from reserpine-induced nerve stimulation, and the membrane-bound dopamine β-hydroxylase might convert dopamine to norepinephrine without the uptake step required in intact vesicles. The relative importance of dopamine vs. norepinephrine in reserpine-resistant pools for acute alleviation of the pharmacological effects of reserpine is unclear, but Carlsson (1965) has suggested that the high levels of dopamine synthesized and released from the mobile pool result in stimulation of central adrenergic receptors without the necessity for conversion to norepinephrine.

Synthesis of serotonin from administered 5-hydroxytryptophan in reserpinized animals is unaffected by blockade of vesicular uptake, since the necessary enzyme is cytoplasmic. However, administration of the precursor does not reverse the pharmacological effects of reserpine in the central nervous system (Carlsson *et al.*, 1957*b*; Everett and Toman, 1959).

3. *Monoamine Oxidase Inhibitors*

Prior administration of a monoamine oxidase inhibitor (such as iproniazid, Fig. 14) markedly alters the pharmacological and biochemical effects of subsequently administered reserpine; excitation is usually seen rather than sedation, along with general sympathetic stimulation, resulting in hyperthermia, hypertension, and piloerection (Carlsson, 1965). The blockade of vesicular uptake by reserpine results in increased leakage of amines from the vesicles into the cytoplasm, but since the amines can no longer be inactivated by monoamine oxidase they can then diffuse out into the synapse and stimulate adrenergic receptors. Thus a sympathomimetic effect is obtained.

On the biochemical level, monoamine oxidase inhibitors also prevent to some extent reserpine-induced amine depletion (Brodie *et al.*, 1956; Pletscher, 1956; Carlsson *et al.*, 1957*a*), most of which represents accumulation of amines in the cytoplasm; however, depletion of vesicular stores may also be slowed (Zbinden *et al.*, 1957; Zbinden and Studer, 1958). This latter effect probably results from at least two separate phenomena:

a. Competition for vesicular uptake sites from the increased cytoplasmic amine concentrations and/or a shift to the reserpine-resistant type of vesicular uptake which operates at higher amine concentrations (Slotkin *et al.*, 1971).

b. Decreased release of amines from adrenergic nerves caused by some monoamine oxidase inhibitors (Axelrod *et al.*, 1961); this action would oppose that part of amine depletion which results from the reserpine-induced increase in neural stimulation.

When monoamine oxidase inhibitors are administered after reserpine has already depleted amine stores, similar but less dramatic effects are obtained (Carlsson, 1965).

4. Other Drugs

Blockade of neuronal uptake of catecholamines by tricyclic antidepressants (Fig. 14) (amitriptyline, imipramine, desmethylimipramine) or cocaine (Fig. 14) results in antagonism of the pharmacological actions of reserpine without altering the course of depletion (Domenjoz and Theobald, 1959; Garattini and Valzelli, 1962; Sulser *et al.*, 1962; Izquierdo *et al.*, 1962). These compounds prolong the period in which released norepinephrine is present in the synapse and thereby increase the net adrenergic effect. Since they do not directly affect amine synthesis, degradation, or release, they cannot alter the reserpine-induced depletion. On the other hand, drugs like bretylium (Fig. 14) which block release of catecholamines interfere with the stimulation-induced phase of depletion by reserpine but are themselves adrenolytic (Callingham and Cass, 1962).

G. Mechanism of Action of Reserpine

The studies already described on the effects of reserpine on biogenic amine synthesis, degradation, uptake, storage, and release all support the concept that reserpine acts to inhibit the ATP-Mg^{2+}-stimulated uptake of amines into storage vesicles. Additional experiments, mostly utilizing adrenal storage vesicles, have been concerned with pinpointing the exact mechanism by which reserpine blocks uptake and with characterizing the nature of the inhibition. The data currently available point toward an interaction of reserpine with a catecholamine transport molecule in the storage vesicle membrane. Before examining this interaction, it is important to establish whether vesicular catecholamine uptake really is a carrier-mediated process. The uptake fulfills most of the requirements for active transport:

1. It requires energy in the form of ATP, and the uptake is linked in some fashion to the activity of a Mg^{2+}-activated ATPase; both the

ATPase and uptake are inhibited by sulfhydryl reagents, such as *N*-ethylmaleimide (Kirshner, 1965).

2. The uptake is saturable, although reported K_ms vary widely; in cow adrenal vesicles Jonasson *et al.* (1964) report a K_m for epinephrine of about 8×10^{-4} M, while Lundborg (1966) reports 4×10^{-4} M; in rat adrenal vesicles the K_m is approximately 4×10^{-5} M (Green and Slotkin, 1973). One reason for the disparities may be difficulties in kinetic interpretation introduced by the second uptake system which operates at higher concentrations (see Section IVE).
3. The uptake displays specificity, since catecholamines are preferred over some noncatecholamines (such as metaraminol) (Slotkin *et al.*, 1971; Slotkin and Kirshner, 1971). However, serotonin, an indoleamine, has the highest affinity for uptake into adrenal storage vesicles (Slotkin and Kirshner, 1971).

It is in the evaluation of the fourth standard parameter for active transport, namely concentration against a gradient, that data are lacking to substantiate such a system in storage vesicles. When uptake is measured *in vitro*, the incorporation of epinephrine and norepinephrine into adrenal storage vesicles is accompanied by spontaneous loss of amines, and at best the addition of ATP and Mg^{2+} leads to a balance of the two processes (Taugner and Hasselbach, 1966; Lishajko, 1969). Furthermore, it is impossible to determine the concentration gradient between the medium and the storage vesicle because the concentration of free amines inside the vesicle cannot be measured; presumably most of the amines are bound in a nondiffusable form. Whether the uptake is active or not, additional data all point toward a carrier-mediated transport:

1. The Q_{10} (3–6) indicates a high degree of temperature dependence (Kirshner, 1962).
2. If adrenal storage vesicles are lysed and the membranes treated such that they reform into empty vesicles, they retain the ability to take up catecholamines, strongly suggesting that there is a carrier in the membrane (Taugner, 1971).
3. Although catecholamines are stored more stably in adrenal storage vesicles, serotonin is taken up more readily, indicating that "uptake" and "storage" are separable processes and that serotonin has a higher affinity for the uptake process, also indicating carrier-mediated transport (Carlsson *et al.*, 1963; Slotkin and Kirshner, 1971).
4. Catecholamines are firmly bound to purified adrenal vesicle membranes, and the binding is inhibited by *N*-ethylmaleimide or by reserpine in the presence of Mg^{2+}; furthermore, the binding of

epinephrine has a K_{diss} of about 10^{-4} M, which is similar to the uptake K_m, and binding has the same specificity as uptake into intact vesicles, *viz. serotonin > epinephrine > metaraminol* (Slotkin and Kirshner, 1973*b*).

Thus there is a considerable body of evidence to support the idea that carrier-mediated transport of amines occurs. Trifaró and Dworkind (1971) have shown that that Mg^{2+}-stimulated ATPase transphosphorylates membrane components and that transphosphorylation, like amine uptake, is inhibited by *N*-ethylmaleimide (but *not* by reserpine; Ferris *et al.*, 1970), and it is tempting to speculate that one step in the uptake process may be phosphorylation of the carrier. Furthermore, Slotkin and Kirshner (1973*b*) have found that ATP actually *decreases* the binding of catecholamines to purified vesicle membranes, suggesting that ATP is utilized to remove catecholamines from the putative carrier. A hypothetical model of vesicular amine transport can be constructed from these data (Fig. 15). A catecholamine molecule (epinephrine, for example) (E) attaches to a carrier (C) at the outside of the membrane and diffuses to the inside surface. The amine–carrier complex (EC) is dissociated enzymatically by an ATPase which also transphosphorylates the carrier, making it unavailable for attachment to catecholamines (C ~ P). The phosphorylated carrier diffuses to the outside of the membrane, where another enzyme dephosphorylates it, making it available for reattachment with another amine molecule. Magnesium may be involved at several steps, and certainly at one point in the functioning of the ATPase, but probably not in the binding of amine to carrier (Slotkin and Kirshner, 1973*b*). While reserpine and *N*-ethylmaleimide do not themselves block binding of catecholamines to the carrier, the addition of the drugs plus Mg^{2+} results in a decrease in binding (Slotkin and

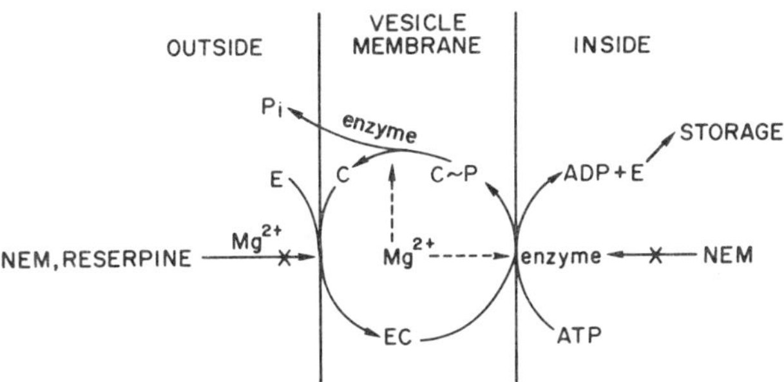

Fig. 15. Hypothetical model of catecholamine transport in storage vesicles, showing possible sites of action of reserpine and *N*-ethylmaleimide (NEM). Abbreviations: E, epinephrine; C. carrier; EC, epinephrine–carrier complex; C ~ P, phosphorylated carrier. From Slotkin (1973).

Kirshner, 1973*b*). This type of pump would give the following behavior:

1. In intact vesicles, amines would be pumped in and ATP would be hydrolyzed; uptake would be stimulated by ATP plus Mg^{2+}.
2. Inhibition of the ATPase with *N*-ethylmaleimide would stop the pump by blocking transphosphorylation as well as blocking attachment of catecholamines to the carrier.
3. Reserpine would stop the pump by blocking attachment of catecholamines, but would not inhibit the ATPase.
4. In isolated membranes, the binding of catecholamines would be reduced both by the addition of ATP or by *N*-ethylmaleimide or reserpine plus Mg^{2+}.

Although all these phenomena are observed, this does not prove or disprove the validity of the model, and such an interpretation should be treated solely as a working hypothesis with which to compare additional results when available.

Since it is likely that carrier-mediated transport occurs and that reserpine interferes with the attachment of catecholamines to the carrier, it is important to ask what the characteristics of inhibition are and why reserpine is so effective. Studies utilizing isolated splenic nerve vesicles (Klein and Lagercrantz, 1971), sympathetic nerve trunk vesicles (Lagercrantz, 1971), and adrenal medullary vesicles (Carlsson *et al.*, 1963; Jonasson *et al.*, 1964; Stjärne, 1964) have all indicated that reserpine produces a competitive inhibition of catecholamine uptake, and, consequently, inhibition may be overcome by increasing the concentration of amines in the medium. However, the inhibition of uptake by reserpine cannot be reversed by washing the treated storage vesicles (Kirshner, 1962; Carlsson *et al.*, 1962, 1963), indicating that the inhibition is irreversible in vesicles exposed *in vitro*.

The question of irreversibility *in vivo* has attracted considerable attention in recent years, and several approaches have been utilized to study the mechanism of recovery after reserpine administration to determine whether

1. Vesicles which are exposed to reserpine can recover their uptake function, or
2. New vesicles must be synthesized.

To some extent, the results obtained have been equivocal, because they appear to vary with species, dose, and tissue studied.

Alpers and Shore (1969) showed that the decline in persistently bound reserpine in rat heart correlates with the degree of norepinephrine depletion, suggesting that recovery would depend on the rate of removal of the drug. However, Häggendal and Dahlström (1971) have shown that the rate of recovery of vesicular uptake in rat sciatic nerve after a large dose of reserpine exactly parallels the transport of new vesicles down the axon, implying that reversibility of reserpine action is not a factor in recovery. Similarly, axotomy in the rat central nervous system results in prolongation of the actions of reserpine, supporting the idea that recovery is due to down transport of new vesicles (Andén and Lundborg , 1970); measurements of dopamine β-hydroxylase and catecholamines in splenic nerve after reserpine indicate a rise in the ratio of enzyme to amine which is probably due to new vesicle formation (Chubb *et al.*, 1972). These data suggest that the inhibition of uptake by reserpine is irreversible in nerve vesicles.

In the adrenal medulla, however, the picture is somewhat more complex. Studies in rabbits (Viveros *et al.*, 1969*b*, 1971) and in rats (Slotkin and Edwards, 1973) have shown that there are species differences in reversibility and that the larger the dose, the greater the degree of irreversibility. Thus, in rabbits, new storage vesicle synthesis (as determined by dopamine β-hydroxylase activity) must occur before recovery of catecholamine uptake is observed. In rats given 2.5 mg/kg of reserpine and pretreated with a ganglionic blocker to prevent reflex stimulation, there was an immediate decrease in catecholamine uptake into adrenal storage vesicles, but recovery was complete in 24 hr (Table I); in this period of time, storage ves-

Table I. Effects of Reserpine on Adrenal Catecholamine and Dopamine β-Hydroxylase Contents and on Uptake of Epinephrine into Isolated Adrenal Storage Vesicles of Rats Pretreated with Chlorisondamine
(10 mg/kg intraperitoneally, 1 hr previously)[a]

	Amount per gland (% of control ± SE)		
Treatment	Catecholamines	Dopamine β-hydroxylase	Epinephrine uptake
Reserpine (2.5 mg/kg)			
1 hr	101 ± 4	—	36 ± 5
4 hr	101 ± 5	114 ± 4	41 ± 6
24 hr	80 ± 6	106 ± 4	86 ± 9
Reserpine (10 mg/kg)			
1 hr	96 ± 1	—	7 ± 1
4 hr	93 ± 4	101 ± 5	13 ± 3
24 hr	56 ± 6	110 ± 7	39 ± 6
72 hr	50 ± 7	143 ± 7	70 ± 6

[a] From Slotkin and Edwards (1973).

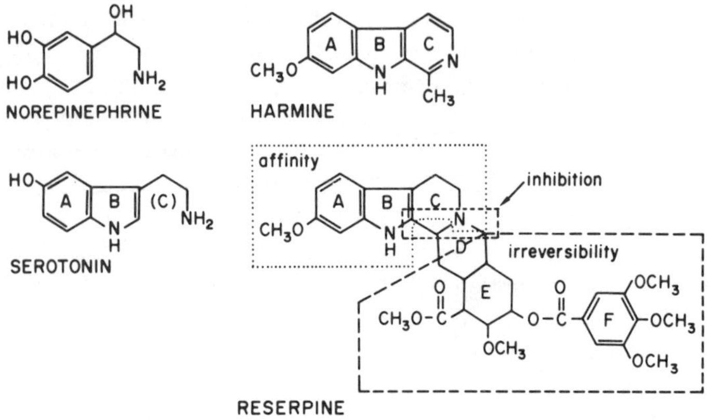

Fig. 16. Structures of some substances with high affinity for the vesicular uptake system, and the relative contributions of different parts of the reserpine molecule to reserpine action. From Green and Slotkin (1973).

icle synthesis did not play a role in recovery, since there was no increase in the levels of dopamine β-hydroxylase. Following administration of a large dose of reserpine, however, some new vesicle synthesis had to occur to permit recovery of uptake, but there was still significant recovery before increases in dopamine β-hydroxylase were evident (Table I). It is noteworthy that the adrenal is relatively more resistant to the actions of reserpine than are sympathetic neurons and that the rat is a more reserpine-resistant species than most others; these factors may play a role in the apparent reversibility of reserpine in the rat adrenal.

Structurally, reserpine does not resemble a catecholamine (Fig. 16) but rather bears a striking similarity to serotonin, which has a higher affinity for vesicular uptake in adrenal catecholamine storage vesicles than do the catecholamines. This suggests that it is the serotonin-like portion of the reserpine molecule which confers the ability to attach to the putative carrier. Some related *Rauwolfia* alkaloids also inhibit amine uptake *in vitro* but reserpic acid does not (Kirshner, 1965), suggesting that the charge on the molecule is also important in establishing blockade of uptake. With these factors in mind, Green and Slotkin (1973) examined the actions of harmine (Fig. 16) on uptake into isolated rat adrenal storage vesicles; this drug was chosen because of its structural resemblance both to serotonin and to reserpine, and because its physicochemical characteristics (pK and lipid solubility) are similar to those of reserpine. Like reserpine, harmine produced a potent, competitive inhibition of ATP-Mg^{2+}-stimulated epinephrine uptake, but with harmine the inhibition was reversible. Unlike serotonin and catecholamines, harmine was not actually transported into the vesicle, so that its effect was purely that of blockade of uptake. Mechanistically, these data suggest that the structure–activity relationships of the reserpine molecule can be divided into three factors: the serotonin-like portion is responsibile for affinity for the vesicular amine pump; the closure of and substitution on the C-ring converts it to a competitive inhibitor of the pump; the remainder of the molecule renders the inhibition long-lasting and potentially irreversible. The reversibility of harmine inhibition of uptake in contrast to the irreversible character of reserpine *in vitro* may indicate that there is an accessory site in the vesicle membrane to which the additional portion of the molecule attaches.

V. BIOCHEMICAL EFFECTS

In view of the complex interplay of direct and reflex actions which follow the acute or chronic administration of reserpine, it is not surprising that a large number of observations have been made concerning biochemical changes which accompany these actions. In many cases, the underlying mechanisms have not yet been elucidated, but most appear to be secondary to the important pharmacological effects of depletion of catecholamines and serotonin. An excellent review by Carlsson (1965) summarizes most of the earlier reports on the various biochemical effects of reserpine.

A. Effects on Other Biogenic Amines and Neurotransmitters

1. *Histamine*

Reserpine has little or no effect on brain histamine levels but produces significant depletion in blood, lung, intestine, and stomach (Waalkes and Weissbach, 1956; Waalkes *et al.*, 1959; Kim and Shore, 1963; Atack, 1971). The mobilization of histamine in rat stomach is probably from a specialized set of enterochromaffin-like cells in the oxyntic gland area, while rat stomach mast cells and another population of stomach enterochromaffin-like cells appear to be somewhat reserpine resistant (Häkonson *et al.*, 1971); the reserpine-sensitive pool of cells also contains vitamin B_{12}–binding proteins (including intrinsic factor) which are depleted by reserpine, although the degree of depletion of intrinsic factor is not high enough to produce vitamin B_{12} deficiency. The histamine released by reserpine may play a role in the production of gastric lesions, since prior degranulation of histamine-containing mucosal cells reduces the incidence of reserpine-induced ulceration (Räsänen and Taskinen, 1967). In addition to release of histamine, reserpine administered *in vivo* produces a decrease in histidine decarboxylase activity in rat stomach which may contribute to histamine depletion (Isaac *et al*., 1971); this effect is indirect, since reserpine does not inhibit the enzyme *in vitro*. Rosengren and Svensson (1969) have also reported decreases in histamine-forming capacity in gastric mucosa and lung of reserpinized rats and have demonstrated that the effect is unrelated to the reserpine-induced release of catecholamines from the adrenal medulla.

Reserpine has the ability to release histamine from isolated rat peritoneal mast cells (Gillespie and Levine, 1969) and blocks the incorporation of histamine and serotonin into both mast cells and isolated mast cell granules (Jansson, 1970; Gripenberg *et al*., 1972). The blockade of uptake bears some similarity to blockade of uptake in neuronal catecholamine storage vesicles in that the subcellular distribution of reserpine follows the distribution of serotonin, suggesting that the reserpine is bound to the granules (Gripenberg *et al*., 1972).

2. *Acetylcholine*

Reserpine administration produces increases in acetylcholine levels in dog heart, ileum, and brain (Malhotra and Pundlik, 1959; Malhotra and Das, 1962) and in rat heart, blood, and brain stem (Malpica *et al*., 1970). In rats, the increase is accompanied by accelerated biosynthesis and catabolism of acetylcholine (Malpica *et al*., 1970). Reserpine has no effect on cholinergic transmission at the neuromuscular junction (Bianchi and Beani, 1966).

3. *Amino Acids*

Reserpine affects the brain levels and turnovers of at least two putative central neurotransmitters, γ-aminobutyric acid (GABA) and glutamate. In reserpinized mice, the decrease in GABA levels is associated with reduction in uptake (Balzer *et al*., 1961*a,b*; Balzer and Palm, 1962); in cats, Berl and Frigyesi (1969) observed a threefold increase in the turnover of GABA and glutamate in the caudate nucleus, thalamus, and sensorimotor cortex. The interpretation of these observations in terms of neurotransmitters is questionable, however, since similar changes are observed in uptake and turnover of amino acids which are not directly involved in neurotransmission (MacLean, 1955; Berl and Frigyesi, 1969).

B. Adenine Nucleotides

ATP is intimately involved in both the uptake and storage of catecholamines. In storage vesicles, in addition to stimulation (along with magnesium) of catecholamine uptake, ATP forms a storage complex with catecholamines (Hillarp, 1960*a*). Because reserpine blocks catecholamine uptake and/or storage, it is extremely important to consider the effects of reserpine on adenine nucleotides.

Studies utilizing adrenal medullary vesicles incubated *in vitro* show a markedly smaller capacity for incorporation of ATP than for catecholamines (Carlsson *et al.*, 1963), despite the fact that the vesicle membrane apparently is permeable to both substances at 0°C (Kirshner *et al.*, 1966). Concentrations of reserpine which completely block catecholamine uptake have a much smaller effect on ATP uptake (Carlsson *et al.*, 1963). These data suggest that the effect of reserpine on catecholamine uptake and storage *in vitro* is not dependent on a primary effect on ATP uptake. On the other hand, reserpine may interact directly with ATP involved in storage; Berneis *et al.* (1970) have demonstrated that the addition of reserpine to solutions containing ATP, norepinephrine, and $CaCl_2$ (conditions under which catecholamines and ATP form complexes) results in the formation of an insoluble, reserpine-containing precipitate. Further studies are required to assess the significance of this finding in reference to possible actions of reserpine on the formation of the catecholamine–ATP storage complex.

After the administration of reserpine *in vivo*, there is a decrease in catecholamines and adenine nucleotides in adrenal medullary storage vesicles, and the percentage of the decrease in catecholamines may be either greater than or equivalent to that of the nucleotides (Schümann, 1958; Kirpekar *et al.*, 1958, 1963; Hillarp, 1960*b*; Burack *et al.*, 1960, 1961; Keswani *et al.*, 1971; Slotkin and Edwards, 1973). The interpretation of most of these experiments is complicated by several factors:

1. Dose–effect relationships vary with species (Muscholl and Vogt, 1958) and strain (Coupland, 1958).
2. Different doses produce different relative degrees of depletion of catecholamines and nucleotides (Schümann, 1958; Burack *et al.*, 1960, 1961).
3. Reserpine has two distinct effects on the intact adrenal medulla:
   a. Reflex stimulation of the splanchnic nerve, which results in exocytotic release of the soluble contents of the vesicles, including catecholamines and nucleotides.

b. Blockade of catecholamine uptake into storage vesicles. Thus in order to detect changes in relative amounts of catecholamines and nucleotides due to *direct* actions of reserpine, the splanchnic nerves must be sectioned or their effects blocked with a ganglionic blocking agent.

4. In many studies, crude vesicle fractions (containing mitochondria, lysosomes, etc.) have been used; these can give misleading ratios of catecholamines to nucleotides.

In a recent study, reserpine was administered to rats which had been pretreated with chlorisondamine, a long-acting ganglionic blocker, and adrenal storage vesicles were then purified and analyzed for catecholamines and ATP (Slotkin and Edwards, 1973). There was an equivalent decrease in both catecholamines and ATP (Table II); since secretion was blocked, these data suggest that reserpine administered *in vivo* may indeed have a direct effect on vesicular ATP, although they do not rule out the possibility that depletion of ATP is in some fashion dependent on depletion of cate-

Table II. Decreases in Catecholamines and ATP in Purified Rat Adrenal Medullary Storage Vesicles Following Intraperitoneal Administration of Chlorisondamine or Chlorisondamine Plus Reserpine[a]

Treatment and time of sacrifice	Percentage decrease ± SE	
	Catecholamines	ATP
Chlorisondamine (10 mg/kg)		
5 hr	−2 ± 2	−6 ± 1
25 hr	−9 ± 9	−12 ± 3
Chlorisondamine + reserpine (2.5 mg/kg)[b]		
4 hr	12 ± 3	11 ± 3
24 hr	34 ± 4	33 ± 4
Chlorisondamine + reserpine (10 mg/kg)[b]		
4 hr	13 ± 5	6 ± 2
24 hr	39 ± 8	37 ± 5
72 hr	27 ± 3	28 ± 3

[a] From Slotkin and Edwards (1973).

[b] Chlorisondamine given 1 hr before reserpine; time listed refers to time after reserpine injection.

cholamines. In this regard, it is important to note that adrenal storage vesicles do *not* require catecholamines in order to contain ATP: during recovery from massive catecholamine depletion evoked by insulin administration, vesicles are formed which are deficient in catecholamines but not in ATP (Slotkin and Kirshner, 1973*a*). Thus after reserpine administration, the loss of catecholamines should not in itself result in depletion of ATP, supporting the concept that reserpine has some direct action on vesicular nucleotides. Clearly, further study is required to elucidate the nature of the reserpine-induced decreases.

In addition to eliciting alterations in adenine nucleotides involved in catecholamine storage, reserpine lowers the ATP/ADP ratio in rat brain and liver (Kirpekar and Lewis, 1959; Kaul and Lewis, 1963), while in mouse brain, ATP, ADP, and AMP are increased slightly (Balzer *et al.*, 1961*b*). Chronic reserpine treatment increases the rate of synthesis of rat brain ATP from labeled acetate (Ahlbaum and Milch, 1962). Reserpine is reported to inhibit cyclic 3′,5′-nucleotide phosphodiesterase at concentrations below 10^{-5} M (Honda and Imamura, 1968); further *in vivo* studies are needed to assess the possible effects of reserpine on cyclic AMP catabolism.

C. Cations

Reserpine produces an increase in the potassium content of cerebral cortex, paleothalamic nuclei, and caudate nuclei of the rabbit brain, but no changes are observed for sodium, calcium, magnesium, or chloride (Hanig and Aprison, 1971). Although reserpine reduces digitalis-induced cardiac arrhythmias, measurements in cat papillary muscle indicate no change in sodium and potassium fluxes (Choi and Roberts, 1970), nor do myocardial potassium levels change in reserpinized rats (Troquet *et al.*, 1966); thus the effect on digitalis arrhythmias does not reflect a local anesthetic action. Cardiac calcium levels are reduced in mice given reserpine (Clower *et al.*, 1969).

In rabbit skeletal muscle, reserpine effectively inhibits the calcium pump in sarcoplasmic reticulum ($ED_{50} = 3 \times 10^{-5}$ M) without affecting calcium storage (Balzer *et al.*, 1968*a*). The effect is accompanied by inhibition of the calcium-stimulated ATPase, but protein phosphorylation is not affected (Balzer *et al.*, 1968*a*). The inhibition of the calcium pump results from temperature-independent binding to the lipids of the membranes of the sarcoplasmic reticulum, which, unlike the binding to membranes of adrenal storage vesicles, is readily reversible (Balzer *et al.*, 1968*b*).

D. Glucose, Carbohydrates, and Lipids

After acute administration, reserpine causes an initial increase in metabolic rate accompanied by elevated blood glucose (Takemoto *et al.*, 1957; Johnson and Sellers, 1961; Rutishauser, 1963); these changes can be prevented by adrenomedullectomy or administration of a ganglionic blocker, indicating that the effect is mediated via catecholamine released by reflex stimulation of the adrenal medulla. Glucagon may also participate in the response (Galansino *et al.*, 1963). Reserpine blocks the hyperglycemic effects of theophylline and caffeine in adrenal demedullated rats, suggesting that xanthine-induced hyperglycemia is catecholamine mediated (Strubelt, 1969).

Reserpine alters the metabolism of glycogen; brain, liver, skeletal muscle, and heart glycogen contents and turnovers are increased in mice and rats administered reserpine (Balzer *et al.*, 1961*b*; Mathé *et al.*, 1961; Balzer and Palm, 1962). Chronic reserpine administration results in decreased percentages of phosphorylase *a* in heart and brain (Belford and Feinleib, 1961).

Reserpine prevents mobilization of free fatty acids in adrenal demedullated rats exposed to cold (Gilgen *et al.*, 1962). Since the mobilization results from sympathetic stimulation, the prevention of free fatty acid mobilization is secondary to catecholamine depletion.

Catecholamines are intimately concerned with the regulation of intermediary metabolism and growth in *Tetrahymena*, and these are markedly altered by reserpine (Blum *et al.*, 1966; Blum, 1967).

E. Prostaglandins

Reserpine is reported to block the release of prostaglandins from isolated guinea pig colon and to noncompetitively antagonize prostaglandin-induced contractions of the colon (Gandini *et al.*, 1972).

F. Mitochondria

Increases in the permeability of mitochondrial membranes have been observed after reserpine (Izumi *et al.*, 1969), and these may in fact lead to fragmentation and disruption of mitochondrial structure (Wilcken *et al.*, 1967). Since the doses of reserpine required to disrupt mitochondria are higher than those which deplete catecholamines, the role of such permeability changes in the actions of reserpine is open to question (Iwayama *et al.*, 1973); however, disruption of mitochondria may represent a significant manifestation of reserpine toxicity.

VI. PHARMACOLOGICAL EFFECTS

The wide interest in the pharmacology of *Rauwolfia* alkaloids has resulted in the publication of a vast number of reports in the past two decades. For detailed reviews, the reader is referred to Bein (1956), Woodson *et al.* (1957), Lewis (1963), Toman (1963), Fawaz (1963), Volle (1963), Gaunt *et al.* (1963), and Carlsson (1965).

As is the case with biochemical effects of reserpine, it is unclear which additional pharmacological effects are secondary to serotonin and catecholamine depletion; the time course of onset of many of the effects is gradual, as is the amine depletion, but most of the readily visible symptoms of reserpine administration disappear far in advance of amine recovery. Furthermore, the various symptoms disappear at different rates, and the rates vary from species to species. Some effects also appear to be secondary to reserpine-induced hypothermia or loss of appetite.

A. Central Nervous System

As the first of the major tranquilizers, reserpine ushered in the modern era of psychopharmacology. The calming effects are distinctly different from those of sedatives and hypnotics (barbiturates, for example) in that reserpine does not induce anesthesia even in high doses; while sleep may be induced, animals are easily aroused and are responsive to external stimuli. While there is generally a decrease in spontaneous activity, motor coordination is not impaired. Normally aggressive monkeys become easy to handle, and "sham rage" in cats is inhibited (see Bein, 1956).

The site of sedative action of reserpine has not been pinpointed; the reticular activating system is not involved (Rinaldi and Himwich, 1955), which is in keeping with the observation that reserpinized animals are readily aroused. Furthermore, few distinctive changes in EEG are observable after treatment with moderate doses, although changes occur after chronic administration of large doses (Bein, 1956). In any case, the sedative action is readily reversed by administration of a catecholamine precursor such as DOPA and by other treatments which increase brain catecholamine levels (Carlsson *et al.*, 1957*b*; Everett and Toman, 1959; Blaschko and Chruściel, 1960; Smith and Dews, 1962; Degkwitz *et al.*, 1960), indicating that sedation results from catecholamine depletion in central adrenergic and/or dopaminergic neurons.

In addition to tranquilization, reserpine has many other effects on the central nervous system:

1. Hypothermia, involving effects on central and peripheral neurons as well as endocrine effects (Bein, 1956; Taylor and Fregly, 1962; Carlsson, 1965).
2. Potentiation of anesthetic agents, possibly secondary to hypothermia (Lessin and Parkes, 1957).
3. Potentiation of analeptics and antagonism toward anticonvulsants, involving both catecholaminergic and serotonergic pathways (Gray *et al.*, 1963; Lessin and Parkes, 1959). This is in contrast to sedatives and minor tranquilizers, which antagonize analeptics.
4. Interference with extrapyramidal motor functions, eliciting a parkinsonism-like condition (tremors, rigidity, hypokinesia), probably due to depletion of dopamine; as in parkinsonism, these signs are reversed by administration of DOPA (Carlsson, 1965). Conversely, reserpine is beneficial in some hyperkinetic syndromes, such as Huntington's chorea and congenital spastic paralysis (Bein, 1956).
5. Interference with consolidation of long-term memory (Dismukes and Rake, 1972).
6. Potentiation of the effects of LSD, perhaps through serotonin depletion (see Hoffer and Osmond, 1967).

B. Peripheral Nervous System

For the most part, the peripheral actions of reserpine can be attributed to catecholamine depletion and the corresponding decrease in sympathetic tone, although parasympathetic stimulation also plays a role. These effects are responsible for a majority of the actions of reserpine on the cardiovascular and gastrointestinal systems (Sections VIC,D) as well. Thus reserpine administration produces profound miosis and relaxation of the nictitating membrane (Woodson *et al.*, 1957) but the miosis persists even after sympathetic denervation (Bogdanski *et al.*, 1961), indicating both sympatholytic and parasympathomimetic actions. Similarly, reserpine can cause nasal stuffiness, increased intestinal motility, peripheral vasodilation, and all other signs of decreased sympathetic and increased parasympathetic tone (Goodman and Gilman, 1970). Bronchospasm has also been reported after reserpine administration in humans (Wise, 1969). High doses of reserpine may produce transient sympathomimetic actions, presumably by reflex effects and/or directly by release of peripheral amine stores (Goodman and Gilman, 1970).

Of particular interest is the development, in adrenergically innervated tissues, of catecholamine supersensitivity after chronic reserpine treatment (see Trendelenburg, 1963, 1966); the effect resembles the supersensitivity seen after catecholamine depletion by other agents, such as guanethidine, or after denervation (Goodman and Gilman, 1970). The enhanced response extends even to the biochemical level; for example, catecholamine activation of cardiac phosphorylase demonstrates reserpine supersensitivity. The enhanced responses may in fact be due to reserpine-induced alterations in intracellular calcium (McNeill, 1969; Carrier and Jurevics, 1973).

In addition to peripheral autonomic effects which result from catecholamine depletion, reserpine affects the permeability of neural membranes. Thus after reserpine administration, there is an enhancement of the efflux of labeled *d*- or *l*-metaraminol from adrenergic neurons which is not related to storage in the vesicles or to the time course of inhibition of vesicular uptake mechanisms (Giachetti and Shore, 1970) but rather reflects increased leakage from the nerve terminal.

C. Cardiovascular System

Reserpine produces hypotension and bradycardia (Woodson *et al.*, 1957), both of which are probably due to the effects on the autonomic nervous system. Intraarterial reserpine causes vasodilatation (Parks *et al.*, 1961), and this has led to the use of reserpine in the treatment of peripheral vascular disorders (Section VIIB). Reserpine has also been used in the treatment of digitalis-induced cardiac arrhythmias.

D. Gastrointestinal System

Reserpine causes a marked increase in gastrointestinal motility, resulting in frequent defecation and diarrhea (Woodson *et al.*, 1957). The effect is complex, consisting of decreased sympathetic tone, increased parasympathetic tone, and possibly direct stimulation of parasympathetic ganglia (Plummer *et al.*, 1955).

Reserpine also causes increased gastric secretion of acid, which results in ulcer formation (Schroeder and Perry, 1955; Hussar and Bruno, 1956); in most cases, the ulcers heal rapidly despite continued reserpine administration (Emås and Fyrö, 1967). The effect is probably vagal in origin: ulcer formation is markedly reduced by truncal vagotomy (Emås and Fyrö, 1967) and ulcers do not form in reserpine-treated neonates, where gastric innervation is incomplete (Reilly *et al.*, 1969). Emås (1968) has suggested that there is also a nonvagal component in ulcer formation and that the vagally induced ulcers result from release of gastrin and/or histamine, while the nonvagal effect is not gastrin mediated. In humans, reserpine-induced secretion of gastric acid can be troublesome in patients with a history of peptic ulcer (Goodman and Gilman, 1970).

E. Endocrine System

Reserpine has a profound effect on endocrine function, but it is unclear which changes are the results of direct actions, which are catecholamine related, and which are secondary (due to hypothermia or changes in body weight, etc.). For instance, reserpine prolongs the menstrual cycle in monkeys (Erickson, 1969) and increases the diestrous phase in rats (Khan and Bernstorf, 1964; Werner and Ganong, 1971), probably due to effects on secretion of gonadotropic hormones. However, the delayed vaginal opening in rats seen after reserpine administration is due instead to changes in maturation secondary to delays in weight gain (Werner and Ganong, 1971). Changes in hypothalamic norepinephrine content may be responsible for the altered release of gonadotropins (Werner and Ganong, 1971). The reserpine-induced inhibition of gonadal function may be related to decreases in release of follice-stimulating hormone (FSH); in hypophysectomized rats, reserpine reduces concentrations of FSH-releasing factor in the hypothalamus (Negro-Villar *et al.*, 1968). On the other hand, reserpine apparently produces a direct inhibition of testosterone uptake by mouse prostate glands (Thomas *et al.*, 1969). Regardless of the origin of the effect, the general depression of gonadal function plays a definite role in the loss of libido and interference with ejaculation and emission seen in patients treated with reserpine (Blair and Simpson, 1966).

Other endocrine effects of reserpine include:

1. Inhibition of insulin-induced release of growth hormone, probably due to catecholamine depletion (Müller *et al.*, 1967*a*); however, high doses of reserpine may elicit secretion of growth hormone (Müller *et al.*, 1967*b*).
2. Prolactin secretion, resulting in alveolar development of the mammary glands and lactation (Khan and Bernstorf, 1964); the effect is probably due to catecholamine depletion, since norepinephrine suppresses prolactin secretion (MacLeod, 1969).
3. Stimulation as well as suppression of antidiuretic hormone secretion (Gaunt *et al.*, 1964; Gabe *et al.*, 1961; Holeček *et al.*, 1957),

probably due to actions in the supraoptic and paraventricular nuclei (Miline *et al.*, 1957); serotonin rather than antidiuretic hormone may actually be involved in the antidiuretic action of reserpine (Khazan *et al.*, 1962); dehydration may also play role.
4. Antagonism of the actions of thyroxine, without altering the plasma half-life of ^{131}I-thyroxine (Watts, 1968); the site of interaction is probably the adrenergic β-receptor, which is sensitized to catecholamines by thyroxine.
5. Stimulation followed by inhibition of ACTH release (Gaunt *et al.*, 1954; Wells *et al.*, 1956; Kitay *et al.*, 1959; Maickel *et al.*, 1962).

In regard to most endocrine effects of reserpine, it is noteworthy that amine levels in brain areas with known endocrine functions, such as the supraoptic and hypothalamic nuclei, are markedly decreased by reserpine (Carlsson, 1965), suggesting that alterations in endocrine function are at least in part due to central catecholamine depletion.

VII. CLINICAL USES AND TOXICITY

Although the first modern report on the pharmacology of reserpine discussed its potential use in the treatment of "insanity and high blood pressure" (Sen and Bose, 1931), the tranquilizing effects were not utilized clinically until the 1950's. The subsequent appearance of the phenothiazines led to the virtually complete abandonment of reserpine in psychiatric therapy simply because the phenothiazines were more effective and easier to control. Consequently, reserpine today is used almost exclusively in the treatment of hypertension and some peripheral vascular diseases.

A. Psychiatric Disorders

Although reserpine was once used for the alleviation of psychoneuroses and in geriatrics, there is no evidence for a beneficial effect (Goodman and Gilman, 1970). However, in the management of psychoses (especially paranoid and manic states), reserpine has a definitely beneficial effect, producing mild tranquilization, improved sociability, fewer assaultive attacks, and less need for restraint, seclusion, and electroshock (see Schlitter and Plummer, 1964). These effects often permit the initiation of psychotherapy and rehabilitation.

The most serious psychiatric side-effect of reserpine administration is the production of mental depression, which can become severe enough to cause suicide. The observation that depletion of brain catecholamines is accompanied by depression, whereas increased catecholamine levels (after administration of monoamine oxidase inhibitors, for example) are associated with elevation of mood, has led to the development of the "catecholamine theory of affective disorders"; the details of the relationships between biogenic amines and mood are beyond the scope of this chapter, and for a detailed discussion the reader should consult the text by Schildkraut (1969).

B. Cardiovascular Disorders

Reserpine is a major therapeutic tool in the management of mild to moderately severe hypertension; the decrease in blood pressure occurs as a consequence of decreased sympathetic tone because of depletion of peripheral catecholamine stores. Similarly, many of the cardiovascular side-effects seen after continued reserpine therapy relate to the sympatholytic actions of the drug: reduced cardiac output, inhibition of cardiovascular reflexes, and postural hypotension (Goodman and Gilman, 1970). In addition, reserpine can cause sodium and water retention, which can progress to congestive heart failure (Goodman and Gilman, 1970).

More recently, reserpine has been used in the treatment of Raynaud's syndrome, in which occlusion of digital vessels occurs. Untreated, the decreased circulation results in ulceration and necrosis of the affected tissue, and until 1967 no consistently reliable therapy had been discovered. In that year, Abboud *et al.* (1967) reported good results using intraarterial reserpine in doses (0.5–1.5 mg) generally higher than the usual oral dose of the drug as utilized in hypertension. Thus, presuming that most of the dose is absorbed by the tissue distal to the point of injection, an extremely large dose is administered directly to the sympathetic nerve endings in the affected area, resulting in long-lasting catecholamine depletion, with consequent vasodilatation and relief of symptoms for periods of months (Abboud *et al.*, 1967; Kontos and Wasserman, 1969; Romeo *et al.*, 1970).

C. Poisoning

Reports of reserpine poisoning in the literature are rare, and neither death nor permanent illness has resulted from ingestion of large doses (Loggie *et al.*, 1967). In experimental animals, lethal doses produce coma and respiratory depression, and death occurs by respiratory arrest (Goodman and Gilman, 1970). In three cases in which children ingested unknown amounts of reserpine (which may have been as high as 25 mg), Loggie *et al.* (1967) observed effects typical of large doses (miosis, tremor, hypothermia, hypotension) but reported a marked hypertensive episode in one child. All three children became comatose, but recovered after 48 hr with no sequelae. Thus it is evident that reserpine poisoning does not represent a serious hazard.

VIII. SUMMARY

Reserpine has a wide variety of pharmacological and biochemical effects, nearly all of which are related to the disruption of adrenergic and serotonergic neurotransmission; consequently, reserpine has been a valuable tool in the evaluation of the role of monoaminergic transmission in central and peripheral nervous function. The primary effect is inhibition of the ATP-Mg^{2+}-stimulated uptake of amines into neuronal storage vesicles and consequent depletion of neurotransmitter. The best model for studying the actions of reserpine is the adrenergic neuron (see Fig. 4), and the principal effects are summarized below:

A. Initial Effects

Blockade of uptake of norepinephrine (step 9) and dopamine (step 5) into storage vesicles results in accumulation of amines in the cytoplasm and consequent inactivation by monoamine oxidase (steps 4 and 8). Synthesis of norepinephrine is inhibited because of blockade of dopamine uptake, and also by direct and feedback inhibition of tyrosine hydroxylase (step 2). Vesicles are not yet depleted, and reflex neural stimulation leads to release into the synapse (step 10), accelerating the onset of depletion. Increased catecholamines in the cytoplasm lead to increased diffusion from the mobile pool into the synapse (step 16); this is accentuated by monoamine oxidase inhibitors, which increase cytoplasmic amines, and may actually result in a sympathomimetic action of reserpine.

B. Later Stages

Vesicles are depleted of catecholamines and neurotransmission is blocked, leading to a decrease in *O*-methylated metabolites (step 13). Persistently bound reserpine in storage vesicle membranes still prevents uptake of amines despite disappearance of most of the drug. The pharmacological characteristics of adrenergic transmission may be recovered transiently by replenishment of the mobile pool by catecholamine precursors, monoamine oxidase inhibitors, or norepinephrine infusion (step 15).

C. Recovery

New vesicles are transported down the axon, leading to recovery from blockade of vesicular uptake. Symptoms of reserpinization disappear prior to reestablishment of amine stores, probably due in part to hypersensitivity of adrenergic receptors (step 12). Catecholamine synthesis is accelerated by trans-synaptic induction of tyrosine hydroxylase (step 2) and dopamine β-hydroxylase (step 6).

ACKNOWLEDGMENT

The author is the recipient of a Faculty Development Award in Pharmacology from the Pharmaceutical Manufacturers Association Foundation.

IX. REFERENCES

Abboud, F. M., Eckstein, J. W., Lawrence, M. S., and Hoak, J. C., 1967, Preliminary observations on the use of intra-arterial reserpine in Raynaud's phenomenon, *Circulation* (Suppl. 2) **36**:49.

Ahlbaum, H. G., and Milch, L. J., 1962, The effect of central nervous system drugs on the incorporation of radioactive carbon into brain adenosine triphosphate (ATP), *Ann. N.Y. Acad. Sci.* **96**:190.

Alpers, H. S., and Shore, P. A., 1969, Specific binding of reserpine—Association with norepinephrine depletion, *Biochem. Pharmacol.* **18**:1363.

Andén, N.-E., and Lundborg, P., 1970, Recovery of the amine uptake–storage mechanism in nerve granules after reserpine treatment: Inhibition by axotomy, *J. Pharm. Pharmacol.* **22**:233.

Andén, N.-E., Roos, B.-E., and Werdinius, B., 1963, 3,4-Dihydroxyphenylacetic acid in rabbit corpus striatum normally and after reserpine treatment, *Life Sci.* **2**:319.

Andén, N.-E., Roos, B.-E., and Werdinius, B., 1964, Effects of chlorpromazine, haloperidol and reserpine on the levels of phenolic acids in rabbit corpus striatum, *Life Sci.* **3**:149.

Atack, C., 1971, Reduction of histamine in mouse brain by N^1-(DL-seryl)-N^2-(2,3,4-trihydroxybenzyl) hydrazine and reserpine, *J. Pharm. Pharmacol.* **23**:992.

Axelrod, J., 1971, Noradrenaline: Fate and Control of its biosynthesis, *Science* **173**:598.

Axelrod, J., Hertting, G., and Patrick, R. W., 1961, Inhibition of H^3-norepinephrine release by monoamine oxidase inhibitors, *J. Pharmacol. Exptl. Therap.* **134**:325.

Axelrod, J., Mueller, R. A. and Thoenen, H., 1970, Neuronal and hormonal control of tyrosine hydroxylase and phenylethanolamine *N*-methyltransferase activity, *Bayer-Symposium* **II**:212.

Balzer, H., and Palm, D., 1962, Über den Mechanismus der Wirkung des Reserpins auf den Glykogengehalt der Organe, *Naunyn-Schmiedeberg's Arch. Pharmakol.* **243**:65.

Balzer, H., Holtz, P., and Palm, D., 1961*a*, Reserpin und γ-Aminobuttersäuregehalt des Gehirns, *Experientia* **17**:38.

Balzer, H., Holtz, P., and Palm, D., 1961*b*, Reserpin und Glykogengehalt der Organe, *Experientia* **17**:304.

Balzer, H., Makinose, M., and Hasselbach, W., 1968*a*, The inhibition of the sarcoplasmic calcium pump by prenylamine, reserpine, chlorpromazine and imipramine, *Naunyn-Schmiedeberg's Arch. Pharmakol.* **260**:444.

Balzer, H., Makinose, M., Fiehn, W., and Hasselbach, W., 1968*b*, The binding of the calcium transport inhibitors reserpine, chloropromazine and prenylamine to the lipids of the membranes of the sarcoplasmic reticulum, *Naunyn-Schmiedeberg's Arch. Pharmakol.* **260**:456.

Barchas, J. D., Ciaranello, R. D., Stolk, J. M., Brodie, H. K. H., and Hamburg, D. A., 1972, Biogenic amines and behavior, in *Hormones and Behavior* (S. Levine, ed.) pp. 235–329, Academic Press, New York.

Bein, H. J., 1956, The pharmacology of *Rauwolfia, Pharmacol. Rev.* **8**:435.

Belford, J., and Feinleib, M. R., 1961, Phosphorylase activity in heart and brain after reserpine, iproniazid and other drugs affecting the central nervous system, *Biochem. Pharmacol.* **6**:189.

Berkowitz, B. A., Tarver, J. H., and Spector, S., 1971, Norepinephrine in blood vessels: Concentration, binding, uptake and depletion, *J. Pharmacol. Exptl. Therap.* **177**:119.

Berl, S., and Frigyesi, T. L., 1969, Effect of reserpine on the turnover of glutamate, glutamine, aspartate and GABA labeled with [1-^{14}C] acetate in caudate nucleus, thalamus and sensorimotor cortex (cat), *Brain Res.* **14**:683.

Berneis, K. H., Pletscher, A., and DaPrada, M., 1969, Metal-dependent aggregation of biogenic amines: A hypothesis for their storage and release, *Nature* (*Lond.*) **224**:281.

Berneis, K. H., Pletscher, A., and DaPrada, M., 1970, Phase separation in solutions of noradrenaline and adenosine triphosphate: Influence of bivalent cations and drugs, *Brit. J. Pharmacol.* **39**:382.

Bertler, Å., 1961, Effect of reserpine on the storage of catecholamines in brain and other tissues, *Acta. Physiol. Scand.* **51**:75.

Bertler, Å., Carlsson, A., and Rosengren, E., 1956, Release by reserpine of catecholamines from rabbits' hearts, *Naturwissenschaften* **22**:521.

Bertler, Å., Hillarp, N.-Å., and Rosengren, E., 1961, Effect of reserpine on the storage of new-formed catecholamines in the adrenal medulla, *Acta Physiol. Scand.* **52**:44.

Bhagat, B., Burke, W. J., and Davis, J. W., 1971, Effect of reserpine on the activity of adrenal enzymes involved in the synthesis of adrenaline, *Brit. J. Pharmacol.* **43**:819.

Bhatia, B. B., 1942, On use of *Rauwolfia serpentina* in high blood pressure, *J. Indian Med. Ass.* **11**:262.

Bianchi, C., and Beani, L., 1966, Reserpine and the neuro-muscular junction, *J. Pharm. Pharmacol.* **18**:757.

Blair, J. H., and Simpson, G. M. 1966, Effect of anti-psychotic drugs on reproductive functions, *Dis. Nerv. Syst.* **27**:645.

Blaschko, H., and Chrúsciel, T. L., 1960, The decarboxylation of amino acids related to tyrosine and their awakening action in mice, *J. Physiol.* (*Lond.*) **151**:272.

Blum, J. J., 1967, An adrenergic control system in *Tetrahymena, Proc. Natl. Acad. Sci.* **58**:81.

Blum, J. J., Kirshner, N., and Utley, J. 1966, The effect of reserpine on growth and catecholamine content of *Tetrahymena, Mol. Pharmacol.* **2**:606.

Boadle-Biber, M. C., and Roth, R. H., 1972, Effect of drugs on the synthesis of noradrenaline in guinea-pig vas deferens, *Brit. J. Pharmacol.* **46**:696.

Bogdanksi, D. F., Sulser, F., and Brodie, B. B., 1961, Comparative action of reserpine, tetrabenazine and chlorpromazine on central parasympathetic activity: Effects on pupillary size and lacrimation in rabbit and salivation in dogs, *J. Pharmacol. Exptl. Therap.* **132**:176.

Brodie, B. B., 1964, Physico-chemical factors in drug absorption, in *Absorption and Distribution of Drugs* (T. B. Binns, ed.) pp. 16–48, Williams and Wilkins, Baltimore.

Brodie, B. B., Pletscher, A., and Shore, P. A., 1956, Possible role of serotonin in brain function, *J. Pharmacol. Exptl. Therap.* **116**:9.

Burack, W. R., Weiner, N., and Hagen, P. B., 1960, The effect of reserpine on the catecholamine and adenine nucleotide contents of adrenal gland, *J. Pharmacol. Exptl. Therap.* **130**:245.

Burack, W. R., Draskóczy, P. R., and Weiner, N., 1961, Adenine nucleotide, catecholamine and protein contents of whole adrenal glands and heavy granules of reserpine-treated fowl, *J. Pharmacol. Exptl. Therap.* **133**:25.

Burn, J. H., and Rand, M. J., 1958, The action of sympathomimetic amines in animals treated with reserpine, *J. Physiol.* (*Lond.*) **144**:314.

Burn, J. H., and Rand, M. J., 1960, The effect of precursors of noradrenaline on the response to tyramine and sympathetic stimulation, *Brit. J. Pharmacol.* **15**:47.

Burn, J. H., and Rand, M. J., 1962, A new interpretation of the adrenergic nerve fiber, *Advan. Pharmacol.* **1**:2.

Callingham, B. A., and Cass, R., 1962, The effects of bretylium and cocaine on noradrenaline depletion, *J. Pharm. Pharmacol.* **14**:385.

Carlsson, A., 1965, Drugs which block the storage of 5-hydroxytryptamine and related amines, *Handbook Exptl. Pharmacol.* **19**:529.

Carlsson, A., and Hillarp, N.-Å., 1956, Release of adrenaline from the adrenal medulla of rabbits produced by reserpine, *Kgl. Fysiogr. Sällsk. Lund. Förh* **26**: No. 8.

Carlsson, A., and Waldeck, B., 1968, Different mechanisms of drug-induced release of noradrenaline and its congeners α-methyl-noradrenaline and metaraminol, *Europ. J. Pharmacol.* **4**:165.

Carlsson, A., Rosengren, E., Bertler, A., and Nilsson, J., 1957*a*, Effect of reserpine on the metabolism of catecholamines, in: *Psychotropic Drugs* (S. Garattini and V. Ghetti, eds.) pp. 363–372, Elsevier, Amsterdam.

Carlsson, A., Lindqvist, M., and Magnusson, T., 1957*b*, 3,4-Dihydroxyphenylalanine and 5-hydroxytryptophan as reserpine antagonists, *Nature* (*Lond.*) **180**:1200.

Carlsson, A., Hillarp, N.-Å., and Waldeck, B., 1962, A Mg^{++}-ATP-dependent storage mechanism in the amine granules of the adrenal medulla, *Med. Exptl.* (*Basel*) **6**:47.

Carlsson, A., Hillarp, N.-Å., and Waldeck, B., 1963, Analysis of the Mg^{++}-ATP dependent storage mechanism in the amine granules of the adrenal medulla, *Acta Physiol. Scand.* **59**:1 (Suppl. 215).

Carlsson, A., Lundborg, P., Stitzel, R., and Waldeck, B., 1967, Uptake storage and release of ^{3}H-α-methylnorepinephrine, *J. Pharmacol. Exptl. Therap.* **158**:175.

Carrier, O., Jr., and Jurevics, H. A., 1973, The role of calcium in "nonspecific" supersensitivity of vascular muscle, *J. Pharmacol. Exptl. Therap.* **184**:81.

Choi, S. J., and Roberts, J., 1970, Effect of reserpine on ^{22}Na and ^{42}K exchange in the cat papillary muscle, *Proc. Soc. Exptl. Biol. Med.* **135**:579.

Chubb, I. W., DePotter, W. P., and De Schaepdryver, A. F., 1972, Influence of reserpine on noradrenaline and dopamine β-hydroxylase in the splenic nerve, *Arch. Int. Pharmacodyn. Therap.* **196**: Suppl. 296.

Clower, B. R., Williams, W. L., and Matheny, J. L., 1969, Effects of reserpine on calcium levels in cardiac tissue of mice. *Cardiovasc. Res.* **3**:64.

Coupland, R. E., 1958, Strain sensitivity of albino rats to reserpine, *Nature* (*Lond*) **181**:930.

DeFelice, F. A., 1957, Plasma disappearance and urinary excretion of reserpine (Serpasil) in the unanesthesized dog, *Experientia* **13**:373.

Degkwitz, R., Frowein, R., Kulenkampff, C., and Mohs, U., 1960, Über die Wirkungen des L-dopa beim Menschen und deren Beeinflussung durch Reserpin, Chlorpromazin, Iproniazid und Vitamin B_1, *Klin. Wschr.* **38**:120.

De Schaepdryver, A. F., Bogaert, M., Delannois, A. L., Bernard, A. L., and Bernard, P., 1963, Peripheral noradrenergic reactivity, *Arch. Int. Pharmacodyn. Therap.* **142**:243.

Dhar, M. M., Kohli, J. D., and Srivastava, S. K., 1955, Studies on the metabolism of reserpine. I. Identification of metabolites, *J. Sci. Ind. Res.* **14C**:179.

Dismukes, R. K., and Rake, A. V. 1972, Involvement of biogenic amines in memory formation, *Psychopharmacologia* **23**:17.

Domenjoz, R., and Theobald, W., 1959, Zur Pharmakologie des Tofranil (*N*-(3-Dimethylaminopropyl)-iminodibenzylhydrochlorid), *Arch. Int. Pharmacodyn. Therap.* **120**:450.

Emås, S., 1968, Mechanisms of action of reserpine on gastric secretion of acid, *Am. J. Digest. Dis.* **13**:572.

Emås, S., and Fyrö, B., 1967, Gastric and duodenal ulcers in cats following reserpine, *Acta Physiol. Scand.* **71**:316.

Enna, S. J., and Shore, P. A., 1971, Regional distribution of persistently bound reserpine in rat brain, *Biochem. Pharmacol.* **20**:2910.

Erickson, L. B., 1969, The comparative effect of reserpine and carbethoxysyringoyl methylreserpate (Su 3118) upon the menstrual cycle of the rhesus monkey, *Can. J. Physiol. Pharmacol.* **47**:99.

Everett, G. M., and Toman, J. E. P., 1959, Mode of action of *Rauwolfia* alkaloids on motor activity, *Biol. Psychiat.* **2**:75.

Falck, B., Hillarp, N.-A., and Högberg, B., 1956, Content and intracellular distribution of adenosine triphosphate in cow adrenal medulla, *Acta Physiol. Scand.* **36**:360.

Farnebo, L.-P., 1971, Effect of reserpine on release of [^{3}H] noradrenaline, [^{3}H] dopamine and [^{3}H] metaraminol from field stimulated rat iris, *Biochem. Pharmacol.* **20**:2715.

Fawaz, G., 1963, Cardiovascular pharmacology, *Ann. Rev. Pharmacol.* **3**:57.

Ferris, R. M., Viveros, O. H., and Kirshner, N., 1970, Effects of various agents on the Mg^{2+}-ATP stimulated incorporation and release of catecholamines by isolated bovine adrenomedullary storage vesicles and on secretion from the adrenal medulla, *Biochem. Pharmacol.* **19**:505.

Gabe, M., Tuchmann-Duplessis, H., and Mercier-Parot, L., 1961, Influence de la réserpine sur la neurosécrétion hypothalamo-hypophysaire du rat albinos, *Compt. Rend. Acad. Sci. (Paris)* **252**:1857.

Gaffney, T. E., Chidsey, C. A., and Braunwald, E., 1963, Study of the relationship between the neurotransmitter store and adrenergic nerve block induced by reserpine and guanethidine, *Circ. Res.* **12**:264.

Galansino, G., Litta-Modignani, R., Berlinger, F., Billinger, D., and Foá, P. P., 1963, Studies on the release of serotonin and catecholamines in the pancreato-duodenal area, *Proc. Soc. Exptl. Biol. Med.* **112**:542.

Gandini, A., Lualdi, P., and Della Bella, D., 1972, Influence of reserpine on the release and effects of prostaglandins, *Arch. Int. Pharmacodyn. Therap.* **196**: Suppl. 179.

Garattini, S., and Valzelli, L., 1962, Biochemistry and pharmacology of serotonin in the central nervous system, in: *Monoamines et Système Nerveux Central* (J. de Ajuriaguerra, ed.) pp. 59–88, George and Company, Geneva.

Gaunt, R., Renzi, A. A., Antonchak, N., Miller, G. J., and Gilman, M., 1954, Endocrine aspects of the pharmacology of reserpine, *Ann. N.Y. Acad. Sci.* **59**:22.

Gaunt, R., Chart, J. J., and Renzi, A. A., 1963, Interactions of drugs with endocrines, *Ann. Rev. Pharmacol.* **3**:109.

Giachetti, A. and Shore, P. A., 1970, Permeability changes induced in the adrenergic neurone by reserpine, *Biochem. Pharmacol.* **19**:1621.

Gilgen, A., Maickel, R. P., Nikodijevic, O., and Brodie, B. B., 1962, Essential role of catecholamines in the mobilization of free fatty acids and glucose after exposure to cold, *Life Sci.* **12**:709.

Gillespie, E., and Levine, R. J. 1969, Histamine release by reserpine from rat peritoneal mast cells *in vitro, Biochem. Pharmacol.* **18**:934.

Glazko, A. J., Dill, W. A., Wolf, L. M., and Kazenko, A., 1956, Studies on the metabolism of reserpine. *J. Pharmacol. Exptl. Therap.* **118**:377.

Glowinski, J., Iversen, L. L., and Axelrod, J., 1966, Storage and synthesis of norepinephrine in the reserpine-treated rat brain, *J. Pharmacol. Exptl. Therap.* **151**:385.

Goodman, L. S., and Gilman, A., 1970, *The Pharmacological Basis of Therapeutics,* 4th ed., Macmillan, New York.

Gray, W. D., Rauh, C. E., and Shanahan, R. W., 1963, The mechanism of the antagonistic action of reserpine on the anticonvulsant effect of inhibitors of carbonic anhydrase, *J. Pharmacol. Exptl. Therap.* **139**:350.

Green, H. O., and Slotkin, T. A., 1973, Reserpine-like effects of harmine on isolated adrenal medullary vesicles, *Mol. Pharmacol.* **9**:748.

Gripenberg, J., Jansson, S.-E., and Partanen, T., 1972, Incorporation of reserpine into isolated rat peritoneal mast cells and mast cell granules *in vitro, Acta Physiol. Scand.* **86**:433.

Häggendal, J., and Dahlström, A., 1971, The functional role of the amine storage granules of the sympathoadrenal system, in: *Subcellular Organization and Function in Endocrine Tissues* (H. Heller and K. Lederis, eds.) pp. 651–669, Cambridge University Press, Cambridge.

Häkonson, R., Lindstrand, K., Nordgren, L., and Owman, C., 1971, Reserpine-induced mobilization of histamine and vitamin B_{12}-binding proteins from a special type of endocrine cells in rat stomach, *Biochem. Pharmacol.* **20**:1259.

Hamberger, B., Malmfors, T., Norberg, K.-A., and Sachs, C., 1964, Uptake and accumulation of catecholamines in peripheral adrenergic neurons of reserpinized animals, studied with a histochemical method, *Biochem. Pharmacol.* **13**:841.

Hanig, R. C., and Aprison, M. H., 1971, The effect of 5-hydroxytryptophan and reserpine administration on the level of sodium, potassium, calcium, magnesium and chloride in five discrete areas of the rabbit brain, *Life Sci.* **10**:279.

Hertting, G., Axelrod, J., and Whitby, L. G., 1961, Effect of drugs on the uptake and metabolism of H^3-norepinephrine, *J. Pharmacol. Exptl. Therap.* **134**:146.

Hess, S. M., Shore, P. A., and Brodie, B. B., 1956, Persistence of reserpine action after the disappearance of drug from brain: Effect on serotonin, *J. Pharmacol. Exptl. Therap.* **118**:84.

Hillarp, N.-Å., 1958, Adenosinephosphates and inorganic phosphate in the adrenaline and noradrenaline containing granules of the adrenal medulla, *Acta Physiol. Scand.* **42**:321.

Hillarp, N.-Å., 1959, Further observations on the state of the catecholamines stored in the adrenal medullary granules, *Acta Physiol. Scand.* **47**:271.

Hillarp, N.-Å., 1960*a*, Different pools of catecholamines stored in the adrenal medulla, *Acta Physiol. Scand.* **50**:8.

Hillarp, N.-Å., 1960*b*, Effect of reserpine on the adrenal medulla of sheep, *Acta Physiol. Scand.* **49**:376.

Hillarp, N.-Å., and Malmfors, T., 1964, Reserpine and cocaine blocking of uptake and storage mechanisms in adrenergic nerves, *Life Sci.* **3**:703.

Hoffer, A., and Osmond, H., 1967, *The Hallucinogens*, Chap. IIA, pp. 83–236. Academic Press, New York.

Holeček, V., Schreiber, V., and Kmentová, V., 1957, The influence of serpasil on the secretion of antidiuretic hormone, *Cas. Lék. Ces.* **96**:1060.

Holtz, P., and Palm, D., 1966, Brenzkatechinamine und andere sympaticomimetische Amine. Biosynthese und Inaktivierung. Freisetzung und Wirkung, in: *Ergebnisse der Physiologie: Biologischen Chemie und experimentellen Pharmakologie*, Vol. 58, Springer, Berlin.

Honda, F., and Imamura, H., 1968, Inhibition of cyclic 3′,5′-nucleotide phosphodiesterase by phenothiazine and reserpine derivatives, *Biochim. Biophys. Acta* **161**:267.

Hussar, A. E., and Bruno, E., 1956, Acute duodenal ulcer associated with reserpine therapy, *Gastroenterology* **31**:500.

Isaac, L., Cho, A. K., and Beaven, M. A., 1971, Decline of histidine decarboxylase activity and histamine levels in rat stomach after reserpine. *Biochem. Pharmacol.* **20**:1453.

Iversen, L. L., Glowinski, J., and Axelrod, J., 1965, The uptake and storage of H^3-norepinephrine in the reserpine-pretreated rat heart, *J. Pharmacol. Exptl. Therap.* **150**:173.

Iwayama, T., Fleming, W. W., and Burnstock, G., 1973, Ultrastructure of mitochondria in atrial muscle associated with depression and supersensitivity produced by reserpine, *J. Pharmacol. Exptl. Therap.* **184**:95.

Izquierdo, J. A., Coussio, J. D., and Kaumann, A. J., 1962, Effect of imipramine on the pressor responses to the afferent vagal stimulation of reserpinized dogs, *Arch. Int. Pharmacodyn. Therap.* **135**:303.

Izumi, F., Oka, M., Yoshida, H., and Imaizumi, R., 1969, Stimulatory effect of reserpine on monoamine oxidase in guinea pig heart, *Biochem. Pharmacol.* **18**:1739.

Jansson, S.-E., 1970, Uptake of 5-hydroxytryptamine by mast cell granules *in vitro*, *Acta Physiol. Scand.* **79**:484.

Johnson, G. E., and Sellers, E. A., 1961, The effect of reserpine on the metabolic rate of rats, *Can. J. Biochem.* **39**:279.

Jonasson, J., Rosengren, E., and Waldeck, B., 1964, Effects of some pharmacologically active amines on the uptake of arylalkylamines by adrenal medullary granules, *Acta Physiol. Scand.* **60**:136.

Jonsson, G., and Sachs, C., 1970, Synthesis of noradrenaline from 3,4-dihydroxyphenylalanine (DOPA) and dopamine in adrenergic nerves of mouse atrium—Effect of reserpine, monoamine oxidase and tyrosine hydroxylase inhibition, *Acta Physiol. Scand.* **80**:307.

Kaul, C. L., and Lewis, J. J., 1963, The effects of reserpine and some related compounds upon the levels of adenine nucleotides, creatine phosphate and inorganic phosphate in the rat brain *in vivo*, *J. Pharmacol. Exptl. Therap.* **140**:111.

Keswani, A., D'Iorio, A., and Mavrides, C., 1971, The fate of catecholamine-containing granules after depletion of the guinea-pig adrenal glands, *Arch. Int. Pharmacodyn. Therap.* **193**:171.

Khan, M. Y., and Bernstorf, E. C., 1964, Effect of chlorpromazine and reserpine upon pituitary function, *Exptl. Med. Surg.* **22**:363.

Khazan, N., Adir, J., Pfeifer, Y., and Sulman, F. G., 1962, Mechanism of antidiuretic action of reserpine, *Proc. Soc. Exptl. Biol. Med.* **109**:32.

Kim, K. S., and Shore, P. A., 1963, Mechanism of action of reserpine and insulin on gastric amines and gastric acid secretion, and the effect of monoamine oxidase inhibition, *J. Pharmacol. Exptl. Therap.* **141**:321.

Kirpekar, S. M., and Lewis, J. J., 1959, Some effects of reserpine and hydrallazine upon tissue respiration and the concentration of adenosine nucleotides in certain tissues, *Brit. J. Pharmacol.* **14**:40.

Kirpekar, S. M., Goodlad, G. A. J., and Lewis, J. J., 1958, Reserpine depletion of adenosine triphosphate from the rat suprarenal medulla, *Biochem. Pharmacol.* **1**:232.

Kirpekar, S. M., Cerroni, P., and Couri, D., 1963, Depletion and recovery of catecholamines and adenosine-triphosphate of rat adrenal medulla after reserpine treatment, *J. Pharmacol. Exptl. Therap.* **142**:71.

Kirshner, N., 1962, Uptake of catecholamines by a particulate fraction of the adrenal medulla, *J. Biol. Chem.* **237**:2311.

Kirshner, N., 1965, The role of the membrane of chromaffin granules isolated from the adrenal medulla, in: *Pharmacology of Cholinergic and Adrenergic Transmission* (G. B. Koelle, W. W. Douglas, and A. Carlsson, eds.) pp. 225–233, Czechoslovak Medical Press, Prague.

Kirshner, N., and Viveros, O. H., 1972, The secretory cycle in the adrenal medulla, *Pharmacol. Rev.* **24**:385.

Kirshner, N., Holloway, C., Smith, W. J., and Kirshner, A. G., 1966, Uptake and storage of catecholamines, in: *Mechanisms of Release of Biogenic Amines* (U.S. von Euler, S. Rosell, and B. Uvnäs, eds.) pp. 109–123, Pergamon Press, New York.

Kirshner, N., Schanberg, S. M., and Ferris, R. M., 1971, Molecular aspects of the storage and uptake of catecholamines, *Advan. Drug Res.* **6**:121.

Kitay, J. I., Holub, D. A., and Jailer, J. W., 1959, "Inhibition" of pituitary ACTH release after administration of reserpine or epinephrine, *Endocrinology* **65**:548.

Klein, R. L., and Lagercrantz, H., 1971, Unidirectional fluxes in isolated splenic nerve vesicles measured by a millipore filter technique: Effects of noradrenaline and competitive reversal of reserpine inhibition, *Acta Physiol. Scand.* **83**:179.

Kontos, H. A., and Wasserman, A. J., 1969, Effect of reserpine in Raynaud's phenomenon, *Circulation* **39**:259.

Kopin, I. J., 1968, Biosynthesis and metabolism of catecholamines, *Anesthesiology* **29**:654.

Kopin, I. J., and Gordon, E. K., 1963, Metabolism of administered and drug-released norepinephrine-7-H^3 in the rat, *J. Pharmacol. Exptl. Therap.* **140**:207.

Lagercrantz, H., 1971, Isolation and characterization of sympathetic nerve trunk vesicles, *Acta Physiol. Scand.*, Suppl. 366.

Lessin, A. W., and Parkes, M. W., 1957, The relation between sedation and body temperature in the mouse, *Brit. J. Pharmacol.* **12**:245.

Lessin, A. W., and Parkes, M. W., 1959, The effects of reserpine and other agents upon leptazol convulsions in mice, *Brit. J. Pharmacol.* **14**:108.

Lewis, J. J., 1963, *Rauwolfia* derivatives, in: *Physiological Pharmacology: A Comprehensive Treatise,* Vol. I: *The Nervous System* (W. S. Root and F. G. Hofmann, eds.) pp. 479–536, Academic Press, New York.

Lindmar, R., and Muscholl, E., 1965, Die Aufnahme von α-Methylnoradrenalin in das isolierte Kaninchenherz und seine Freisetzung durch Reserpin und Guanethidin *in vivo, Naunyn-Schmiedeberg's Arch. Pharmakol.* **249**:529.

Lishajko, F., 1969, Release, reuptake and net uptake of dopamine, noradrenaline and adrenaline in isolated sheep adrenal medullary granules, *Acta Physiol. Scand.* **76**:159.

Lishajko, F., 1971, Studies on catecholamine release and uptake in adrenomedullary storage granules, *Acta Physiol. Scand.*, Suppl. 362.

Loggie, J. M. H., Saito, H., Kahn, I., Fenner, A., and Gaffney, T. E., 1967, Accidental reserpine poisoning: Clinical and metabolic effects, *Clin. Pharmacol. Therap.* **8**:692.

Lucas, R. A., 1963, The chemistry and pharmacology of the *Rauwolfia* alkaloids, *Prog. Med. Chem.* **3**:146.

Lundborg, P., 1966, Uptake of metaraminol by the adrenal medullary granules, *Acta Physiol. Scand.* **67**:423.

Lundborg, P., and Stitzel, R., 1967*a*, Uptake of biogenic amines by two different mechanisms present in adrenergic granules, *Brit. J. Pharmacol.* **29**:342.

Lundborg, P., and Stitzel, R., 1967*b*, Effect of reserpine and protriptyline on the subcellular distribution of ^{3}H-metaraminol in the mouse heart, *Brit. J. Pharmacol.* **30**:379.

Lundborg, P., and Waldeck, B., 1971, On the mechanism of amphetamine induced release of reserpine-resistant ^{3}H-noradrenaline and ^{3}H-α-methylnoradrenaline, *Acta Pharmacol. Toxicol.* **30**:339.

Maass, A. R., Jenkins, B., Shen, Y., and Tannenbaum, P., 1969, Studies on absorption, excretion and metabolism of ^{3}H-reserpine in man, *Clin. Pharmacol. Therap.* **10**:366.

MacLean, P. D., 1955, Hippocampal studies: Their possible bearing on neuropsychiatry, *Arch. Neurol. Psychiat.* (*Chicago*) **74**:219.

MacLeod, R. M., 1969, Influence of norepinephrine and catecholamine-depleting agents on the synthesis and release of prolactin and growth hormone, *Endocrinology* **85**:916.

MacPhillamy, H. B., Huebner, C. F., Schlittler, E., St. André, A. F., and Ulshafer, P. R., 1955, *Rauwolfia* alkaloids. XIX. The constitution of deserpidine and reserpine, *J. Am. Chem. Soc.* **77**:4335.

Maggiolo, C., and Haley, T. J., 1964, Brain concentration of reserpine-H^3 and its metabolites in the mouse, *Proc. Soc. Exptl. Biol. Med.* **115**:149.

Maickel, R. P., Westermann, E. O., and Brodie, B. B., 1962, Effects of reserpine and cold-exposure on pituitary adrenocortical function in rats, *J. Pharmacol. Exptl. Therap.* **134**:167.

Malhotra, C. L., and Das, P. K.,1962, Effect of reserpine on the acetylcholine content of the heart, the ileum and the hypothalamus of the dog, *Brit. J. Pharmacol.* **18**:190.

Malhotra, C. L., and Pundlik, P. G., 1959, The effect of reserpine on the acetylcholine content of different areas of the nervous system of the dog, *Brit. J. Pharmacol.* **14**:46.

Malpica, J. F., Jurupe, H., and Campos, H. A., 1970, Actions of reserpine and tyramine on the acetylcholine content of brain stem, heart and blood of the rat, *Arch. Int. Pharmacodyn. Therap.* **185**:13.

Manara, L., and Garattini, S., 1967, Time course of ^{3}H-reserpine levels in brains of normal and tetrabenazine-pretreated rats, *Europ. J. Pharmacol.* **2**:139.

Manara, L., Carminati, P., and Mennini, T., 1972, *In vivo* persistent binding of ^{3}H-reserpine to rat brain subcellular components, *Europ. J. Pharmacol.* **20**:109.

Mathé, V., Kassay, G., and Hunkár, K., 1961, Die Wirkung des Reserpins auf den Gehalt des Rattengehirns an gesamtreduzierenden Stoffen und Glykogen, *Z. Ges. Exptl. Med.* **134**:249.

McNeill, J. H., 1969, Reserpine supersensitivity to catecholamine-induced cardiac phosphorylase activation, *Can. J. Physiol. Pharmacol.* **47**:515.

Miline, R., Stern, P., Serstnev, E., and Muhibic, M., 1957, Effet de la réserpine et de la réserpine associée au luminal sur le complexe hypothalamohypophysaire, in: *Psychotropic Drugs* (S. Garattini and V. Ghetti, eds.) pp. 332–349, Elsevier, Amsterdam.

Müller, E. E., Sawano, S., Arimura, A., and Schally, A. V., 1967*a*, Blockade of release of growth hormone by brain norepinephrine depletors, *Endocrinology* **80**:471.

Müller, E. E., Saito, T., Arimura, A., and Schally, A. V., 1967*b*, Hypoglycemia, stress and growth hormone release: Blockade of growth hormone release by drugs acting on the central nervous system, *Endocrinology* **80**:109.

Müller, J. M., Schlittler, E., and Bein, H. J., 1952, Reserpin, der sedative Wirkstoff aus *Rauwolfia serpentina* Benth., *Experientia* **8**:338.

Muscholl, E., 1960, Die Hemmung der Noradrenalin-Aufnahme des Herzens durch Reserpin und die Wirkung von Tyramin, *Naunyn-Schmiedeberg's Arch. Pharmakol.* **240**:234.

Muscholl, E., 1972, Adrenergic false transmitters, *Handbook Exptl. Pharmacol.* **33**:618.

Muscholl, E., and Sprenger, E., 1966, Vergleichende Untersuchung der Blutdruckwirkung, Aufnahme und Speicherung von Dihydroxyephedrin (α-Methyladrenalin) und Dihydroxypseudoephedrin, *Naunyn-Schmiedeberg's Arch. Pharmakol.* **254**:109.

Muscholl, E., and Vogt, M., 1958, The action of reserpine on the peripheral sympathetic system, *J. Physiol.* (*Lond.*) **141**:132.

Nasmyth, P. A., 1962, An investigation of the action of tyramine and its interrelationship with the effects of other sympathomimetic amines, *Brit. J. Pharmacol.* **18**:65.

Negro-Vilar, A., Dickerman, E., and Meites, J., 1968, Removal of plasma FSH-RF activity in hypophysectomized rats by testosterone propionate or reserpine, *Endocrinology* **83**:1349.

Norn, S., and Shore, P. A., 1971*a*, Further studies on the nature of persistent reserpine binding: Evidence for reversible and irreversible binding, *Biochem. Pharmacol.* **20**:1291.

Norn, S., and Shore, P. A., 1971*b*, Failure to affect tissue reserpine concentrations by alteration of adrenergic nerve activity, *Biochem. Pharmacol.* **20**:2133.

Numerof, P., Gordon, M., and Kelly, J. M., 1955, The metabolism of reserpine. I. Studies in the mouse with C^{14}-labeled reserpine, *J. Pharmacol. Exptl. Therap.* **115**:427.

Numerof, P., Virgona, A. J., Cranswick, E. H., Cunningham, T., and Kline, N. S., 1958, The metabolism of reserpine. II. Studies in schizophrenic patients, *Psychiat. Res. Rep.* **9**:139.

Oka, M., Ohuchi, T., Yosida, H., and Imaizumi, R., 1966, Selective release of noradrenaline and adrenaline from isolated adrenal medullary granules, *Life Sci.* **5**:433.

Parks, V. J., Sandison, A. G., Skinner, S. L., and Whelan, R. F., 1961, The mechanism of the vasodilator action of reserpine in man, *Clin. Sci.* **20**:289.

Patrick, R. L., and Kirshner, N., 1971, Acetylcholine-induced stimulation of catecholamine recovery in denervated rat adrenals after reserpine-induced depletion, *Mol. Pharmacol.* **7**:389.

Pepinsky, R., Turley, J. W., Okaya, Y., Doyne, T., Vand, V., Shimada, A., Lovell, F. M., and Sogo, Y., 1957, X-ray analysis of some biochemically important compounds, *Acta Crystallog.* **10**:811.

Philippu, A., and Schümann, H. J., 1966, Uber die Bedeutung der Calcium- und Magnesiumionen für die Speicherung der Nebbenierenmarkhormone, *Naunyn-Schmiedeberg's Arch. Pharmakol.* **252**:339.

Pletscher, A., 1956, Beeinflussung des 5-Hydroxytryptamin-Stoffwechsels im Gehirn durch Isonikotinsaüre-hydrazide, *Experientia* **12**:479.

Pletscher, A., Shore, P. A., and Brodie, B. B., 1955, Serotonin release as a possible mechanism of reserpine action, *Science* **122**:374.

Pletscher, A., Besendorf, H., and Bächtold, H. P., 1958, Benzo[*a*]chinolizine, eine neue Körperklasse mit Wirkung auf den 5-Hydroxytryptamin- und Noradrenalin-Stoffwechsel des Gehirns, *Naunyn-Schmiedeberg's Arch. Pharmakol.* **232**:499.

Pletscher, A., DaPrada, M., and Berneis, K. H., 1971, Aggregation of biogenic monoamines and nucleotides in subcellular storage organelles, in: *Subcellular Organization and Function in Endocrine Tissues* (H. Heller and K. Lederis, eds.) pp. 767–783, Cambridge University Press, Cambridge.

Plummer, A. J., Barrett, W. E., and Rutledge, R., 1955, The action of reserpine on the motility of the digestive tract, *Am. J. Digest. Dis.* **22**:337.

Plummer, A. J., Sheppard, H., and Schulert, A. R., 1957, The metabolism of reserpine, in: *Psychotropic Drugs* (S. Garattini and V. Ghetti, eds.) pp. 350–362, Elsevier, Amsterdam.

Poisner, A. M., and Trifaró, J. M., 1967, The role of ATP and ATPase in the release of catecholamines from the adrenal medulla. I. ATP-evoked release of catecholamines, ATP, and protein from isolated chromaffin granules, *Mol. Pharmacol.* **3**:561.

Quinn, G. P., Shore, P. A., and Brodie, B. B., 1959, Biochemical and pharmacological studies of Ro 1-9569 (tetrabenazine), a non-indole tranquilizing agent with reserpine-like effects, *J. Pharmacol. Exptl. Therap.* **127**:103.

Räsänen, T., and Taskinen, E., 1967, Protection of the gastric mucosa against lesions caused by reserpine through degranulation of mucosal mast cells, *Acta Physiol. Scand.* **71**:96.

Raymond-Hamet, M., 1939, Le "Rauwolfia vomitoria" Afzelius possède-t-il réellement les vertus thérapeutiques que lui attribuent les guérisseurs indigènes?, *Bull. Acad. Med.* **122**:30.

Reilly, J. F., Ahlstrom, A. P., Watts, J. S., Cassidy, P. S., and Lusky, L. M., 1969, Influence of age, sex, and cold exposure on susceptibility to reserpine-induced gastric lesions, *Toxicol. Appl. Pharmacol.* **15**:97.

Rieppel, F. W., 1955, Leonhard Rauwolf. Ein Beitrag zu seiner Biographie, *Deutsch. Med. Wschr.* **80**:653.

Rinaldi, F., and Himwich, H. E., 1955, A comparison of effects of reserpine and some barbiturates on the electrical activity of cortical and subcortical structures in the brain of rabbits, *Ann. N.Y. Acad. Sci.* **61**:27.

Robison, M. M., Lucas, R. A., MacPhillamy, H. B., Dziemian, R. L., Hsu, I., Kiesel, R. J., and Morris, M. J., 1961, The development of non-hypotensive sedative drugs from methyl-reserpate, in: *139th American Chemistry Society Meeting Abstracts*, p. 3N.

Romeo, S. G., Whalen, R. E., and Tindall, J. P., 1970, Intra-arterial administration of reserpine, *Arch. Int. Med.* **125**:825.

Rosecrans, J. A., 1967, Effects of route of administration on the chronic toxicity of reserpine, *Psychopharmacologia* **10**:452.

Rosen, W. E., and O'Conner, J. M., 1961, *Rauwolfia* alkaloids. XXXVII. Methyl neoreserpate, an isomer of methyl reserpate, *J. Org. Chem.* **26**:3051.

Rosengren, E., and Svensson, S. E., 1969, Histamine formation in rat gastric mucosa and lung after injecting reserpine or adrenaline, *Brit. J. Pharmacol.* **37**:659.

Roth, R. H., and Stone, E. A., 1968, The action of reserpine on noradrenaline biosynthesis in sympathetic nerve tissue, *Biochem. Pharmacol.* **17**:1581.

Rumpf, G. E., 1755, *Herbarii Amboinensis Auctuarium* Uytwerf and Schouten, Amsterdam.

Rutishauser, M., 1963, Beeinflussung des Kohlenhydratstoffwechsels des Rattenhirns durch Psychopharmaka mit sedativer Wirkung, *Naunyn-Schmiedeberg's Arch. Pharmakol.* **245**:396.

Rutledge, C. O., and Weiner, N., 1967, The effect of reserpine upon the synthesis of norepinephrine in the isolated rabbit heart, *J. Pharmacol. Exptl. Therap.* **157**:290.

Saxton, J. E., 1960, The indole alkaloids, in: *The Alkaloids* (R. H. F. Manske, ed.) Vol. 7, pp. 1–199, Academic Press, New York.

Schildkraut, J. J., 1969, *Neuropsychopharmacology and the Affective Disorders*, Little, Brown, Boston.

Schlitter, E., and Plummer, A. J., 1964, Tranquilizing drugs from *Rauwolfia*, in: *Psychopharmacological Agents* (M. Gordon, ed.) Vol. 1, pp. 9–34, Academic Press, New York.

Schroeder, H. A., and Perry, H. M., 1955, Psychosis apparently produced by reserpine, *J. Am. Med. Ass.* **159**:839.

Schümann, H. J., 1958, Die Wirkung von Insulin und Reserpin auf den Adrenalin-und ATP-Gehalt der chromaffinen Granula des Nebennierenmarks, *Naunyn-Schmiedeberg's Arch. Pharmakol.* **233**:237.

Schümann, H. J., Grobecker, H., and Schmidt, K., 1965, Über die Wirkung von α-Methyl-Dopa auf den Brenzcatechinamingehalt von Meerschweinchenorganen, *Naunyn-Schmiedeberg's Arch. Pharmakol.* **251**:48.

Seiden, L. S., and Carlsson, A., 1963, Temporary and partial antagonism by -DOPA of reserpine-induced suppression of a conditioned avoidance response, *Psychopharmacologia* **4**:418.

Seiden, L. S., and Carlsson, A., 1964, Brain and heart catecholamine levels after -DOPA administration in reserpine treated mice: Correlations with conditioned avoidance response, *Psychopharmacologia* **5**:178.

Sen, G., and Bose, K. C., 1931, *Rauwolfia serpentina*, a new Indian drug for insanity and high blood pressure, *Indian Med. World* **2**:194.

Sheppard, H., Lucas, R. A., and Tsien, W. H., 1955, The metabolism of reserpine-C^{14}, *Arch. Int. Pharmacodyn. Therap.* **103**:256.

Sheppard, H., Tsien, W. H., Sigg, E. B., Lucas, R. A., and Plummer, A. J., 1957, The metabolism of reserpine-C^{14}. III. C^{14}-concentration vs. time in the brains and other tissues of rats and guinea pigs, *Arch. Int. Pharmacodyn. Therap.* **113**:160.

Sheppard, H., Tsien, W. H., Plummer, A. J., Peets, E. A., Giletti, B. J., and Schulert, A. R., 1958, Brain reserpine levels following large and small doses of reserpine-H^3, *Proc. Soc. Exptl. Biol. Med.* **97**:717.

Shore, P. A., 1972, Transport and storage of biogenic amines, *Ann. Rev. Pharmacol.* **12**:209.

Shore, P. A., Silver, S. L., and Brodie, B. B., 1955, Interaction of reserpine, serotonin, and lysergic acid diethylamide in brain, *Science* **122**:284.

Shore, P. A., Pletscher, A., Tomich, E., Carlsson, A., Kuntzman, R., and Brodie, B. B., 1957, Role of brain serotonin in reserpine action, *Ann. N.Y. Acad. Sci.* **66**:609.

Slotkin, T. A., 1973, Hypothetical model of catecholamine uptake into adrenal medullary storage vesicles, *Life Sci.* **13**:675.

Slotkin, T. A., and Edwards, K., 1973, Effects of reserpine on the content and properties of rat adrenal medullary storage vesicles, *Biochem. Pharmacol.* **22**:549.

Slotkin, T. A., and Kirshner, N., 1971, Uptake, storage, and distribution of amines in bovine adrenal medullary vesicles, *Mol. Pharmacol.* **7**:581.

Slotkin, T. A., and Kirshner, N., 1973*a*, Recovery of rat adrenal amine stores after insulin administration, *Mol. Pharmacol.* **9**:105.

Slotkin, T. A., and Kirshner, N., 1973*b*, Binding of amines to purified bovine adrenal medullary storage vesicle membranes, *Biochem. Pharmacol.* **22**:2492.

Slotkin, T. A., DiStefano, V., and Au, W. Y. W., 1970, Blood levels and urinary excretion of harmine and its metabolites in man and rats, *J. Pharmacol. Exptl. Therap.* **173**:26.

Slotkin, T. A., Ferris, R. M., and Kirshner, N., 1971, Compartmental analysis of amine storage in bovine adrenal medullary granules, *Mol. Pharmacol.* **7**:308.

Smith, A. D., 1968, Biochemistry of adrenal chromaffin granules, in: *The Interaction of Drugs and Subcellular Components in Animal Cells* (P. N. Campbell, ed.) pp. 239–292, Churchill, London.

Smith, C. B., and Dews, P. B., 1962, Antagonism of locomotor suppressant effects of reserpine in mice, *Psychopharmacologia* **3**:55.

Smith, E. R., 1963, The effect of norepinephrine infusions upon some responses of reserpine-treated spinal cats to tyramine, *J. Pharmacol. Exptl. Therap.* **139**:321.

Stitzel, R. E., Wagner, L. A., and Swartz, R. J., 1972, Studies on the microsomal metabolism of ^{3}H-reserpine, *J. Pharmacol. Exptl. Therap.* **182**:500.

Stjärne, L., 1964, Studies of catecholamine uptake storage and release mechanisms, *Acta Physiol. Scand.* 62: Suppl. 288.

Stjärne, L., 1972, The synthesis, uptake, and storage of catecholamines in the adrenal medulla: The effect of drugs, *Handbook Exptl. Pharmacol.* **33**:231.

Stjärne, L., and Lishajko, F., 1966, Drug-induced inhibition of noradrenaline synthesis *in vitro* in bovine splenic nerve tissue, *Brit. J. Pharmacol.* **27**:398.

Strubelt, O., 1969, The influence of reserpine, propranolol, and adrenal medullectomy on the hyperglycemic actions of theophylline and caffeine, *Arch. Int. Pharmacodyn. Therap.* **179**:215.

Sulser, F., Bickel, M. H., and Brodie, B. B., 1962, On mechanism of the antidepressant action of imipramine, in: *Proceedings of the First International Pharmacology Meeting* (W. D. M. Paton and P. Lindgren, eds.) Vol. 8, pp. 123–129, Pergamon Press, Oxford.

Sulser, F., Owens, M. L., Strada, S. J., and Dingell, J. V., 1969, Modification by desipramine (DMI) of the availability of norepinephrine released by reserpine in the hypothalamus of the rat *in vivo*, *J. Pharmacol. Exptl. Therap.* **168**:272.

Takemoto, Y., Shore, P. A., Tomich, E. G., Kuntzman, R., and Brodie, B. B., 1957, Studies on the mechanism of reserpine-induced epinephrine release and hyperglycemia, *J. Pharmacol. Exptl. Therap.* **119**:188.

Taugner, G., 1971, The membrane of catecholamine storage vesicles of adrenal medulla, *Naunyn-Schmiedeberg's Arch. Pharmakol.* **270**:392.

Taugner, G., and Hasselbach, W., 1966, Über den Mechanismus der Catecholamine-Speicherung in den "chromaffinen Granula" des Nebennierenmarks, *Naunyn-Schmiedeberg's Arch. Pharmakol.* **255**:266.

Taylor, R. E., Jr., and Fregly, M. J., 1962, Effect of reserpine on body temperature regulation of the rat, *J. Pharmacol. Exptl. Therap.* **138**:200.

Thomas, J. A., Knych, E. T., and Mawhinney, M. G., 1969, Effect of reserpine on the uptake of 1,2-^{3}H-testosterone by mouse prostate glands, *Europ. J. Pharmacol.* **8**:361.

Toman, J. E. P., 1963, Some aspects of central nervous pharmacology, *Ann. Rev. Pharmacol.* **3**:153.

Trendelenburg, U., 1963, Supersensitivity and subsensitivity to sympathomimetic amines, *Pharmacol. Rev.* **15**:225.

Trendelenburg, U., 1966, Mechanisms of supersensitivity and subsensitivity to sympathomimetic amines, *Pharmacol. Rev.* **18**:629.

Trendelenburg, U., 1972, Factors influencing the concentration of catecholamines at the receptors, *Handbook Exptl. Pharmacol.* **33**:726.

Trifaró, J. M., and Dworkind, J., 1971, Phosphorylation of membrane components of adrenal chromaffin granules by adenosine triphosphate, *Mol. Pharmacol.* **7**:52.

Troquet, J., Colinet-Lagneaux, D., and Hermann-Gedang, I., 1966, Influence of reserpine on myocardial content of potassium in the rat, *Arch. Int. Pharmacodyn. Therap.* **163**:232.

Udenfriend, S., Weissbach, H., and Bogdanski, D. F., 1957, Increase in tissue serotonin following administration of its precursor 5-hydroxytryptophan, *J. Biol. Chem.* **224**:803.

Vakil, R. L., 1949, A clinical trial of *Rauwolfia serpentina* in essential hypertension, *Brit. Heart J.* **11**:350.

Viveros, O. H., Arqueros, L., and Kirshner, N., 1969*a*, Mechanism of secretion from the adrenal medulla. V. Retention of storage vesicle membranes following release of adrenaline *Mol. Pharmacol.* **5**:342.

Viveros, O. H., Arqueros, L., Connett, R. J., and Kirshner, N., 1969*b*, Mechanism of secretion from the adrenal medulla. IV. The fate of the storage vesicles following insulin and reserpine administration, *Mol. Pharmacol.* **5**:69.

Viveros, O. H., Arqueros, L., and Kirshner, N., 1971, Mechanism of secretion from the adrenal medulla. VI. Effect of reserpine on the dopamine β-hydroxylase and catecholamine content and on the buoyant density of adrenal storage vesicles, *Mol. Pharmacol.* **7**:434.

Volle, R. L., 1963, Pharmacology of the autonomic nervous system, *Ann. Rev. Pharmacol.* **3**:129.

von Euler, U. S., 1972, Synthesis, uptake and storage of catecholamines in adrenergic nerves, the effect of drugs, *Handbook Exptl. Pharmacol.* **33**:186.

Waalkes, T. P., and Weissbach, H., 1956, *In vivo* release of histamine from rabbit blood by reserpine, *Proc. Soc. Exptl. Biol. Med.* **93**:394.

Waalkes, T. P., Coburn, H., and Terry, L. L., 1959, The effect of reserpine on histamine and serotonin, *J. Allergy* **30**:408.

Wagner, L. A., and Stitzel, R. F., 1972, The relation between the subcellular distribution of (^{3}H)-reserpine and its proposed site of action, *J. Pharm. Pharmacol.* **24**:396.

Watts, C. C., 1968, Effects of reserpine on the plasma half-time of [^{131}I]thyroxine, *J. Pharm. Pharmacol.* **20**:487.

Weiner, N., Cloutier, G., Bjur, R., and Pfeffer, R. I., 1972, Modification of norepinephrine synthesis in intact tissue by drugs and during short-term adrenergic nerve stimulation, *Pharmacol. Rev.* **24**:203.

Wells, H., Briggs, N., and Munson, P. L., 1956, The inhibitory effect of reserpine on ACTH secretion in response to stressful stimuli, *Endocrinology* **59**:571.

Werner, R. I., and Ganong, W. F., 1971, Effect of the depletion of brain catecholamines on puberty and the estrous cycle in the rat, *Neuroendocrinology* **8**:125.

Wilchen, D. E. L., Brender, D., Macdonald, G. J., Shorey, C. D., and Hinterberger, H., 1967, Effect of reserpine on the structure of heart mitochondria and the relation to catecholamine depletion, *Circ. Res.* **21**:203 (Suppl. III).

Wise, J. R., 1969, Inquiry: Bronchospasm after reserpine? *New Engl. J. Med.* **281**:563.

Woodson, R. E., Jr., Youngken, H. W., Schlittler, E., and Schneider, J. A., 1957, *Rauwolfia: Botany, Pharmacognosy, Chemistry and Pharmacology,* Little, Brown, Boston.

Woodward, R. B., Bader, F. E., Bickel, H., Frey, A. J., and Kierstead, R. W., 1956*a*, The total synthesis of reserpine, *J. Am. Chem. Soc.* **78**:2023.

Woodward, R. B., Bader, F. E., Bickel, H., Frey, A. J., and Kierstead, R. W., 1956*b*, A simplified route to a key intermediate in the total synthesis of reserpine, *J. Am. Chem. Soc.* **78**:2657.

Zbinden, G., and Studer, A., 1958, Histochemische Untersuchungen über den Einfluss von Iproniazid (Marsilid) auf die durch Reserpin erzeugte Freisetzung von Adrenalin und Noradrenalin aus dem Nebennierenmark, *Experientia* **14**:201.

Zbinden, G., Pletscher, A., and Studer, A., 1957, Hemmung der Reserpinbedingten 5-Hydroxytryptamin-Freisetzung im enterochromaffinen System durch Isopropyl-isonicotinsäurehydrazid, *Klin. Wschr.* **33**:565.

Chapter 2

Nicotine

Ronald W. Ryall

Department of Pharmacology
University of Cambridge
Cambridge, England

I. CHEMISTRY

Nicotine is 1-methyl-2-(3-pyridyl)pyrrolidine. It has an empirical formula $C_{10}H_{14}N_2$ and a molecular weight of 162.23. Its structural formula is shown in Fig. 1, from which it will be seen that nicotine can exist as two optically active isomers, with the asymmetrical carbon atom at position 2 in the pyrrolidine ring. The natural (−) isomer has an *S*-configuration and is more potent that the (+)-R isomer (Barlow, 1968).

Nicotine is a colorless to pale yellow, oily volatile liquid which turns brown on exposure to air. The boiling point is 247°C at 745 mm Hg and 123°C at 17 mm Hg. The liquid is highly hygroscopic and forms an alkaline solution: a 0.05 M solution has a *p*H of 10.2. The pK_1 at 15°C is 6.16 and the pK_2 is 10.96. Nicotine is very soluble in a variety of organic solvents, including alcohol, chloroform, ether, petroleum ether, kerosene, and various oils. It forms salts with almost any acid and double salts with

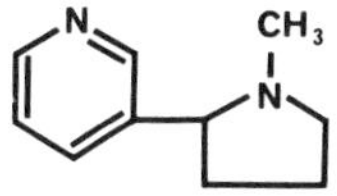

N CH₃ N

NICOTINE

Fig. 1. Structure of nicotine.

metals and acid. Examples of double salts are nicotine aurichloride ($C_{10}H_{14}N_2 \cdot 2HCl \cdot 2AuCl_3$) and nicotine zinc chloride ($C_{10}H_{14}N_2 \cdot 2HCl \cdot ZnCl_2 \cdot H_2O$). Nicotine has an acrid, burning taste and smells of pyridine.

II. METHODS OF ASSAY

Bioassay techniques were used extensively in the past. These included procedures for assay on the blood pressure of various species, on isolated intestine, adrenal grafts, the pupil, nictitating membrane, skeletal muscle, frog heart, and invertebrate muscles. Nicotine was also assayed by its effects on the behavior of a number of animal species ranging from water fleas to mice. Maximum sensitivity is obtained by amounts of the order of 0.1 μg/ml (0.6×10^{-6} M) on isolated tissues. However, amounts ranging upward to milligram quantities may be required to elicit effects when systemically administered to intact animals.

A major disadvantage with bioassay procedures is that they are generally tedious to perform, require experience for successful and repeatable assays, and are subject to the normal sources of variation and error in biological experiments. They have therefore been to a large extent superseded by chemical techniques which are usually relatively easily standardized and are therefore more reliable, reproducible, and less demanding in operator time and skills. Sensitive chemical procedures may be highly sensitive to interference by contaminants, and elaborate purification procedures may be required. Since nicotine is a volatile liquid, it may be partially purified by distillation, preferably under reduced pressure since some decomposition occurs at the high temperatures required for distillation at normal atmospheric pressures. It may also be separated by chromatography or electrophoresis, which may be employed in the identification of nicotine. A variety of chemical methods may be used for the determination of nicotine, including gravimetric, colorimetric, ultraviolet absorption, spectrophotometric, and turbidmetric techniques (see Larson *et al.*, 1961). Nicotine in ethanol emits a phosphorescence at 390 mμ when excited at 270 mμ. This may be used to detect quantities as small as 0.01 μg/ml (0.6×10^{-7} M) (Udenfriend, 1969), and the test is therefore one of the most sensitive available for the detection of minute amounts.

III. OCCURRENCE

Linnaeus in 1753 named the genus *Nicotiniana* after Jean Nicot (1530–1600), a French ambassador to Portugal who is said to have been the first to present tobacco to the courts of those two countries. Tobacco is a member of the family *Solanaceae*. There are approximately 600 species of *Nicotiniana*, most of them native to the Americas, especially South America, with a few Australian species, e.g., *N. suaveoleus*. The common tobacco plant is *N. tabacum*, the only species grown commercially in America; it has not been found growing in the wild since the time of Columbus. *N. rustica* is grown commercially in some other countries, for example, in the U.S.S.R. and in parts of Asia and Australia. It is cultivated not only for use in smoking but also as a source of nicotine sulfate for agricultural use. The dried leaves of *N. tabacum* and *N. rustica* contain from 0.5 to 8% nicotine, and some strains may contain relatively large amounts of nornicotine. Nicotine may also be present in considerable quantities in other plants which do not belong to the genus *Nicotiniana*. In western Queensland, Western and central Australia, *Duboisia hopwoodii* grows wild and contains up to 5.3% of nicotine and up to 1.1% of nornicotine. Nicotine or nornicotine is also found in *Asclepias syriaca* (Asclepiadaceae), *Equisetum, Lycopodium, Sedum acre* (Crassulaceae), and *Eclipta alba* (Compositae).

Although the leaves of the tobacco plant contain the highest concentration of nicotine, the alkaloid is present in all parts, including the seeds. In commercially prepared tobacco, the quantity of nicotine varies greatly. In cigarette tobacco, the concentration ranges from 0.3 to 3% (Goodman and Gilman, 1970), and even "denicotinized" cigarettes may contain relatively large amounts.

IV. USES

Although nicotine has no therapeutic applications in man, Larson *et al.* (1961) present an impressive list of case histories purporting to demonstrate the efficacy of nicotine in the treatment of various illnesses ranging from disorders of the nervous system and the cardiovascular, respiratory, genitourinary, gastrointestinal, and endocrine systems to treatment of allergic, collagen, skin, and infectious diseases. Nicotine no longer occurs in either the British Pharmacopoeia or the Pharmacopoeia of the United States. Many of the claims made for its therapeutic effectiveness remain either unsubstantiated or superseded by the rapid development in the last 30 years of modern pharmacological agents with a lower toxicity than nicotine.

Nicotine still has some application in veterinary medicine as a cheap anthelmintic in large animals and poultry, but again its use has been largely superseded by the advent of less toxic, and more expensive, substances, especially in the treatment of infections in pet animals such as dogs and cats.

The major agricultural use of nicotine is as an insecticide in the form of a solution of the sulfate, or as a fumigant, when solutions of the free base may be employed, or as a contact poison, often in the form of a soap. The amount of nicotine used as an insecticide is over 500 tons per year in the United States alone (*Merck Index*, 1968).

The major use of nicotine, of course, is in the form of tobacco; it is used mainly for social purposes in modern society and to a lesser extent for ritual purposes in the less "advanced" societies. Most of the tobacco used is smoked either as cigarettes or as cigars, but some is chewed. The taking of tobacco in the form of snuff is now rare. About 90% of the nicotine in tobacco smoke is absorbed when inhaled into the lungs, but even when only taken into the mouth about 25–50% is absorbed. Since the smoke from a cigarette may contain from 6 to 8 mg of nicotine and the smoke from a cigar may contain up to 40 mg, it is evident that considerable amounts of nicotine are absorbed by smokers of tobacco.

Finally, nicotine has proved to be useful as a scientific tool in physiological and pharmacological studies of the nervous system.

V. TOXICOLOGY

Nicotine is highly toxic to most species, from protozoa to mammals. As a tertiary amine, it can easily penetrate membranes of all types and is therefore well absorbed not only when taken into the alimentary tract but also when it comes into contact with the skin. Its high solubility in both aqueous and organic solvents assures it of easy passage to peripheral structures and to the central nervous system of higher vertebrates.

Although there are exceptions, toxic effects of nicotine can usually be obtained on invertebrate animals at concentrations in the medium of the order of 10^{-3} to 10^{-5} M. Of particular relevance to the treatment of platyhelminth and nematode infestations in mammals is the observation that worms such as *Fasciola, Taenia,* and *Ascaris* are paralyzed or killed by nicotine concentrations of 3×10^{-5} to 3×10^{-4} M *in vitro*. For comparison, if one examines the LD_{50} for an intravenous injection of nicotine in a number of mammals (Table I), it is evident that, despite some variation, a "good average" LD_{50} is about 5 mg/kg. If one assumes a blood volume of 70 ml/kg body weight, an injection of 5 mg/kg represents a concentration of 4×10^{-4} M. This concentration is clearly close to the concentration required to affect the parasites, and the comparison indicates the probable basis of the low therapeutic index for the use of nicotine as an anthelmintic. This low ratio of toxic to therapeutic dose will become even smaller if one takes, not the LD_{50}, but the doses producing minimal toxic reactions as the

Table I. Toxicity of Nicotine in Small Mammals[a]

Route	LD_{50} (mg/kg)					
	Mouse	Rat	Rabbit	Guinea pig	Cat	Dog
Intravenous	0.5	3	7	4.5[b]	2	5
Subcutaneous	30	40	30	80[b]	1[b]	—
Per os	30	190	200	—	—	10[b]
Intramuscular	8[b]	15[b]	30	15[b]	6[b]	15[b]
Intraperitoneal	10	20[b]	14	30[b]	—	—

[a] The figures in the table are approximate figures obtained by averaging diverse figures quoted in the literature.

[b] Not LD_{50}s but doses which are quoted as having lethal effects in some animals. They may therefore range from minimal to maximal lethal doses and cannot be considered to be accurate (see Larson *et al.*, 1961, for references).

basis for comparison. Admittedly, accurate determinations of LD_{50} have not been made in those animals in which nicotine is most used as an anthelmintic. Nevertheless, the recommended dose of nicotine sulfate as an anthelmintic in ruminants is 30 ml of a 1% solution per 35 lb body weight (*Merck Index*, 1968), corresponding to 19 mg/kg *per os* and an estimated blood concentration, assuming rapid and complete absorption and a blood volume of 70 ml/kg, of 6×10^{-4} M.

An approximate LD_{50} of 11 mg/kg for nicotine sulfate in young lambs given the drug by mouth can be deduced from the observations of Crawshaw (1944). This again emphasizes the lack of safety in attempted therapy with nicotine.

Feurt *et al.* (1958) have compared the toxicity of nicotine administered by intramuscular injection in a number of large species including horses, goats, deer, swine, chinchillas, and monkeys. Minimum paralytic doses ranged from 3 to 10 mg/kg, and fatal doses from 6 to 18 mg/kg, in the different species. It may be seen that these figures are not vastly different from those given for smaller species in Table I. This again draws attention to the fact that nicotine is similarly toxic in a wide range of species.

The agricultural use of nicotine as an insecticide spray raises the question of its toxicity in birds. In pigeons, the minimum lethal dose of nicotine (subcutaneous) is about 5 mg/kg (Meyer, 1891), which is similar to the lethal dose when administered intravenously (Hanzlik and Wood, 1929), and not greatly different from the lethal intramuscular dose of 9 mg/kg (Feurt *et al.*, 1958). Quantities of 1 mg or less intravenously or subcutaneously are lethal for hens (Hofstatter-Von, 1923), and the LD_{50} in canaries is 29 mg/kg subcutaneously (Gaede, 1940).

It may be thought that the unpleasant taste of nicotine might deter animals, including birds, from ingesting toxic amounts of nicotine, but this is not definitely known. There is the additional risk that spraying crops with relatively high concentrations of nicotine sulfate may inadvertently lead to the absorption of toxic quantities through the skin, and this route of absorption may be as important, toxicologically, as any other.

Acute toxic effects may also follow accidental percutaneous absorption of nicotine from insecticide sprays in man. However, the accidental ingestion of nicotine is more common. This is no doubt related to the exceedingly high incidence of tobacco smoking, leading to a significant incidence of accidental ingestion of tobacco by adults or even deliberate ingestion by children. Since the use of tobacco for therapeutic purposes is now largely restricted to folk medicine (Larson *et al.*, 1961), such use, for example, as an enema, presumably now has little toxicological significance. The fatal dose of nicotine for a man is about 60 mg orally, or just a bit more than the nicotine content of some 10-g cigars. However, children have ingested cigarettes with little ill effect. This may possibly be due to the vomiting induced.

It should be remembered that tobacco contains many other substances besides nicotine, which may contribute to or possibly ameliorate to a degree some of the effects of nicotine itself. In general, it is difficult to determine the specific role of nicotine in chronic tobacco poisoning for this reason. At the present time, the major toxicological effects of tobacco smoking pertain to an increased predisposition to a number of diseases, including cancers of various descriptions, bronchitis, emphysema, ischemic heart disease, peptic ulcers, and tuberculosis (Fletcher and Horn, 1971), which are probably unrelated to the nicotine content *per se* of the tobacco. Single puffs of tobacco smoke from a cigarette or small cigar may contain as much as 0.3 mg of nicotine, 11% by volume of carbon monoxide, 13% by volume of carbon dioxide, 90 μg of hydrogen cyanide, and sundry other constituents (Hoffmann and Wynder, 1972). Thus the acute toxic effects of tobacco smoke are not entirely due to the nicotine content.

Although a fatal dose of nicotine is probably about 60 mg for a man, much smaller amounts in the region of 1–2 mg by mouth may produce toxic effects in nonsmokers, whereas larger amounts up to about 8 mg are tolerated by smokers. On application to the skin, 3 mg per day is believed to be dangerous (Lehman, 1948), but somewhat smaller amounts will be tolerated on multiple exposure.

Nicotine is very rapidly absorbed, and, given a sufficient quantity, death ensues within a few minutes. A number of factors may slow absorption and so decrease the toxic action. This may explain why swallowed tobacco often seems to be less toxic than would be expected from the nicotine content of the tobacco. Thus if absorption from the gastrointestinal tract is slowed, sufficient nicotine may be absorbed to induce vomiting, which would expel the remaining nicotine from the stomach before absorption could be completed.

The basic pharmacological action of nicotine on nerve cells and terminals, which will be considered in detail in later sections, should lead to the expectation that the symptoms of acute nicotine poisoning would involve most bodily functions, by actions both at the periphery and on the central nervous system, as indeed they do. Thus there are changes in sensation which may be attributable partly to changes in sensory endings and partly to effects on the central nervous system. Signs of changed activity in the autonomic nervous system appear. These include effects on the heart, on the gastrointestinal tract, on the pupil, and on salivary and sweat glands. There are changes in the activity of skeletal muscle which may lead to respiratory paralysis in severe poisoning. These may be due partly to peripheral and partly to central actions of nicotine. There may be other effects attributed mainly to an action on the central nervous system. These could include changes in subjective phenomena such as concentration, confusion, tiredness, anxiety, and nausea, and more objective effects, for example, vomiting, fainting, and convulsions.

Since the acute toxic effects of nicotine are all attributable to its major mechanism of pharmacological action, an interaction with cholinoceptive receptors at many sites in the body, the symptoms differ mainly in degree and not in kind with different doses: paralysis is here being considered merely the result of an interaction of large amounts of nicotine with the receptors which are at first activated. Therefore, any manifestation of the pharmacological action of nicotine could be considered to be a manifestation of toxicity, and these symptoms are readily produced by cigarette smoking either in the novice with his first cigarette or in the habitual smoker after bouts of excessive smoking.

The treatment of severe acute nicotine poisoning is mainly conservative. If ingestion has been recent, then gastric lavage may be of some use, but if ingestion occurred some time previously, especially of nicotine or nicotine salts rather than of tobacco, then the rapid absorption will render such procedures of little help. Fortunately, nicotine is quickly detoxified either by excretion of about 10% unchanged in urine, and to a lesser extent in bile and feces, or by metabolism of the remainder, chiefly by the liver. A large proportion of the nicotine is probably eliminated within the first few hours and most within a day. Therefore, maintenance of respiration by artificial ventilation is the chief form of therapy, which should be given first priority but should be necessary for only a relatively brief period. Stimulants are contraindicated. It is the rapid absorption and action of nicotine which render this form of poisoning so effective and difficult to counteract. Central anticholinergic drugs, such as ethopropazine, trihexyphenidyl, and diethazine, may be of some value, and maintenance of body temperature may be necessary.

The literature is replete with descriptions of the effect in man of the chronic use of tobacco. However, little is known of the chronic effects of nicotine itself in man. No doubt there are reactions to nicotine which occur only with repeated exposure to mild doses, as in experimental animals, but those probably pale in relation to the far more important chronic toxicological effects of other constituents of tobacco smoke. Nevertheless, it is pertinent to mention in this brief survey of the toxicology of nicotine that it is unlikely that any marked degree of tolerance to or of physical dependence on the pharmacological action of nicotine accrues with repeated exposure. Such habituation as occurs is related to a psychic dependence on the ritual and perhaps to some degree on the physiological reactions associated with the habit.

VI. PHARMACOLOGY

There is a vast literature describing the pharmacological actions of nicotine. Larson *et al.* (1961) in a book of nearly 1000 pages review the data on nicotine or tobacco reported in about 6000 papers published before 1960. This short chapter will make no attempt to repeat the exercise. Instead, the pharmacology of nicotine will be examined from a very limited viewpoint which reflects not only the interests of the author but also those of many contemporary investigators: the actions of nicotine will be examined as they relate to its use as a research tool in physiological and pharmacological studies.

Nicotine has two basic sites of action. The first is on acetylcholine-sensitive (cholinoceptive) receptors at cholinergic synapses associated with both the peripheral and central components of the nervous system. These effects are best understood, and since they involve the somatic motor system, the sympathetic and parasympathetic parts of the autonomic nervous system, and, to some degree, most parts of the central nervous system, the great variety and complexity in the action of nicotine should not be unexpected. This complexity of action is further compounded by the fact that at each of these sites there may be first excitation and then depression.

The second site of action is on the terminals of afferent nerve fibers, and possibly also on the terminals of efferent nerve fibers and on extrasynaptic regions of nerve and effector cells. The physiological significance of these actions is not so readily obvious, but they may contribute to some of the general pharmacological and toxicological properties of nicotine.

Since the actions of nicotine are to a large extent similar in their sensitivity to drug antagonists, it is reasonable to assume that they are related to interactions with membrane receptors which have similar, although not necessarily identical, stereochemical properties. Because acetylcholine invariably interacts with these receptors, nicotine has been instrumental in mapping the location of these sites throughout the body. Indeed, the response to nicotine has been incorporated into our pharmacological definitions of cholinoceptive sites.

A. Historical

Despite the fact that the pioneering studies of Langley and his colleagues with nicotine were carried out at the end of the nineteenth and the beginning of this century (Langley, 1890*a,b,* 1896, 1899–1900, 1901, 1905, 1906, 1907–1908, 1908*a,b,* 1909, 1910*a,b,c,* 1911, 1911–1912, 1912–1913, 1913, 1914, 1918–1919; Langley and Anderson, 1894, 1895; Langley and Dickinson, 1889*a,b,* 1890; Langley and Sherrington, 1891), his studies are still relevant today as the basis of our understanding of the anatomical structure of the autonomic nervous system. He formulated quite clearly the concept of a "receptive substance" for nicotine and curare (Langley, 1905, 1906, 1907–1908, 1908*a,b,* 1909, 1910*a*) quite separate from the component of muscle giving rise to contraction. It is therefore of some interest to look back on his findings in a little more detail and to study the impact they have had on current concepts in physiology and pharmacology.

The earliest studies (Langley and Dickinson, 1899*a,b,* 1890; Langley, 1890*a,b*; Langley and Sherrington, 1891; Langley and Anderson, 1894, 1895; Langley, 1896, 1899–1900, 1901) were concerned chiefly with the location of nerve cells along the courses of peripheral autonomic nerves and the site of action of nicotine. This analytical approach to the interpretation of drug actions, as opposed to straightforward reporting of miscellaneous drug effects, is instructive. It was found, for instance, that the salivary secretion evoked by stimulation of the chorda tympani nerve was blocked by an intravenous injection of nicotine, but secretion was produced when the nerves in the hilus of the gland were stimulated. From this, it was concluded that there were nerve cells along the course of the chorda tympani nerve which were blocked by nicotine. After the injecton of massive doses of 500 mg of nicotine in the cat or 800 mg in the dog, the secretion with direct stimulation of the gland was not affected. The analysis was then taken a stage further by painting nicotine solutions over various structures and noting the effect. A 1% solution of nicotine blocked secretion in the cat only when it was applied directly to the submaxillary ganglion. An important conclusion in 1890 from these experiments was that secretory terminals in the gland were not affected.

Noting some differences between the effects obtained on local and intravenous injection, Langley (1890*b*) considered that intravenous injection was more relevant, bearing in mind the possibility that 1% solutions could be exerting indirect effects such as changes in local blood supply. This lesson could well be noted even by some contemporary investigators.

It was soon found that nicotine paralyzed all nerve cells in autonomic ganglia. In fact, on reading the early papers the impression is gained that Langley believed that this action of nicotine would be exerted on all nerve cells and that nicotine could be used as a diagnostic test, so to speak, for a nerve cell. Clearly, even if Langley believed this at first, he had modified his ideas by 1918, when he concluded that nicotine had no specific paralyzing action on anterior horn cells because it did not prevent strychnine from causing clonic contractions of muscle. Although nicotine paralyzed all autonomic neurons, there appeared to be some differences in sensitivity. Thus secretory cells on the course of the cervical sympathetic nerve were more easily paralyzed than cells on the chorda tympani in the cat, whereas the reverse was true in the dog and some of the effects of stimulating the cervical sympathetics were blocked before others (Langley and Dickinson, 1889*b*). In decreasing order of ease of paralysis by nicotine, these effects are:

1. Secretion from the submaxillary gland.
2. Opening of the eye.
3. Dilation of the pupil.
4. Constriction of blood vessels in the conjunctiva.
5. Constriction of blood vessels of the mouth.
6. Constriction of blood vessels of the ear.
7. Withdrawal of the nictitating membrane.

In attempting to explain these differences, the authors noted that the differences were sometimes not particularly great, and might be explained in part by unequal tonic stimulation reaching the parts by nerve fibers other than sympathetic. However, they clearly believed that the more marked differences were due to unequal sensitivities of different ganglion cells to nicotine. This may be correct, particularly since it is now recognized that nicotinic receptors are not necessarily everywhere identical, but this still remains to be demonstrated conclusively. The difference may lie not so much in a difference in effectiveness of nicotine on the receptors as in differences in the effectiveness of transmission from pre- to postganglionic neurons in the different populations of nerve cells.

Langley and Dickinson in 1890 compared the pharmacological properties of pituri and nicotine and arrived at the conclusion that the active ingredient of pituri was in fact nicotine. Pituri was used by Australian aborigines for chewing and was derived from *Duboisia hopwoodii*, which is known to contain a relatively high percentage of nicotine. However, before 1890, others had claimed that the active ingredient was atropine or hyoscyamine. Again, Langley was able to demonstrate the importance of careful observation in deducing chemical identity from pharmacological action.

Many of Langley's observations with nicotine led to conclusions which are today axioms of physiology. For example, he and Sherrington (1891) showed that there are nerve cells on the course of pilomotor fibers to hair cells. With Dickinson (1889*a*) he demonstrated that motor fibers of the vagus nerve do not end in the nerve cells of the solar plexus, and in 1896 he suggested that ganglion cells may be located more peripherally than the more obvious ganglionic masses of the coeliac ganglion. Langley and Anderson (1899–1900) also concerned themselves with the question of local reflexes in autonomic ganglia, and by combining pharmacological experiments on nicotine with experiments involving section and degeneration of preganglionic nerves they arrived at the conclusion that "no reflexes save axon reflexes occur from the ganglia of the sympathetic system." Similar axon reflexes are thought to occur in the sacral parasympathetic pelvic nerve outflow (de Groat and Ryall, 1969), even though some investigators persist in the belief that Langley's conclusion is incorrect, at least in the sacral outflow (Purinton *et al.*, 1971). In 1895, Langley and Anderson demonstrated that nicotine did not prevent the visceral effects of stimulating fibers in the inferior mesenteric plexus and concluded that the nerve cells of Meisner's and Auerbach's plexus were not cells of the sympathetic nervous system. In a paper in 1901, Langley gave what must be one of the earliest precise considerations of possible sites of drug action on a system of nerves and synapses. He considered the possibility that nicotine action in ganglia could be due to (1) an effect on preganglionic fibers, (2) an effect on the nerve endings of preganglionic fibers (3), an effect on the nerve cell or its dendrites, or (4) an effect on the postganglionic fibers. He ruled out the first and last explanations by showing that local applications of nicotine to pre- and postganglionic fibers did not cause blockade. Since the drug still worked after denervation and degeneration of the terminals, he concluded that the site of action must therefore be on the postganglionic cells.

Langley was aware of the fact that the actions of nicotine on ganglion cells were blocked by curare, although it was chiefly from his experiments on skeletal muscle that he drew his conclusion that the action of curare was also on the postsynaptic structure. In this context, it is curious that to this day these conclusions are still supported by many but that there are a few who believe that the major effects could be on the nerve terminals rather than on the postsynaptic structure. Suffice it for us to note in this historical perspective that Langley was aware of the problems, and on good evidence had rejected the latter possibility. The idea that terminals are a more important site of drug action than postsynaptic structures is not new but represents a full circle of the wheel which Langley was turning at the end of the nineteenth century.

If Langley's experiments on ganglia were of major importance in delineating anatomical features of the autonomic outflow, his studies of the effects of nicotine and curare on skeletal muscle (Langley, 1905, 1906, 1907–1908, 1908*a,b,* 1909, 1910*a*, 1911, 1913, 1914) were to introduce pharmacology to some new ideas which today are still under extensive investigation. As already mentioned, he coined the term "receptive substance" to describe the part of the cell with which nicotine interacts. Today we would call it, more tersely, the "receptor."

Langley was aware from his experiments on ganglia that the paralyzing effect of nicotine was preceded by a brief phase of stimulation and that subsequent doses produced less paralysis than previous doses. These dual actions of nicotine were seen more clearly in skeletal muscle. In the fowl, nicotine in a dose of 0.5–1 mg intravenously caused a tonic extensor rigidity, and this peripheral effect was blocked by curare. He concluded (1905) that "the mutual antagonism can only mean that the two poisons act on the same protoplasmic substance or substances. Curare in combining leads to diminished excitability, nicotine in combining also leads to diminished excitability but it stimulates in combining." This is not only a concise statement of a mechanism for drug antagonism at the receptor level, but it could also be considered as a forerunner of the much more sophisticated "rate theory" of drug–receptor interaction proposed many years later by Paton (1961).

In noting the difference between the muscles of mammals, amphibia, and birds in their reaction to nicotine, Langley concluded that there may be differences in the receptors at different sites, and even suggested that the first nerve connections to form tend to fix the character of the receptive substance in the immediate neighborhood of the nerve ending. Here we have an early suggestion of trophic influences, now a subject of intense interest. Using what would now be considered a rather crude technique, he was able to show that sensitivity to nicotine was up to 1000 times greater at points on the muscle fiber closest to the nerve terminal. With far more elegant techniques, this has now been shown to be also true for acetylcholine sensitivity (Miledi, 1960). He demonstrated that the sensitivity to nicotine increased after denervation, a phenomenon we would now call "denervation supersensitivity." Langley also noted the differences between muscles of the frog in the manner in which they responded to nicotine by twitches or tonic contraction. He noted that twitches were produced only when nicotine was applied to the nerve terminal region, although he was not aware of the difference between conducted action potentials and graded depolarizations in muscle fibers. In the rectus abdominis muscle, he noted that nicotine gave a contraction wherever it was applied but that in sartorius muscle the site of action was localized to the nerve terminal region. Langley looked for but did not find any evidence of axon reflexes set up by nicotine in motor nerve fibers which he knew to be branched. High concentrations (greater than 0.1%) of nicotine also caused a delayed and prolonged contracture of muscle. Langley (1908*b*) believed this to be due to the interaction of nicotine with "contractile substances" in the muscle fiber. This effect of high concentrations was not confined to the innervated region of the muscle and was not blocked by curare (Langley, 1909, 1914). This observation is still difficult to explain, but it may be relevant to recent discussions of the question of the nature of the cholinoceptive receptors normally present in muscle and those appearing away from end-plate regions after denervation (Beránek and Vyskočil, 1967).

B. Mechanism of Action of Nicotine

The end product of the interaction of nicotine with receptive substances within a tissue is, broadly speaking, either excitation or depression, resulting in an increase or a decrease in a measured response. The measured response may be a phenomenon as complex in mechanism as the electroencephalogram or as relatively simple as a change in membrane potential in reaction to a given simple input. From the beginning, it has been a consistent observation that the depressant effects of nicotine are preceded by a phase, however transient, of excitation, and the controversial concept of depolarization blockade has become part of our pharmacological vocabulary. In this section, the mechanism of action of nicotine will be examined at each of its major sites of action in ganglia, at the neuromuscular junction, on nerve terminals, and in the central nervous system. The validity of the concept of depolarization blockade with respect to nicotine will also be examined.

In general, the stimulant effect of nicotine is produced by lower doses or concentrations than the depressant effects, and it has been considered that it is probable that the blood concentrations achieved by smoking tobacco are sufficient to produce only the initial stimulating phase (Larson *et al.*, 1961). Nevertheless, many of the effects produced by nicotine require such small amounts that it may be unwise to assume that depressant effects are never produced at any site as the result of inhaling nicotine from tobacco smoke (see Section VIB4). In this connection, it would be as well to remember that although the action of nicotine has been studied in great detail at the ganglion and neuromuscular junction, and its direct action on single neurons in the central nervous system has been studied in a few instances, for the vast majority of central neurons we know nothing of its action. Furthermore, depending on one's concept of the processes involved in the depressant actions of nicotine, one could consider that the processes of excitation and desensitization are inseparable. In terms of overall, gross behavioral change, it may nevertheless be possible to agree with Larson *et al.* (1961) that only "stimulation" results from the absorption of nicotine from tobacco smoke.

1. Autonomic Ganglia

The action of nicotine on autonomic ganglia has been studied more intensively than any other. The effects are probably the most important among the peripheral actions of nicotine, and they form the basis of many of the reported actions on the cardiovascular system, the gastrointestinal tract, etc. Together with the effect on the neuromuscular junction, they are probably also of most importance in the toxicological effects of nicotine. However, the most important effects from the point of view of smoking tobacco are clearly those on the central nervous system. Nevertheless, there are many similarities at each of the major sites of action of nicotine, and the effects on ganglia are highly relevant to effects on the central nervous system.

In autonomic ganglia, the most important transmitter mediating transmission from the preganglionic fibers to the postganglionic neurons is acetylcholine (ACh). However, the effect of acetylcholine is quite complex. There is an early, short-lasting phase of excitation which is due to interaction of the transmitter with a postsynaptic receptor with which nicotine-like substances interact. There is also a later, more prolonged phase of excitation resulting from the interaction of ACh with muscarine-sensitive receptors, also located postsynaptically (see reviews by Volle, 1966*a,b*, 1969; Volle and Hancock, 1970).

Langley, of course, had described the action of nicotine on ganglia at the turn of the century, and had noted that the effect was blocked by curare. However, it was not until 1956 that the first indication that all ACh receptors in ganglia are not nicotinic appeared. Ambache *et al.* (1956) showed that ganglia were sensitive to muscarine, as well as to nicotine, and that in denervated ganglia the sensitivity to muscarine but not to nicotine increased. They found that hexamethonium selectively blocked the action of nicotine, but not that of muscarine or of acetylcholine, in denervated ganglia. Thus there were other acetylcholine receptors present which were blocked by atropine. Curiously, in innervated ganglia hexamethonium blocked not only the response to preganglionic stimulation, as was well known, but also those of ACh and of muscarine. Thus it appears that the action of ACh switches from a mainly nicotinic action in innervated ganglia to a mainly muscarinic action in denervated ganglia. Electrophysiological evidence for the presence of nicotinic and muscarinic receptors in sympathetic ganglia was later provided by Eccles and Libet (1961) and by Volle and his collaborators.

In previous experiments, Ambache and Edwards (1951) had shown that atropine, in a concentration of $1\text{–}5 \times 10^{-7}$ g/ml, abolished nicotine-evoked contractions of isolated intestine or stomach strips taken from kittens or guinea pigs but that the nicotine responses of rabbit ileum were not blocked. This action of atropine in kittens and guinea pigs is at the postganglionic nerve–smooth muscle junction and is distinct from the site of action of nicotine in the parasympathetic ganglia: despite much speculation, the atropine-resistant effects are still without a definite explanation, but the possibility of noncholinergic transmission must be borne in mind (Burnstock, 1972). Ambache and Edwards (1951) also noted that after atropine treatment nicotine elicited an inhibition of the gut which could be attributed to a stimulation of sympathetic inhibitory ganglion cells because the inhibition was blocked by hexamethonium or by ephedrine. Similarly, treatment of mice with botulinum toxin (Ambache, 1951) caused a loss of peristaltic activity and motor response to nicotine. In the rabbit, a local injection of botulinum toxin into the intestinal wall again blocked the motor response to nicotine and revealed an inhibition which was blocked in turn by ephedrine. These experiments provided strong evidence for the predilection of the toxin for cholinergic nerve terminals.

Feldberg and Vartiainen (1935) and Feldburg and Gaddum (1934) provided the first experimental proof of cholinergic transmission in a sympathetic ganglion. They showed that not only was ACh released into the perfusate when the preganglionic nerve was stimulated in the presence of physostigmine but also that paralytic doses of physostigmine, which blocked transmission, did not reduce the release of ACh but abolished the stimulant action of nicotine. Furthermore, they made the important observation that the amount of ACh released from the preganglionic terminals, as measured on the blood pressure of the chloralose cat, was not increased by nicotine. This provides strong evidence against a site of action of nicotine on preganglionic elements. These studies supported the previous conclusions made by Langley based on the observation that nicotine still affected denervated ganglia. Although Langley showed that nicotine applied locally clearly blocked transmission, it was not certain that the paralytic effects on isolated gut in an organ bath were due to the same mechanism. However, Ambache and Rocha e Silva (1951) showed that after nicotine paralysis of guinea pig ileum, a response to bradykinin was still elicited. Thus smooth muscle is not depressed by nicotine. In isolated rabbit ganglia (Eccles, 1956), nicotine added to the bathing fluid causes a maintained depolarization. At low concentrations (6×10^{-7} M), there is a slight diminution in the size of the synaptic potentials elicited by a preganglionic nerve volley, and the time constant of decay is slightly shortened from 85 to 60 msec. At higher concentrations despite the presence in the bath of 7×10^{-5} M dihydro-β-erythroidine, nicotine (6×10^{-6} M) causes discharges in response to stimulation of the preganglionic nerve, and this is blocked by doubling the concentration of dihydro-β-erythroidine. The higher concentration of nicotine causes a further reduction in the time constant of decay of the membrane. This effect on the time constant of decay of the synaptic potential is attributed to the increase in membrane conductance due, in all probability, to an increase in the permeability of the membrane to all small ions (Eccles, 1956). While this may be a partial explanation of the block of transmission by nicotine in isolated rabbit ganglia, where nicotine causes a maintained depolarization, it is probably not a major factor in other situations. In the superior cervical ganglion of the cat *in vivo*, nicotine administered intraarterially (Paton and Perry, 1951, 1953) causes a depolarization which is not maintained. At the same time, there is a block of transmission. In contrast, tubocurarine causes a block without first depolarizing (Paton and Perry, 1951). Paton and Perry (1953) obtained evidence that the block of transmission by nicotine was not attributable solely to the depolarization and the associated conductance change. During the onset of block, the reduction of transmission, as indicated by the reduction in the compound action potential recorded postganglionically in response to a preganglionic volley, was less for a given level of depolarization than during recovery from the block: the curves relating depolarization and block of transmission for onset and offset of drug effect showed hysteresis. Second, the depolarization produced by nicotine in these experiments was more transient than that produced by ACh or tetramethylammonium, and yet the block of transmission was more profound. Thus nicotine causes desensitization by a process which is not simply related to the conductance change leading to depolarization. It is this desensitization which explains the diminished response to a second injection of nicotine.

Lundberg and Thesleff (1953) also noted that the ganglionic blockade by nicotine outlasted the period of depolarization and showed that the blockade could be partly relieved by repetitive stimulation of the preganglionic nerve. Working on the hypothesis that the block could have been due to epinephrine liberated from the adrenals by nicotine, they tested dihydroergotamine on the response, but with negative results. They concluded that the block was therefore unlikely to be due to activation of an adrenergic mechanism by nicotine. The block is unlikely to be due to activation by nicotine of an intraganglionic adrenergic (or dopaminergic) mechanism because this mechanism is blocked by α-adrenergic receptor antagonists (Eccles and Libet, 1961), and the cholinoceptive receptor involved is blocked by atropine, not by hexamethonium. Gebber (1968) showed that tetanic stimulation of the preganglionic nerve antagonized nicotine blockade, even during the depolarizing phase of its action. In contrast to these results in cat ganglia where nicotine or acetylcholine causes a depolarization of short duration, in rat ganglia (Krivoy and Willis, 1956) acetylcholine causes a prolonged depolarization but a relatively short-lasting block of transmission.

Others have also confirmed the lack of correlation between depolarization and block by nicotine. In cat ganglia, depolarization by nicotine abolishes the response, measured by the contraction of the nictitating membrane, to the ganglionic stimulant effect of the polypeptides angiotensin and bradykinin. However, during the late, nondepolarizing phase of block by nicotine, the response to angiotensin is increased while that to bradykinin remains depressed (Trendelenburg, 1966). Tubocurarine antagonizes the depolarization produced by nicotine, but intensifies the block (Gebber, 1968). In frogs, nicotine causes a depolarization which subsides despite a persistent block (Ginsborg and Guerro, 1964), as in the cat. In contrast, succinylcholine and decamethonium, which depolarize and block at the skeletal neuromuscular junction, block transmission in frog sympathetic ganglia without causing an initial depolarization (Ginsborg and Guerro, 1964). Riker (1968), confirming that ACh blocked transmission far outlasting depolarization in frog ganglia, noted that some cells were not depolarized but that transmission to them was nevertheless blocked. Restoring the membrane potential by passing current through the membrane did not relieve the block, and depolarization of the membrane by current did not cause block.

Riker's experiments confirm the lack of correlation between depolarization and blockade, but he proposed the conclusion that the site of action of the acetylcholine was presynaptic. We have already considered some of the evidence which negates this conclusion. Thus nicotine and acetylcholine are effective in denervated ganglia, and, as Feldberg and Vartiainen (1935) showed, nicotine does not increase the release of ACh in normal ganglia.

There is now more recent evidence which makes the suggestion that nicotine and acetylcholine produce their effects via presynaptic mechanisms even more unlikely. Gebber (1968) showed that an intravenous infusion of nicotine evoked a continuous postganglionic discharge, even when transmission was completely blocked. Brown *et al.* (1970) loaded ganglia with tritium-labeled ACh. Stimulation of the preganglionic nerve evoked a release, but neither nicotine, carbachol, ACh, tetramethylammonium, nor methacholine caused any release. Similarly negative results were obtained by Collier and Katz (1970) with ACh and carbachol. Ginsborg (1971) recorded extracellularly from presynaptic terminals in frog sympathetic ganglia and showed that ACh or carbachol attenuated or even abolished the action potential, but that these effects were transient in comparison with the prolonged block of transmission.

Autoradiographic studies with C^{14}-labeled nicotine (Applegren *et al.*, 1963) demonstrated that nicotine was selectively taken up by the ganglion cells, with very little appearing in the satellite cells or connective tissue. It was of some interest that some cells took up far more nicotine than others, although the percentage seemed to be different from that which stained deeply for cholinesterase.

In conclusion, nicotine has a biphasic action on most autonomic ganglionic neurons. The first depolarizing phase is probably due to a nonselective increase in the ion permeability of the postsynaptic membrane, as the result of interaction with a special receptor which is competitively blocked by substances such as curare or hexamethonium. Depolarization of ganglia by nicotine is accompanied by a small decrease in intracellular *p*H (Brown and Halliwell, 1972), which may be the consequence of the inward movement of sodium ions. The second blocking phase is unrelated to the depolarization, but its origin is not clear. It too is almost certainly a postsynaptic action of nicotine. Brown and Halliwell (1972) have recently demonstrated that nicotine is concentrated intracellularly in rat sympathetic ganglia. The ratio of intracellular to extracellular concentrations may be of the order of five times, and the uptake is reduced in the presence of hexamethonium. The nicotine is only slowly washed out (Brown and Scholfield, 1972). Thus we must consider the possibility that the blocking action of nicotine may be produced by some intracellular mechanism yet to be elucidated. However, it seems a more attractive proposition for the moment to account for the blocking action in terms of membrane receptors. In particular, the explanation may well lie within the realm of the intermediate receptor hypothesis of Katz and Thesleff (1957) and the concepts of metaphilic antagonism proposed by Rang and Ritter (1969, 1970*a,b*).

Since the chromaffin cells of the adrenal medulla may be considered to be modified adrenergic postganglionic neurons and their innervation is cholinergic, nicotine causes excitation and the release of epinephrine into the circulation. However, Armitage and Milton (1965) consider that it is unlikely that sufficient nicotine is absorbed from tobacco smoke by the majority of smokers to produce such an effect on the adrenals, although they do admit that such a response is possible in sensitive individuals.

2. Skeletal Neuromuscular Junction

In its essential aspects, the mode of action of nicotine at the neuromuscular junction is similar to that in autonomic ganglia. There are some minor differences which should be mentioned here. The most important difference concerns the probable nature of the receptor with which nicotine interacts on the postsynaptic membrane. In autonomic ganglia, the nicotinic receptor is blocked, not only by typical ganglionic blocking agents such as hexamethonium or pentamethonium, but also by classical neuromuscular blocking agents such as tubocurarine or dihydro-β-erythroidine. At the neuromuscular junction, hexamethonium and similar drugs are relatively ineffective. There is also a difference in the affinity of the receptors for different agonists. In comparison with its potency relative to acetylcholine in the ganglion, the effect of nicotine on skeletal muscle is "surprisingly weak" (Bacq and Brown, 1937). In the ganglion, the nicotinic receptor interacts not only with nicotine but also with acetylcholine or dimethylphenylpiperazinium (DMPP), but it does not interact with phenyltrimethylammonium (PTMA). In contrast, the receptor at the neuromuscular junction interacts with PTMA, but not with DMPP. It is not improbable that the nicotinic receptor differs slightly at each type or part of cell on which it is located. Thus we should anticipate differences between receptors on muscle, on nerve terminals, and on nerve cells and conceivably even between different major types of neurons.

Langley described the major aspect of nicotine action at the neuromuscular junction in amphibia and birds. Later work has largely confirmed his findings in other species, including mammals, and has added a great deal of sophistication to his data and a greater insight into the mechanism of action. Some important contributions were made by Dale and Gasser (1926), Bacq and Brown (1937), Kuffler (1943), and Thesleff (1955). Much of the earlier work is reviewed by Gasser (1930), and some of the later work is reviewed by Fischer *et al.* (1960).

In small doses given either intravenously or intraarterially to a muscle, nicotine causes twitchings or tremors in mammals, followed, at higher doses, by neuromuscular paralysis. In the chicken, Langley showed that nicotine produced a prolonged contracture, not evident in the mammal. Similar prolonged contractures are produced by other "depolarizing" neuromuscular blocking agents such as decamethonium and succinylcholine in chickens.

Langley (1908*b*) noted that in frogs the local application of nicotine caused quick contractions when administered near the nerve terminals, but a slow contraction when applied elsewhere along the muscle fibers. The concentration of nicotine required to elicit an effect was much higher outside the neural region. Furthermore, curare did not appreciably antagonize the action of nicotine at nonneural regions (Langley, 1914). The explanation of this observation is not clear, although Langley (1908*b*) suggested that nicotine may act directly on contractile elements in addition to its more marked effect at the end plate. The idea of two receptors is reiterated in a paper by Ariens and Van Rossum (1956). However, nicotine apparently does not cause isolated actomyosin threads to contract (McIntyre and Braverman, 1947). Although it is well established that the sensitivity to ACh and to nicotine increases markedly after denervation, the sensitivity to curare decreases a little (Beránek and Vyskočil, 1967). Thus the possibility of a curare-resistant action of nicotine on normal and denervated muscle remains a possibility, but such an action would clearly contribute very little if any to the overall action of nicotine, which is exerted predominantly at the end plate. After denervation, the sensitivity of muscle increases to other excitants such as caffeine, as well as to ACh or nicotine (Kuffler, 1943). Thus the changes occurring after denervation are not specific for acetylcholine receptors.

After the initial excitation, nicotine readily causes a paralysis of the neuromuscular junction. If anything, this paralysis is more readily obtained, relative to excitation, than it is at ganglionic synapses. However, the mechanism of the block appears to resemble that in ganglia. Thesleff (1955), using both intracellular and extracellular recordings from frog sartorius muscle, showed that ACh, nicotine, decamethonium, and succinylcholine cause a brief depolarization of the end-plate region which rapidly returns to the normal resting potential, despite the continued presence of the agonist. The depolarizing action of nicotine is more prolonged than that of the other agents: ACh (10^{-5} g/ml) depolarization recovered in 10 min, nicotine (1.5×10^{-5} g/ml) in 25 min, decamethonium (4×10^{-5} g/ml) in 15 min, and succinylcholine (2×10^{-5} g/ml) in 15 min. Block of transmission occurs as the membrane potential is recovering to normal, and maximal block occurs just before the membrane has returned to the resting level. During the block, the end plates are insensitive to acetylcholine, showing that the effect appears to be postsynaptic. Paralysis develops earlier with nicotine than with acetylcholine. As in ganglia, the mechanism of paralysis is therefore independent of depolarization. Whether the mechanism is explained in terms of rate theory (Paton, 1961), intermediate receptors (Katz and Thesleff, 1957), or metaphilic antagonisms (Rang and Ritter, 1969, 1970*a,b*) is largely a matter for personal preference at the present state of our knowledge, but Riker and Okamoto (1969) take the unorthodox view that the block may be due to a depressant effect on the motor nerve terminals.

The neuromuscular paralysis brought about by nicotine may be particularly important in relation to its acute toxicity. Toxic doses exert effects on the respiratory system at all levels, but the action on the neuromuscular junction has been considered to be of prime importance as the cause of death in respiratory paralysis due to nicotine, with paralysis of the respiratory center requiring larger doses than those required to paralyze the respiratory muscle (see Larson *et al.*, 1961).

In connection with the effects of nicotine on respiration, it should be recalled that, in addition to its effects on the respiratory muscles, nicotine also has effects on the muscles of the trachea and bronchi (see Larson *et al.*, 1961). These effects may vary somewhat in different species. They seem to be produced in man as a consequence of tobacco smoking, but the reported effects are variable. Many of these actions are probably due to effects on autonomic ganglia, since they are prevented by treatment with ganglionic blocking agents. For example, nicotine causes bronchostriction in the guinea pig and this effect is blocked by atropine or hexamethonium (Herxheimer, 1956). Other effects may be due to the actions of nicotine on the afferent terminals of sensory fibers involved in respiratory reflexes or to effects on the central nervous system.

3. *Nerve Terminals*

In 1940, Coon and Rothman described a pilomotor response to the intradermal injection of acetylcholine or nicotine (1:20,000–1:500,000). This effect in the cat was not confined to the site of injection, nor was it abolished by atropine. It was prevented by the local administration of a local anesthetic, but not by an acute section of the nerve trunk. In the cat's tail, there was no response after sympathectomy or after blockade of adrenergic receptors by ergotamine. The authors therefore suggested that the reaction was due to a local axon reflex, set up by the stimulation of adrenergic nerve terminals by the nicotinic agents. In this instance, the terminals belonged to autonomic postganglionic nerves.

The situation regarding skeletomotor nerve terminals is probably similar. At the skeletomotor neuromuscular junction, acetylcholine and related nicotinic ions have been said to excite the terminals and to cause a decrease in the resting potential and a decrease in the action potential of unmyelinated axons (Riker and Okamoto, 1969). It has been considered that in this respect there is nothing special about the unmyelinated nerve terminal (Riker and Okamato, 1969; Dettbarn, 1966). However, Langley (1907, 1908) could find no evidence that nicotine could evoke axon reflexes in the terminal branches of motor nerves, but it is possible that the concentrations he used were inappropriate.

The effect of nicotine-like substances on the endings of afferent nerve fibers is well documented (see reviews by Paintal, 1964, 1971; Gray and Diamond, 1957). Brown and Gray (1948) obtained evidence for excitation of sensory fibers by acetylcholine-like substances. They demonstrated that cutaneous receptors and receptors in the mesentery were excited when exposed to the intraarterial administration of nicotine (0.2 ml of 1:10,000 of the tartrate) or acetylcholine (0.2 ml of 1:10,000 of the chloride). The discharge recorded in sensory fibers was not blocked by atropine or by sympathectomy. Acetyl-β-methylcholine was inactive, and carbamylcholine was 1000 times less effective. The concentration required to excite the sensory terminals was far less than that required to affect axons directly. Large doses of nicotine caused a blockade of responses to small doses of nicotine and acetylcholine. Nicotine applied topically to sensory ganglia in concentrations of 0.1–1% (Langley, 1901) causes neither reflexes nor a reduction of reflex action. Nicotine also stimulates a variety of receptors with afferent fibers in the vagus, for example, those involved in pulmonary and cardiovascular reflexes (Paintal, 1955; Armitage and Hall, 1969), and stretch receptors in the stomach (Paintal, 1954). All of these nicotine-sensitive cutaneous and visceral receptors appear to be similar to those on A and C fibers in cutaneous nerves (Douglas and Ritchie, 1960) and are invariably blocked by hexamethonium or tubocurarine, but not by atropine. Similar nicotinic receptors are present on pain nerve endings in man (Keele and Armstrong, 1964). It is likely that the receptors are located on the regenerative region of the receptor, rather than on the generator region (Paintal, 1964, 1971). With regard to the visceral stretch receptors, it is considered that the receptors are located on the nerve terminals themselves and that the excitation is not due to indirect effects caused by the contraction of smooth muscle (Paintal, 1954).

The afferent endings in muscle spindles are excited by nicotine and succinylcholine (Hunt, 1952; Verhey and Voorhoeve, 1963; Ginzel *et al.*, 1969). The discharge occurs mainly in group IA fibers, but there is some discharge in group II fibers. Muscarine has no effect (Verhey and Voorhoeve, 1963). The discharge is blocked by *d*-tubocurarine (Hunt, 1952). Hunt believed that nicotine exerted its effect directly on the nerve terminal in the spindle. Such an action is quite consistent with the effect of nicotine elsewhere, but in the specific example of the muscle spindle, with its own cholinergic innervation and postsynaptic nicotinic, curare-sensitive receptors on the intrafusal muscle fibers, it is difficult to be certain that the effects are not indirect and attributable to contraction of the intrafusal fibers.

Finally, nicotine and related drugs excite chemoreceptors in the carotid body (Douglas, 1952; Byck, 1961; Eyzaguirre and Koyano, 1965; Eyzaguirre *et al.*, 1972; Sampson, 1971) and pressure receptors in the carotid sinus (Heymans *et al.*, 1931). The effects of acetylcholine and nicotine on carotid body chemoreceptors are blocked by hexamethonium or mecamylamine (Sampson, 1971), as they are at other sensory receptors. However, the role of the cholinoceptive receptors in the carotid body is a matter of some debate. On the basis that the blocking agents blocked not only the action of ACh on the receptors but also the evoked discharges in their experiments, Eyzaguirre and his colleagues have postulated a cholinergic link in normal physiological excitation of the receptors. In contrast, Douglas (1952) and Sampson (1971) have not been able to block any discharge in the sensory nerve, except those caused by ACh and related substances, in their experiments. On this evidence, the view has been advanced that the nicotinic receptors on the chemoreceptors of the carotid body are not functional in the physiological activation of the receptors (Sampson, 1971).

In conclusion, it may be said that nicotinic receptors occur on the terminals and axons of many sensory and motor nerver fibers, but the physiological significance of these receptors is obscure, since blockade of the nicotinic receptors by hexamethonium does not lead to a loss of sensation.

4. Central Nervous System

Systemic administration of nicotine, or topical application to exposed parts of the central nervous system, causes profound changes in the gross behavior of animals. In general, these may be summarized by saying that small doses "stimulate" while large doses "depress" the activity of the CNS (see review by Silvette *et al.*, 1962). The effects include tremors, which are observed both in man and in other animals, or even convulsions after large doses. There may be increases or decreases in "spontaneous" activity, depending on the dose, and decreases in conditioned reflexes and learning ability. There may be marked changes in the electrical potentials recorded from the surface of the brain and changes in the function of sensorimotor areas of the cerebral cortex, where it has been considered (Silvette *et al.*, 1962) that the concentrations of nicotine used in many of the reported experiments were so high as to cause tissue damage, and where there is doubt that "such experiments should be given serious consideration." Nicotine also causes nausea and vomiting. This action is particularly prominent in man, and is a common experience of smoking novitiates. There are marked effects on spinal reflexes, generally resulting in a reduction of monosynaptic reflexes and little change or even facilitation of polysynaptic reflexes (see Goldfarb, 1971).

In many of these studies, attempts have been made to determine the site and mechanism of action of nicotine. However, conclusions drawn from such studies are often particularly hazardous. It is not even certain to what extent the actions are due to an effect on central structures and to what extent they are due to stimulation of afferent nerve endings. For example, the emetic effect of nicotine is probably due mainly to an effect on the emetic chemoreceptor trigger zone in the medulla (Laffan and Borison, 1957), but nicotine excites the terminals of many vagal afferent fibers that may form part of the pathway involved in emesis. In cats, but not in dogs, the emetic response to nicotine persists after ablation of the chemoreceptor trigger zone. Similarly, monosynaptic reflexes are usually inhibited by nicotine in cats (Schweitzer and Wright, 1938; Ginzel *et al.*, 1953; Curtis *et al.*, 1957; Goldfarb, 1971). Occasionally, the monosynaptic reflex is augmented after nicotine, and this has been attributed to stimulation of peripheral afferent nerve terminals (Curtis *et al.*, 1957). In contrast, the facilitation of polysynaptic reflexes after nicotine has been considered to be due entirely to central actions (Goldfarb, 1971). These examples are probably sufficient to illustrate the difficulties which lie in the way of interpretation of the effects of systemically administered nicotine on the central nervous system. Others are easily found in considering cardiovascular and respiratory actions. This analysis can be taken even further. In the examples considered above, an attempt was made to differentiate between peripheral and central actions. The spatial separation of these structures allows a certain degree of experimental manipulation in differentiating between central and peripheral loci. Within the central nervous system, experimental manipulation is not only difficult but also often crude, nonselective, and sometimes impossible. Central neurons are of varied types, even within the same anatomical location. Nicotine, as will be discussed below, acts on some but not other central neurons. It should not be considered a nonselective stimulant (or depressant) of nervous tissue, even though it may be just that in a sufficiently high concentration. The concept of a "center" is not today as scientifically acceptable as it was in former times, and to crudely apply nicotine to a particular locus of cells, designated as a particular "center," probably has little interpretative value. To speak of a selective activation of the reticular formation or of the cerebral cortex, hippocampus, or any other structure after a systemic administration of nicotine is to ignore the vast complexity of the system and the certainty that the nicotine is acting simultaneously on cells in many parts of the nervous system. The end product, whether it be a change in an electroencephalogram, a change in cell firing in one part of the system, or a modification of a reflex, is likely to be somewhat variable and will depend on the many factors which go to make the living physiological substrate on which the drug is acting. Thus it is not surprising that some reflexes are depressed, while the others are facilitated. Such observations do not necessarily mean that nicotine is exciting some cells but inhibiting others. They merely show that the neuronal connections are different and that the balance of excitation versus inhibition is in one case decreased and in the other increased.

From the above, it will be clear that experiments of the type which have been described do not serve much purpose other than as purely descriptive accounts of the action of systemically administered nicotine. They cannot by themselves give much information about the locus or mechanism of action. They are of some value in enumerating the symptomatology of nicotine administration, and careful comparisons with the effects of smoking may yield valuable information on the pharmacological relevance of nicotine in the toxicology of the tobacco-smoking habit (for example, Armitage *et al.*, 1968; Hall, 1970). Conversely, a detailed knowledge of the mechanism and site of action at the cellular level will probably be of little help in toxicology, but it will aid in our basic understanding of the physiological operation of the nervous system. It is in this sense of the use of nicotine as a research tool that discussion will continue of the action of nicotine on the central nervous system.

With regard to the use of nicotine as a research tool in the study of the central nervous system, three factors must be borne in mind. The first is the action of nicotine on the postsynaptic structure, where the effect is to mimic that of the transmitter, acetylcholine. Such an effect is to be expected only where there are cholinoceptive receptors of the appropriate type. The distribution of cholinoceptive sites and the action of nicotine on them will be discussed below, and particular care must be taken not to equate cholinoceptivity with cholinergicity. The second factor is that nicotine may exert an action on nerve terminals in the CNS, as it does at the periphery. At the outset, it must be admitted that there is little evidence which bears directly on this problem; it is clearly an area for future research. The third factor, which may be indirectly related to the others, is the ability of nicotine to release transmitters from their storage sites.

At the periphery, claims have sometimes been made that nicotine causes the release of acetylcholine from the nerve terminals. In general, recent work with radioactive labeling has failed to confirm these suggestions (see previous sections) that the release is due to a direct action on the cholinergic nerve terminals. Great caution should therefore be used in interpreting the action of nicotine on acetylcholine release in the central nervous system. Although nicotine, tetramethylammonium, choline, and carbamylcholine cause the release of acetylcholine from synaptic vesicles *in vitro* isolated from cerebral cortex (Chiou *et al*., 1970), there is no evidence that a similar mechanism operates *in vivo*. Nicotine, injected intravenously in cats, usually causes an increase in the resting release of acetylcholine from the exposed surface of the cerebral cortex into a plastic cup containing Ringer's solution with physostigmine (Armitage *et al*., 1968, 1969), but sometimes the output of acetylcholine is decreased. These effects are associated with characteristic changes in the pattern of the electroencephalogram, an increase in release being associated with cortical "desynchronization" and a decrease in release with an increase in the amplitude of slow waves. The amount of nicotine administered (2 μg/kg every 30 sec for 20 min) was considered by Armitage *et al*. to be roughly equivalent to the nicotine intake of a smoker who smoked two cigarettes, inhaling deeply. Identical effects on the EEG were produced by the introduction of cigarette smoke into the lungs (Hall, 1970). Despite the fact that similar effects have not yet been noted in man, the action on ACh release and on cortical activity must be taken into consideration in interpreting the central actions of nicotine. However, accepting this, it seems to the reviewer to be unlikely that the mechanism of ACh release entails a direct action on the nerve terminals. Nicotine has a sufficient variety of effects, which can be well substantiated, to obviate the need to postulate a releasing action on the stores of acetylcholine. The change in release is then seen as a consequence of the state activation of the cortex, rather than the cause.

Similarly, the increased release of ^{3}H-norepinephrine into the perfused third cerebral ventricle of the cat after intravenous injections of 2 μg/kg every 30 sec for 30 min (Hall and Turner, 1972), or after the inhalation of cigarette smoke, or after perfusion of the cerebral ventricles with a solution of nicotine may also be due to an action of nicotine on postsynaptic neuronal sites rather than to an effect on the nerve terminals *per se*. Nicotine also caused a specific release of norepinephrine from perfused rat hypothalamic slices *in vitro* (Hall and Turner, 1972). The concentration required to produce an effect *in vitro* was fairly high (1×10^{-4} M), and the relevance to *in vivo* effects is not certain. This is important because it is unlikely that the *in vitro* preparations were capable of propagating action potentials, and a direct effect on the terminals is more likely under these circumstances. In view of the action of nicotine on peripheral nerve terminals, some direct action at a sufficient concentration of nicotine is not improbable. However, it would be desirable to have more information on the effects of antagonists on transmitter release by nicotine. The observation that the effect of nicotine on the EEG is blocked by mecamylamine (Yamamoto and Domino, 1965; Hall, 1970), an antagonist of acetylcholine at "nicotinic" receptor sites, and also by atropine (Hall, 1970), an antagonist of acetylcholine at "muscarinic" sites, indicates that the effect on the EEG may be on classical postsynaptic receptors. The drug–receptor interaction may then lead to excitation of cholinergic pathways terminating in the cerebral cortex at synapses where the action of acetylcholine is muscarinic in type and so blocked by atropine. Since it has been noted that the acetylcholine-releasing effect of nicotine is associated with changes in the EEG, it is not an unreasonable extrapolation to suggest that the release of acetylcholine from the cerebral cortex may be due to the activation of extracortical neurons.

Attention can now be given to the precise mode of action of nicotine at the cellular level. To do this, it will be necessary to consider mainly those studies in which nicotine has been administered microelectrophoretically into the immediate environment of a single nerve cell from which simultaneous recording of its electrical activity has been obtained. Only in this way can problems be overcome which are associated with the simultaneous activation of many receptors, both central and peripheral, when the substance is administered systemically, or the indirect effects produced on a single neuron under observation when the drug is applied topically or by perfusion of a relatively large mass of nervous tissue.

The first use of the microelectrophoretic technique for the study of the action of nicotine on central neurons was in an investigation of the Renshaw cell by Curtis and Eccles (1958); this was subsequently investigated in greater detail by Curtis and Ryall (1966*a*,*b*). Nicotine was about ten times as potent as acetylcholine in terms of the relative electrophoretic currents required to produce a similar increase in the firing frequency of Renshaw cells. The effects with nicotine took longer to reach a maximum, and the time to recovery of the original firing rate was also prolonged. This is presumably a reflection of the fact that the administered acetylcholine is hydrolyzed by cholinesterase before it has diffused far from the site of application. In contrast, nicotine, which is not hydrolyzed, can affect a larger proportion of the cell membrane but will take longer to reach a maximum concentration at distant sites which are inaccessible to the administered acetylcholine. The action of nicotine on Renshaw cells is clearly similar to that in autonomic ganglia, because the excitation is blocked by dihydro-β-erythroidine or tetraethylammonium, but not by atropine. In contrast, the action of acetyl-β-methylcholine on the Renshaw cell is blocked by atropine but not by the antagonists of the nicotinic action of acetylcholine. "Depolarization blockade" at the Renshaw cell was not evident with the cholinomimetics (Curtis and Ryall, 1966*a*). This would have been revealed, had it been present, as a reduction in the amplitude of the extracellularly recorded action potentials. Nevertheless, despite the continued administration of nicotine, the increase in firing level declined from its initial peak to a lower value; that is, the response showed "fade." The fade is attributable both to a nonspecific desensitization of the cell, in which the sensitivity to all excitants is reduced, and to a specific desensitization of the nicotinic receptor, in which there is a selective depression of the excitatory response to acetylcholine but not to an excitant amino acid.

These observations on the Renshaw cell show that nicotine can be used as a tool in investigations of the central nervous system, even when more than one type of acetylcholine receptor is present. In this particular instance, intraarterial injections of nicotine cause a similar excitation of Renshaw cells (Eccles *et al.*, 1956), but it would be unwise to assume that such a parallelism would invariably be found.

The nicotinic receptors on Renshaw cells are well known to be involved in the "early" synaptically evoked discharges which ensue when the Renshaw cells are excited through motor axon collaterals by antidromic volleys in motor nerves (see Curtis and Ryall 1966*c*) or via monosynaptic excitation of predominantly large α-motoneurons by stimulation of group IA afferent fibers from the muscle spindles (Ryall *et al.*, 1972). In contrast, the rather weak depressant effects of nicotine on some other spinal interneurons (Curtis *et al.*, 1966) are not known to be related to any known cholinergic pathways. Nevertheless, even if these nicotinic receptors on the interneurons are only pharmacological curiosities, they should not be neglected in a consideration of the effects of systemically administered nicotine on spinal reflexes.

The effects of intravenous nicotine on spinal reflexes are quite complicated (Ginzel *et al.*, 1969; Goldfarb, 1971; Goldfarb and Sharpless, 1971). Low doses (20–40 μg/kg) of nicotine blocked the monosynaptic reflex without influencing the activity of muscle spindles (Ginzel *et al.*, 1969). Succinylcholine similarly blocked the reflex but only at doses eliciting a discharge from the spindles. The effect of nicotine could be explained by an excitatory effect on Renshaw cells because it was antagonized by mecamylamine, which antagonizes the nicotinic action of acetylcholine at this site, but mecamylamine did not antagonize the effect of succinylcholine, which appeared therefore to be mediated via the action on the spindle. At higher doses of nicotine, effects on the monosynaptic reflex appeared to be mediated via changes in fusimotor activity or by a direct action on the spindle. These effects are blocked by gallamine, as are those of succinylcholine. Goldfarb (1971) similarly attributed the depressant effects of nicotine in rather large doses to effects on the Renshaw cells in cats paralyzed by gallamine. However, there was also a reduction in recurrent inhibition and an increase in polysynaptic reflexes. It is far more difficult to explain these latter effects in terms of a simple action of nicotine on Renshaw cells. This example illustrates once again that, even at a site (the Renshaw cell) where we know a great deal about the mechanism of action of nicotine and the neurophysiology of the system, so many effects occur when the drug is injected intravenously that interpretation becomes exceedingly complicated.

There are other sites in the central nervous system at which nicotine may exert its effect. Since, in common parlance, the mechanism involved in the production of the pleasurable effects of smoking tobacco may be thought to be associated with an action on the "higher centers" of the nervous system, it is natural to consider the action of nicotine on the cerebral cortex. Although electrophoretic administration of nicotine has some excitatory actions on cerebral cortical neurons, they are much weaker than those of acetylcholine (Krnjević and Phillis, 1963; Crawford and Curtis, 1966; Curtis and Crawford, 1969), and the excitation by acetylcholine is predominantly muscarinic in nature and therefore blocked by atropine. It therefore seems unlikely that these weak excitations could be of much relevance to the central actions of nicotine. However, nicotine depresses the activity of some cortical neurons which are also depressed by acetylcholine (Phillis and York, 1968*a*) and by acetyl-β-methylcholine. The action of nicotine is blocked effectively by dihydro-β-erythroidine or by hexamethonium, but atropine also surprisingly shows some antagonistic action. Thus Phillis and York (1968*a*) concluded that this particular receptor for nicotine does not show the usual muscarinic–nicotinic receptor specificity when tested with antagonists. Since the action of acetylcholine was more powerfully affected by atropine than by dihydro-β-erythroidine, Jordan and Phillis (1972) concluded that the receptor was more muscarinic than nicotinic in character. Either intraarterial or intravenous injections of nicotine (Phillis and York, 1968*b*) similarly reduced the excitability of cortical neurons, and these effects were mimicked by the administration of cigarette smoke. It was noted that since the effects of acetylcholine in these experiments were weaker than those of nicotine, the effects could not be due to the release of acetylcholine from the nerve terminals. This argument is clearly invalid, because, however unlikely, it must be admitted that it is not known how much acetylcholine would be released under the conditions of these experiments, nor is the actual concentration of any released acetylcholine known at the subsynaptic receptors.

There are further observations which should be considered in relation to the mechanisms involved in the central effects of systemically administered nicotine or tobacco smoke. One of these is the fact that at least two constituents of tobacco smoke, nicotine and carbon monoxide, cause an increase in cerebral blood flow (Hall, 1972*a*), and this could lead to very indirect effects on cerebral function. Another is a rise in cerebrospinal fluid pressure (Hall, 1968), which could be due to the change in blood flow. In addition, nicotine may cause hyper- or hypothermic effects, probably via cholinergic mechanisms in the hypothalamus (Hall and Myers, 1972). It has been postulated (Hall, 1972b) that the hypothermic action of intraventricularly injected nicotine in the anesthetized cat is due to interaction with a nicotinic receptor in the hypothalamus which is blocked by hexamethonium or by mecamylamine. In recent experiments (Knox *et al.*, 1973), it was found that unit activity in the rostral hypothalamus, which increased when heat was applied to the rat's tail, also increased when nicotine or acetylcholine was administered either locally by microinjection or systemically by intravenous injection.

Elsewhere in the central nervous system, the electrophoretic administration of nicotine excites many neurons, depresses others, and is inactive on some, for instance, in the basal ganglia and dorsal column nuclei (see review by Curtis and Crawford, 1969).

In the cerebellum, the potency of nicotine is about equal to that of acetylcholine on Purkinje cells (Crawford *et al.*, 1966), but granule cells and basket cells have been found to be insensitive to cholinomimetics (but see McCance and Phillis, 1968). Crawford *et al.* (1966) considered the acetylcholine receptors to be muscarinic in nature, based on the relative potency of cholinomimetics and the ability of intravenous atropine to antagonize the effects. The not inconsequential activity of nicotine and the ability of dihydro-β-erythroidine to antagonize the action of acetylcholine on some cells (Crawford *et al.*, 1966; McCance and Phillis, 1968) indicate that an action on typical nicotinic receptors may well be involved in any cerebellar effects of systemically administered nicotine. Nevertheless, it seems unlikely at this time that any of these actions are of more than pharmacological as opposed to physiological relevance.

In the brain stem, nicotine and other cholinomimetic substances such as 1,1-dimethyl-4-phenylpiperazinium and choline phenylether excited neurons which were excited by acetylcholine (Bradley, 1968). In contrast, both inhibitory and excitatory effects were produced by substances with a muscarine-like action. Since dihydro-β-erythroidine antagonized only excitatory responses to acetylcholine and some antagonism was also shown by atropine, it was suggested that the receptors may have mixed nicotinic and muscarinic properties.

Nicotine has rather weak effects (or is inactive) compared with acetylcholine in many other parts of the central nervous system, for example, in the thalamus and geniculate nuclei, where both excitatory and inhibitory effects may be encountered (Phillis, 1971), in the rhinencephalon, basal ganglia, and dorsal column nuclei (see Curtis and Crawford, 1969).

VIII. CONCLUSIONS

These studies with nicotine on many different types of neurons in the central nervous system have helped to elucidate the nature of the cholinoceptive receptor at many sites. It has become clear that the receptor often appears not to conform to the relatively simple pattern which obtains in the peripheral nervous system and that occasional paradoxical effects are observed. This leads one to suspect that perhaps there are many types of "nicotinic" receptors on central neurons, just as there appear to be at least two at the periphery. Alternatively, it is possible that "nicotinic" and "muscarinic" receptors are dispersed in different proportions on different neurons. The difficulty with this hypothesis is the fact that the receptors would sometimes appear to differ in their relative affinities for nicotine and antagonistic drugs. This is by no means impossible but seems unlikely. Finally, the variety of sites at which nicotine acts in the central nervous system reemphasizes what has been a repetitive theme in this chapter, that extreme caution must be employed in attempting to interpret the results of systemic administration. It is clear that there are many "nicotinic" receptors in the central nervous system to which we can as yet attribute no physiological function. It is to be hoped that future research will give replies to some of these unanswered questions.

VIII. REFERENCES

Ambache, N., 1951, Unmasking, after cholinergic paralysis by botulinum toxin, of a reversed action of nicotine on the mammalian intestine, revealing the probable presence of local inhibitory ganglion cells in the enteric plexus, *Brit. J. Pharmacol.* **6**:51.

Ambache, N., and Edwards, J., 1951, Reversed nicotine action on the intestine by atropine, *Brit. J. Pharmacol.* **6**:311.

Ambache, N., and Roche e Silva, M., 1951, Analysis of certain interactions of nicotine with bradykinin and histamine, *Brit. J. Pharmacol.* **6**:68.

Ambache, N., Perry, W. L. M., and Robertson, R. A., 1956, The effect of muscarine on perfused superior cervical ganglia of cats, *Brit. J. Pharmacol.* **11**:442.

Applegren, L. E., Hansson, E., and Schmitterlow, C. G., 1963, Localization of radio-activity in the superior cervical ganglion of cats following injection of C^{14} labelled nicotine, *Acta Physiol. Scand.* **59**:330.

Ariens, E. J., and van Rossum, J. M., 1956, Nicotine induced contracture of the rectus abdominis muscle of the frog, *Acta Physiol. Pharmacol. Neerl.* **5**:259.

Armitage, A. K., and Hall, G. H., 1969, Mode of action of intravenous nicotine in causing a fall of blood pressure in the cat, *Europ. J. Pharmacol.* **7**:23.

Armitage, A. K., and Milton, A. S., 1965, The release of adrenaline by nicotine from the adrenal medulla, in: *Tobacco Alkaloids and Related Compounds*, Proceedings of Fourth International Symposium at Wenner-Gren Center, Stockholm, 1964, Pergamon Press, Oxford.

Armitage, A. K., Hall, G. H., and Morrison, C. F., 1968, Pharmacological basis for the smoking habit, *Nature* (*Lond.*) **217**:331.

Armitage, A. K., Hall, G. H., and Sellers, C. M., 1969, Effects of nicotine on electrocortical activity and acetylcholine release from the cat cerebral cortex, *Brit. J. Pharmacol.* **35**:152.

Bacq, Z. M., and Brown, G. L., 1937, Pharmacological experiments on mammalian voluntary muscle, in relation to the theory of chemical transmission, *J. Physiol.* (*Lond.*) **89**:45.

Barlow, R. B., 1968, *Introduction to Chemical Pharmacology*, Methuen, London.

Beránek, R., and Vyskočil, F., 1967, The action of tubocurarine and atropine on the normal and denervated rat diaphragm, *J. Physiol.* (*Lond.*) **188**:53.

Bradley, P. B., 1968, Synaptic transmission in the central nervous system and its relevance for drug action, *Internat. Rev. Neurobiol.* **11**:1.

Brown, D. A., and Halliwell, J. V., 1972, Intracellular *p*H in rat isolated superior cervical ganglia in relation to nicotine depolarization and nicotine uptake, *Brit. J. Pharmacol.* **45**:349.

Brown, D. A., and Scholfield, C. N., 1972, Nicotine washout rates from isolated rat ganglia in relation to recovery from nicotine depolarization, *Brit. J. Pharmacol.* **45**:29.

Brown, D. A., Jones, K. B., Halliwell, J. V., and Quilliam, J. P., 1970, Evidence against a presynaptic action of acetylcholine during ganglionic transmission, *Nature* (*Lond.*) **226**:958.

Brown, G. L., and Gray, J. A. B., 1948, Some effects of nicotine-like substances and their relation to sensory nerve endings, *J. Physiol.* (*Lond.*) **107**:306.

Burnstock, G., 1972, Purinergic nerves, *Pharmacol. Rev.* **24**:509.

Byck, R., 1961, The effect of hexamethonium on the carotid chemoreceptor response to nicotine and cyanide, *Brit. J. Pharmacol.* **16**:15.

Chiou, C. Y., Long, J. P., Potrepka, R., and Spratt, J. L., 1970, The ability of various nicotinic agents to release acetylcholine from synaptic vesicles, *Arch. Int. Pharmacodyn. Therap.* **187**:88.

Collier, B., and Katz, H. S., 1970, The release of acetylcholine by acetylcholine in the cat's superior cervical ganglion. *Brit. J. Pharmacol.* **39**:428.

Coon, J. M., and Rothman, S., 1940, The nature of the pilomotor response to acetylcholine; some observations on the pharmacodynamics of the skin, *J. Pharmacol. Exptl. Therap.* **68**:301.

Crawford, J. M., and Curtis, D. R., 1966, Pharmacological studies on feline Betz cells, *J. Physiol.* (*Lond.*) **186**:121.

Crawford, J. M., Curtis, D. R., Voorhoeve, P. E., and Wilson, V. J., 1966, Acetylcholine sensitivity of cerebellar neurones in the cat, *J. Physiol.* (*Lond.*) **186**:139.

Crawshaw, H. A., 1944, Nicotine poisoning in lambs, *Vet. Rec.* **56**:276.

Curtis, D. R., and Crawford, J. M., 1969, Central synaptic transmission—Microelectrophoretic studies, *Ann. Rev. Pharmacol.* **9**:209.

Curtis, D. R., and Eccles, R. M., 1958, The excitation of Renshaw cells by pharmacological agents applied electrophoretically, *J. Physiol.* (*Lond.*) **141**:435.

Curtis, D. R., and Ryall, R. W., 1966*a*, The excitation of Renshaw cells by cholinomimetics, *Exptl. Brain Res.* **2**:49.

Curtis, D. R., and Ryall, R. W., 1966*b*, The acetylcholine receptors of Renshaw cells, *Exptl. Brain Res.* **2**:66.

Curtis, D. R., and Ryall, R. W., 1966*c*, The synaptic excitation of Renshaw cells, *Exptl. Brain Res.* **2**:81.

Curtis, D. R., Eccles, J. C., and Eccles, R. M., 1957, Pharmacological studies on spinal reflexes, *J. Physiol.* (*Lond.*) **136**:420.

Curtis, D. R., Ryall, R. W., and Watkins, J. C., 1966, The action of cholinomimetics on spinal interneurones, *Exptl. Brain Res.* **2**:97.

Dale, H. H., and Gasser, H. S., 1926, The pharmacology of denervated mammalian muscle. Part I. The nature of the substances producing contracture, *J. Pharmacol. Exptl. Therap.* **29**:53.

de Groat, W. C., and Ryall, R. W., 1969, Reflexes to sacral parasympathetic neurones concerned with micturition in the cat, *J. Physiol* (*Lond.*) **200**:87.

Dettbarn, W. D., 1966, in: *Biochemistry and Pharmacology of the Basal Ganglia*, (E. Costa, L. J. Cote, and M. D. Yahr, eds.) pp. 57–61, Raven Press, New York.

Douglas, W. W., 1952, The effect of a ganglion-blocking drug, hexamethonium, on the response of the cat's carotid body to various stimuli, *J. Physiol.* (*Lond.*) **118**:373.

Douglas, W. W., and Ritchie, J. M., 1960, The excitatory action of acetylcholine on cutaneous non-myelinated fibrers, *J. Physiol.* (*Lond.*) **150**:501.

Eccles, J. C., Eccles, R. M., and Fatt, P., 1956, Pharmacological investigations on a central synapse operated by acetylcholine, *J. Physiol.* (*Lond.*) **131**:154.

Eccles, R. M., 1956, The effect of nicotine on synaptic transmission in the sympathetic ganglion, *J. Pharmacol. Exptl. Therap.* **118**:26.

Eccles, R. M., and Libet, B., 1961, Origin and blockade of the synaptic responses of curarized sympathetic ganglia, *J. Physiol.* (*Lond.*) **157**:484.

Eyzaguirre, C., and Koyano, H., 1965, Effects of some pharmacological agents on chemoreceptor discharges, *J. Physiol.* (*Lond.*) **178**:410.

Eyzaguirre, C., Nishi, K., and Fidone, S., 1972, Chemoreceptor synapses in the carotid body, *Fed. Proc.* **31**:1385.

Feldberg, W., and Gaddum, J. H., 1934, The chemical transmitter at synapses in a sympathetic ganglion, *J. Physiol.* (*Lond.*) **81**:305.

Feldberg, W., and Vartiainen, A., 1935, Further observations on the physiology and pharmacology of a sympathetic ganglion, *J. Physiol.* (*Lond.*) **83**:103.

Feurt, S. D., Jenkins, J. H., Haynes, F. A., and Crockford, H. A., 1958, Pharmacology and toxicology of nicotine with special reference to species variation, *Science* **127**:1054.

Fischer, E., Silvette, H., Larson, P., and Haag, H. B., 1960, Effect of nicotine and tobacco on muscle function, *Am. J. Phys. Med.* **39**:63.

Fletcher, C. M., and Horn, D., 1971, *Smoking and Health* World Health Organization (WHO). Printed for Her Majesty's Stationery Office by J. W. Arrowsmith Ltd., Bristol, England.

Gaede, D,. 1940, Über die Wirkung fortgesetzer Nikotininjektionen bei Kanarienvögeln, *Arch. Exptl. Pathol. Pharmakol.* **196**:164.

Gasser, H. S., 1930, Contractures of skeletal muscle, *Physiol. Rev.* **10**:35.

Gebber, G. L., 1968, Dissociation of depolarization and ganglionic blockade induced by nicotine, *J. Pharmacol. Exptl. Therap.* **160**:124.

Ginsborg, B. C., 1971, On the presynaptic acetylcholine receptors in sympathetic ganglia of the frog, *J. Physiol* (*Lond.*) **216**:237.

Ginsborg, B. C., and Guerro, S. J., 1964, On the action of depolarizing drugs on sympathetic ganglion cells of the frog, *J. Physiol.* (*Lond.*) **172**:189.

Ginzel, K. H., Eldred, E., and Sasaki, Y., 1969, Comparative study of the actions of nicotine and succinylcholine on the monosynaptic reflex and spindle afferent activity, *Internat. J. Neuropharmacol.* **8**:515.

Ginzel, K. H., Klupp, H., Sotrmann, H., and Werner, G., 1953, Hemmung des Patellarsehnen-reflexes durch zentral und peripher wirkende Stoffe, *Arch. Exptl. Pathol. Pharmakol.* **218**:308–312.

Goldfarb, J., 1971, Action of nicotine on reflexes in spinal cats, *Neuropharmacology* **10**:399.

Goldfarb, J., and Sharpless, S. K., 1971, Effects of nicotine and recurrent inhibition on monosynaptic reflexes in acute and chronic spinal cats, *Neuropharmacology* **10**:413.

Goodman, L. S., and Gilman, A., 1970, *The Pharmacological Basis of Therapeutics*, 4th ed., Macmillan, London.

Gray, J. A. B., and Diamond, J., 1957, Pharmacological properties of sensory receptors and their relation to those of the autonomic nervous system, *Brit. Med. Bull.* **13**:185.

Hall, G. H., 1968, Influence of nicotine on intraventricular cerebrospinal fluid pressure in the anaesthetized cat, *Internat. J. Neuropharmacol.* **7**:365.

Hall, G. H., 1970, Effects of nicotine and tobacco smoke on the electrical activity of the cerebral cortex and olfactory bulb, *Brit. J. Pharmacol.* **38**:271.

Hall, G. H., 1972*a*, Effects of nicotine, carbon monoxide and tobacco smoke on regional blood flow in the cerebral cortex, *Europ. J. Pharmacol.* **19**:385.

Hall, G. H., 1972*b*, Changes in body temperature produced by cholinomimetic substances injected into the cerebral ventricles of unanaesthetized cats, *Brit. J. Pharmacol.* **44**:634.

Hall, G. H., and Myers, R. D., 1972, Temperature changes produced by nicotine injected into the hypothalamus of the conscious monkey, *Brain Res.* **37**:241.

Hall, G. H., and Turner, D. M., 1972, Effects of nicotine on the release of ^{3}H-noradrenaline from the hypothalamus, *Biochem. Pharmacol.* **21**:1829.

Hanzlik, P. J., and Wood, D. A., 1929, The mechanism of digitalis-emesis in pigeons, *J. Pharmacol. Exptl. Therap.* **37**:67.

Herxheimer, N., 1965, Bronchoconstrictor agents and their antagonists in the intact guinea-pig, *Arch. Int. Pharmacodyn. Therap.* **106**:371.

Heymans, C., Bouckaert, J. J., and Dautrebande, L., 1931, Sinus carotidien et réflexes respiratoires. III. Sensibilité des sinus carotidiens aux substances chimiques. Action stimulante respiratoire réflexe du sulfure de sodium, du cyanure du potassium, de la nicotine et de la lobeline, *Arch. Int. Pharmacodyn. Therap.* **40**:54.

Hoffman, D., and Wynder, E. C., 1972, Smoke of cigarettes and little cigars: An analytical comparison, *Science* **178**:197.

Hofstatter-Von, R., 1923, Experimentelle Studie über die Einwirkung des Nicotins auf die Keimdrüsen und auf die Fortpflanzung, *Virchow's Arch.* **244**:183.

Hunt, C. C., 1952, Drug effects on mammalian muscle spindles, *Fed. Proc.* **11**:75.

Jordan, L. M., and Phillis, J. W., 1972, Acetylcholine inhibition in the intact and chronically isolated cerebral cortex, *Brit. J. Pharmacol.* **45**:584.

Katz, B., and Thesleff, S., 1957, A study of desensitization produced by acetylcholine at the motor and plate, *J. Physiol.* (*Lond.*) **138**:63.

Keele, C. A., and Armstrong, D., 1964, *Substances Producing Pain and Itch*, Edward Arnold, London.

Knox, G. V., Campbell, C., and Lomax, P., 1973, The effects of acetylcholine and nicotine on unit activity in the hypothalamic thermoregulatory centres of the rat, *Brain Res.* **51**:215.

Krivoy, W. A., and Willis, J. H., 1956, Adaptation to constant concentrations of acetylcholine, *J. Pharmacol. Exptl. Therap.* **116**:220.

Krnjević, K., and Phillis, J. W., 1963, Pharmacological properties of acetylcholine-sensitive cells in the cerebral cortex, *J. Physiol.* (*Lond.*) **166**:328.

Kuffler, S. W., 1943, Specific excitability of the end plate region in normal and denervated muscle, *J. Neurophysiol.* **6**:99.

Laffan, R. J., and Borison, H. L., 1957, Emetic action of nicotine and lobeline, *J. Pharmacol. Exptl. Therap.* **121**:468.

Langley, J. N., 1890*a*, On the physiology of salivary secretion. Part VI. Chiefly upon the connection of peripheral nerve cells with the nerve fibres which run to the sub-lingual and sub-maxillary glands, *J. Physiol.* (*Lond.*) **11**:123.

Langley, J. N., 1890*b*, Action of various poisons upon nerve fibres and peripheral nerve cells, *J. Physiol.* (*Lond.*) **11**:509.

Langley, J. N., 1896, On the nerve cell connections of the splanchnic nerve fibres, *J. Physiol.* (*Lond.*) **20**:223.

Langley, J. N., 1899–1900, On axon reflexes in the preganglionic fibres of the sympathetic system, *J. Physiol.* (*Lond.*) **25**:364.

Langley, J. N., 1901, On the stimulation and paralysis of nerve cells and of nerve endings. Part I, *J. Physiol* (*Lond.*) **27**:224.

Langley, J. N., 1905, On the reaction of cells and of nerve endings to certain poisons, chiefly as regards the reaction of striated muscle to nicotine and to curari, *J. Physiol.* (*Lond.*) **33**:374.

Langley, J. N., 1906, On nerve endings and on special excitable substances in cells, *Proc. Roy. Soc. Lond. Ser. B* **78**:170.

Langley, J. N., 1907–1908, On the contraction of muscle, chiefly in relation to the presence of "receptive" substances. Part I, *J. Physiol.* (*Lond.*) **36**:347.

Langley, J. N., 1908*a*, On the contraction of muscle, chiefly in relation to the presence of "receptive" substances. Part II, *J. Physiol.* (*Lond.*) **37**:165.

Langley, J. N., 1908*b*, On the contraction of muscle, chiefly in relation to the presence of "receptive" substances. Part III. The reaction of frog's muscle to nicotine after denervation, *J. Physiol.* (*Lond.*) **37**:285.

Langley, J. N., 1909, On the contraction of muscle, chiefly in relation to the presence of "receptive" substances. Part IV. The effect of curari and of some other substances on the nicotine response of the sartorius and gastrocnemius muscles of the frog, *J. Physiol.* (*Lond.*) **39**:235.

Langley, J. N., 1910*a*, Note on the action of nicotine and curari on the receptive substance of the frog's rectus abdominis muscle, *J. Physiol. Lond.* **40**:lix.

Langley, J. N., 1910*b*, Inhibitory fibres for the bladder in the pelvic nerve: Antagonism by curare of the nicotine stimulations of nerve cells, *J. Physiol.* (*Lond.*) **40**:lxii.

Langley, J. N,. 1910*c*, The sympathetic innervation of the skin of the frog, *J. Physiol.* (*Lond.*) **40**:lxiii.

Langley, J. N., 1911, The action of salts on the neural and non-neural regions of muscle, *J. Physiol.* (*Lond.*) **42**:xxiv.

Langley, J. N., 1911–1912, The effect of various poisons upon the response to nervous stimuli chiefly in relation to the bladder, *J. Physiol.* (*Lond.*) **43**:125.

Langley, J. N., 1912–1913, Observations on vascular reflexes chiefly in relation to the effect of strychnine, *J. Physiol.* (*Lond.*). **45**:239.

Langley, J. N., 1913, The protracted contraction of muscle caused by nicotine and other substances chiefly in relation to rectus abdominis muscle of the frog, *J. Physiol.* (*Lond.*) **47**:159.

Langley, J. N., 1914, The antagonism of curari and nicotine in skeletal muscle, *J. Physiol.* (*Lond.*) **48**:73.

Langley, J. N., 1918–1919, Persistence of the central somatic effect of strychnine after a large dose of nicotine, *J. Physiol.* (*Lond.*) **52**:xliv.

Langley, J. N., and Anderson, H. K., 1894, On reflex action from sympathetic ganglia, *J. Physiol.* (*Lond.*) **14**:410.

Langley, J. N., and Anderson, H. K., 1895, The innervation of the pelvic and adjoining viscera, Part V. Position of nerve cells on the course of the efferent nerve fibres. *J. Physiol.* (*Lond.*) **19**:131.

Langley, J. N., and Dickinson, W. L., 1889*a*, On the local paralysis of peripheral ganglia, and on the connexion of different classes of nerve fibres with them, *Proc. Roy. Soc. Lond.* **46**:432.

Langley, J. N., and Dickinson, W. L., 1889*b*, On the progressive paralysis of the different classes of nerve cells in the superior cervical ganglion, *Proc. Roy. Soc. Lond.* **47**:379.

Langley, J. N., and Dickinson, W. L., 1890, Pituri and nicotine, *J. Physiol.* (*Lond.*) **11**:265.

Langley, J. N., and Sherrington, C. S., 1891, On pilo-motor nerves, *J. Physiol.* (*Lond.*) **12**:278.

Larson, P. S., Haag, H. B., and Silvette, H., 1961, *Tobacco: Experimental and Clinical Studies*, Williams and Wilkins, Baltimore.

Lehman, A. J., 1948, The toxicology of the newer agricultural chemicals, *Bull. Ass. Food Drug Officials* **12**:82.

Lundberg, A., and Thesleff, S., 1953, Dual action of nicotine on the sympathetic ganglion of the cat, *Acta Physiol. Scand.* **28**:218.

McCance, I., and Phillis, J. W., 1968, Cholinergic mechanisms in the cerebellar cortex, *Internat. J. Neuropharmacol.* **7**:447.

McIntyre, A. R., and Braverman, I., 1947, The action of certain drugs on an actomyosin–ATP system, *Fed. Proc.* **6**:158.

Merck Index, 1968, 8th ed., Merck & Co., Rahway, N.J.

Meyer, J., 1891, Beitrag zur Kenntnis der Wirkung des Nicotins, Inaugural Dissertation Kiel. Quoted by Larson *et al.* (1961).

Miledi, R., 1960, The acetylcholine sensitivity of frog muscle fibres after complete or partial denervation, *J. Physiol.* (*Lond.*) **151**:1.

Paintal, A. S., 1954, The response of gastric stretch receptors and certain other abdominal and thoracic vagal receptors to some drugs, *J. Physiol.* (*Lond.*) **126**:271.

Paintal, A. S., 1955, Impulses in vagal afferent fibres from specific pulmonary deflation receptors: The response of these receptors to phenyl diguanide, potato starch, 5-hydroxytryptamine, and nicotine, and their role in respiratory and cardiovascular reflexes, *Quart. J. Exptl. Physiol.* (*Lond.*) **40**:89.

Paintal, A. S., 1964, Effects of drugs on vertebrate mechanoreceptors, *Pharmacol. Rev.* **16**:341.

Paintal, A. S., 1971, Action of drugs on sensory nerve endings, *Ann. Rev. Pharmacol.* **11**:231.

Paton, W. D. M., 1961, A theory of drug action based on the rate of drug–receptor combination, *Proc. Roy. Soc. Lond. B* **154**:21.

Paton, W. D. M., and Perry, W. L. M., 1951, Depolarization and transmission block in the cat's superior cervical ganglion, *J. Physiol.* (*Lond.*) **112**:48P.

Paton, W. D. M., and Perry W. L. M., 1953, The relationship between depolarization and block in the cat's superior cervical ganglion, *J. Physiol.* (*Lond.*) **119**:43.

Phillis, J. W., 1971, The pharmacology of thalamic and geniculate neurons, *Internat. Rev. Neurobiol.* **14**:1.

Phillis, J. W., and York, D. H., 1968*a*, Pharmacological studies on a cholinergic inhibition in the cerebral cortex, *Brain Res.* **10**:297.

Phillis, J. W., and York, D. H., 1968*b*, Nicotine, smoking and cortical inhibition, *Nature* (*Lond.*) **219**:89.

Purinton, T., Fletcher, T., and Bradley, W., 1971, Sensory perikarya in autonomic ganglia, *Nature New Biol.* **231**:63.

Rang, H. R., and Ritter, J. M., 1969, A new kind of drug antagonism: Evidence that agonists cause a molecular change in acetylcholine receptors, *Mol. Pharmacol.* **5**:394.

Rang, H. R., and Ritter, J. M., 1970*a*, On the mechanism of desensitization at cholinergic receptors, *Mol. Pharmacol.* **6**:357.

Rang, H. R., and Ritter, J. M., 1970*b*, The relationship between desensitization and the metaphilic effect at cholinergic receptors, *Mol. Pharmacol.* **6**:383.

Riker, W. K., 1968, Ganglion cell depolarization and transmission block by ACH: Independent events, *J. Pharmacol. Exptl, Therap.* **159**:345.

Riker, W. F., and Okamoto, M., 1969, Pharmacology of motor nerve terminals, *Ann. Rev. Pharmacol.* **9**:173.

Ryall, R. W., Piercey, M. F., Goldfarb, J., and Polosa, C., 1972, Excitation of Renshaw cells in relation to orthodromic and antidromic excitation of motoneurones, *J. Neurophysiol.* **35**:137.

Sampson, S. R., 1971, Effects of mecamylamine on responses of carotid body chemoreceptors *in vivo* to physiological and pharmacological stimuli, *J. Physiol.* (*Lond.*) **212**:655.

Schweitzer, A., and Wright, S., 1938, Action of nicotine on the spinal cord, *J. Physiol.* (*Lond.*) **94**:136.

Silvette, H., Hoff, E. C., Larson, P. S., and Haag, H. B., 1962, The actions of nicotine on the central nervous system functions, *Pharmacol. Rev.* **14**:137.

Thesleff, S., 1955, The mode of neuromuscular block caused by acetylcholine, nicotine, decamethonium and succinylcholine, *Acta Physiol. Scand.* **34**:218.

Trendelenburg, U., 1966, Observations on the ganglion stimulating action of angiotensin and bradykinin, *J. Pharmacol. Exptl. Therap.* **154**:418.

Udenfriend, S., 1969, *Fluorescence Assay in Biology and Medicine*, Vol. II, Academic Press, New York and London.

Verhey, B. A., and Voorhoeve, P. E., 1963, Activation of group IA and group II muscle spindle afferents by succinylcholine and other cholinergic drugs, *Acta Physiol. Pharmacol. Neerl.* **12**:23.

Volle, R. L., 1966*a*, Muscarinic and nicotine stimulant actions at autonomic ganglia, in: *International Encyclopedia of Pharmacology and Therapeutics*, Sect. 12, Vol. 1, Pergamon Press, Oxford.

Volle, R. L., 1966*b*, Modification by drugs of synaptic mechanisms in autonomic ganglia, *Pharmacol. Rev.* **18**:839.

Volle, R. L., 1969, Ganglionic transmission, *Ann. Rev. Pharmacol.* **9**:135.

Volle, R. L., and Hancock, J. C., 1970, Transmission in sympathetic ganglia, *Fed. Proc.* **29**:1913.

Yamamoto, K., and Domino, E. F., 1965, Nicotine-induced EEG and behavioural arousal, *Internat. J. Neuropharmacol.* **4**:359.

Chapter 3

Curare

Jose del Castillo

Laboratory of Neurobiology
and
Department of Pharmacology
University of Puerto Rico
San Juan, Puerto Rico, U.S.A.

and

Margaret Anderson

Department of Biological Sciences
Smith College
Northampton, Massachusetts, U.S.A.

I. INTRODUCTION

The word *curare*, like its synonyms *curari, huareli, woorari,* and *woorali*, stems from the native names given to plant extracts that Indians of the Amazon and Orinoco valleys and the Guianas have used for centuries as arrow poisons. Small bamboo darts, whose tips are coated with a brownish layer of "flying death," are shot from blowguns. The typical result is rapid paralysis and death of the animals that are hit. There are several advantages to curare as an arrow poison for hunting. For example, it is highly potent, and its effects are rapid. Furthermore, meat from animals killed with it can be eaten without danger, because the active principles of the poison are not absorbed from the digestive tract.

The first reference to curare appeared in a letter written in 1504 by

Pedro Martir de Angleria. This and subsequent letters were compiled by Antonio de Nebrija and published under the title *De Orbe Novo Decades*, a book translated into English by MacNutt (1912). This was the beginning of a long and fascinating history, often mixed with legend and lore. The interested reader is referred to Gill (1940), McIntyre (1947), Granier-Doyeux (1951), Marsh (1951), Miguel and Vela (1953), Waser (1953), and Kreig (1964).

For many years, curare was regarded as a toxicological curiosity. It was occasionally used as a medicine to treat spastic paralysis and tetanus. In the fourteenth century, curare received the attention of prominent physiologists. Their findings, emphasizing that a drug-sensitive link is involved in the transfer of excitation from nerve to muscle, can be regarded as one of the sources of the chemical theory of synaptic transmission.

In our century, the potential clinical use of curare as a muscle relaxant greatly stimulated research on its chemistry and pharmacology, as well as the synthesis of new molecules with curare-like actions. Today curare and its synthetic analogues have become powerful and indispensable tools for the investigation of problems involving acetylcholine-sensitive cellular surfaces. Studies dealing directly with the effects of curare, or with curare as a pharmacological tool, are numerous and increasing at a steady rate. This chapter does not pretend to be exhaustive. Our aim is to offer an overall view of the actions of curare, and their possible mechanisms, within the framework of the present ideas on cholinergic synaptic transmission. Although this chapter concerns the pharmacology of curare and its alkaloids, we shall also mention synthetic curare-like compounds. A number of reviews on curare can be found in the literature (Boehm, 1920; McIntyre, 1947; Cheymol, 1949; Paton, 1949; Hunt and Kuffler, 1950; Miner *et al.*, 1951; Craig, 1955; Bovet *et al.*, 1959; deReuck, 1962; Fänge, 1962; Khromov-Borisov and Michelson, 1966; Koelle, 1970). We have borrowed heavily from them, and they should be consulted for further information and additional bibliographical references.

The arrow poison curare is prepared from a number of plant species belonging to the families Menispermaceae and Loganiaceae. The actual combinations of plants and methods of preparation originally used by natives are unknown, since the recipes were secrets guarded by each tribe. It was not until the eighteenth century that explorers witnessed the preparation of the poison. In the early nineteenth century, samples of the plants used in the preparation of curare were obtained, and many of them were identified and catalogued. In the nineteenth century, samples of curare were studied by Claude Bernard and Francois Magendie in France and by A. Kölliker in Germany. Bernard, in particular, established the peripheral locus of action of curare. He observed that if the hind leg of a frog was ligatured so that its circulation was stopped, and curare was injected into the lymph sac, the effects of the drug appeared in all parts of the animal except in the ligatured leg. In this leg, electrical stimulation of the sciatic nerve still produced contraction; however, the opposite leg with its circulation intact was paralyzed. Furthermore, afferent stimulation of the central end of the sciatic nerve of the paralyzed limb elicited cross-reflex responses in the unpoisoned leg. This showed that curare must reach the muscle to produce paralysis. Bernard was able to localize more precisely the action of curare by showing that the poisoned muscle contracts normally following direct stimulation and that the sciatic nerve soaked in a solution of curare is still capable of conducting impulses (Bernard, 1857). These results definitely established that curare blocks or paralyzes a functional link between nerve and muscle—the process of neuromuscular transmission.

The word *curare* was used originally to refer to the crude plant extract; *curarines* and *toxiferines* are the alkaloids responsible for the biological activity of curare. Since true curare preparations are no longer used for scientific purposes, we shall use the words *curare* and *curarine* interchangeably, unless otherwise indicated. The term "curare-like drug" applies to any drug that blocks neuromuscular transmission without impairing either nerve conduction or twitch tension elicited by direct stimulation of muscle.

II. SOURCES AND CHEMISTRY

A. Natural Curare Alkaloids

1. Boehm's Classification of Curares

Boehm (1920) first showed that the active principles of curare are quaternary ammonium compounds, and he classified the curare extracts into three groups according to the containers in which they were exported.

a. The curares that came from western Amazonia were prepared from several species of the Menispermaceae family, in particular *Chondodendron tomentosum* (Ruiz and Pavon), which is the chief source of the curare prepared in Peru and Ecuador. This curare was exported in bamboo tubes and was called "tubocurare," from which Boehm isolated the principle *tubocurarine*. For lists of the members of the Menispermaceae family used in the manufacture of curare, the reader should consult Krukoff and Moldenke (1938) and Barneby and Krukoff (1971).

b. The main source of curares of the eastern Amazon valley are the climbing vines of the genus *Strychnos*, of which *S. toxifera* is the most active. This curare came in gourds and was called "calabash curare," from which Boehm isolated *curarine*.
c. Other curares were stored in earthenware jars. These were the "pot curares," from which Boehm isolated *protocurarine*.

Although Preyer isolated an alkaloid from a crude extract of curare as early as 1865, it was not until much later that King (1935), using a museum sample of unknown origin, determined the structure of one of its alkaloids. This was a bis-quaternary ammonium compound, which became known as *d*-tubocurarine (dTC), and happened to be one of the most important active principles of curare. Since then, almost 50 different alkaloids have been isolated either from crude extracts or directly from plants, and the structures of most of them have been determined.

2. *Alkaloids from the Genus Chondodendron*

Wintersteiner and Dutcher (1943) reported the structure of an alkaloid identical to dTC which they isolated from a crude extract prepared from *C. tomentosum.* A further step in establishing the origin of dTC was the introduction into the United States by Gill (1940) of 30 lb of an authenticated curare preparation from *C. tomentosum*. The availability of the substance made possible chemical and pharmacological studies as well as the development of bioassay methods. A standardized preparation of curare from *C. tomentosum* was developed by Squibb for clinical purposes. One unit of this preparation (Intocostrin) is equivalent to 0.15 mg of dTC.

dTC is a white, odorless powder widely available for both clinical and experimental applications. It has a molecular weight of 695.67; it exists in the form of various hydrates, the most common one of which contains five molecules of water; it crystallizes in hexagonal and pentagonal microplates from water, and its solubility in water has been reported variously as from 25 to 50 mg/ml.

From the viewpoint of its chemistry and structure–activity relationships, the most important features of the dTC molecule (Fig. 1) are the two quaternary ammonium groups, the distance of about 14 Å between them, and the presence of a ring system between the onium groups. The quaternary ammonium groups are completely ionized, and the unit positive charge is uniformly distributed and highly concentrated in the nitrogen atom. Replacement of the methyl group by an ethyl group, which reduces the charge concentration, weakens the energy of the electrostatic bonding

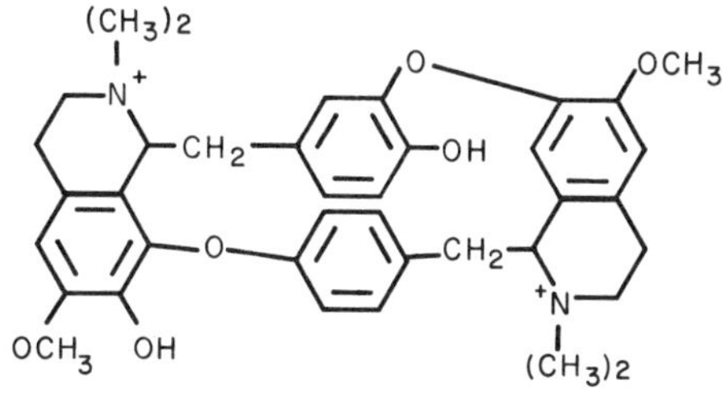

Fig. 1. Structure of *d*-tubocurarine.

that the onium group forms with the negative sites of the cell receptors (Taylor and Nedergaard, 1965) and also increases the radius of this group.

Although dTC is poorly, if at all, metabolized in the body, the two phenolic hydroxyl groups in its molecule may be important from a pharmacodynamic viewpoint, since they offer a starting point for metabolic degradation. The activity of dTC can be increased by replacing these two —OH groups by CH_3—O—groups. The dimethyl ether of dTC (Metubine) is about 33% more potent than dTC, perhaps because it is more hydrophobic.

Other quaternary alkaloids isolated from *C. tomentosum* are *l*-tubocurarine, which is the levorotatory enantiomorph of dTC and has from one-tenth to one-sixtieth of the activity of dTC, *d*-chondrocurarine, which is four or five times more potent than dTC but occurs only in very small amounts, and *l*-tomentocurarine. In the same plants there are many other alkaloids devoid of curariform activity.

3. *Alkaloids of the Genus Strychnos*

The most potent curare alkaloids appear to be those isolated from calabash curare, especially from the curare made from *Strychnos toxifera*. There are at least 30 very similar alkaloids in calabash curare and at least 12 different ones in *S. toxifera* (Craig, 1955). Two of these alkaloids are curarine I, and a closely related alkaloid, toxiferine I, which is the most active of all curare alkaloids and has approximately the same potency in all species tested in terms of mg/kg. Its activity is at least 15–30 times greater than that of dTC, although its mechanism of action seems to be the same (van Maanen, 1948; Paton and Perry, 1951). These alkaloids share with dTC their bis-quaternary character and the presence of a complex ring system (Fig. 2). Active curarines that possess only a single quaternary ammonium group, such as curarine III (fluorocurarine), have also been isolated from calabash curare.

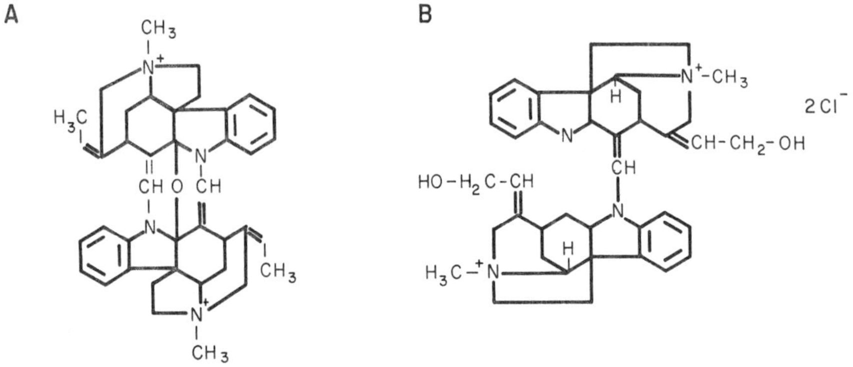

Fig. 2. Structures of curarine I(A) and toxiferine I (B).

4. Alkaloids of the Genus Erythrina

Another source of curare-like alkaloids that possess a single nitrogen atom is the seeds of plants of the genus *Erythrina*, which grow in most of the subtropical regions of the world, including Australia and South America. There are no records that these plants were used for arrow poisons, but the mechanism of their paralytic action is similar to that of curare (Lehman, 1935–1936; Paton and Perry, 1951).

The curare-like alkaloids from *Erythrina* are unique in that they are tertiary bases with a relatively high curarizing potency that is greatly diminished by quaternization. The tertiary nature of these alkaloids causes them to be active by mouth, to cross the blood–brain barrier, and to have effects on the central nervous system such as depression of spinal interneurons, which may cause muscle relaxation (see Section XI). They also depress blood pressure and respiration, they may have some hypnotic effects, and, although the reports are conflicting, they are believed not to liberate histamine. The alkaloids from *Erythrina* important from an experimental viewpoint are dihydro-β-erythroidine and β-erythroidine (Fig. 3).

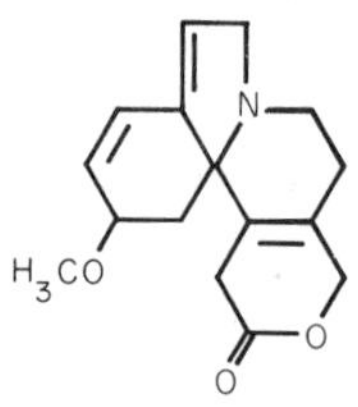

Fig. 3. Structure of β-erythroidine.

5. *Other Curarizing Alkaloids*

Quinine has long been known to exert a number of complex pharmacological actions on muscle, and among these is a weak curare-like action (Harvey, 1939). Conversion of quinine into a quaternary salt, such as quinine methochloride, reduces most of its actions but considerably enhances its curare-like activity (Harvey, 1940).

The quaternary salts of other alkaloids have also been found to exhibit curarizing-like activity (see Craig, 1955, for details). Recently, new curare-like agents of plant origin have been found in certain species of *Delphinium*, especially *D. crassifolium*, growing in Transbaikalia (Mats, 1972).

B. Synthetic Curare-like Agents

Crum-Brown and Fraser (1868, 1869) are credited with the discovery of the curare-like action of quaternary ammonium salts and quaternary derivatives of alkaloids. The synthesis of new curare-like agents was achieved in the 1940s, mainly through the work of Bovet *et al.* (1946), Barlow and Ing (1948*a,b*), and Paton and Zaimis (1948, 1949). The first attempts to synthesize curare-like molecules involved imitations of curare that were bis-quaternary derivatives of the quinoline and isoquinoline series. Since these efforts were highly successful, simpler molecules were synthesized. In Bovet's (1951) own words, "the investigations have proceeded through a series of repeated simplifications of the molecule. They have arrived on the one hand at such a schematically simple model as decamethonium iodide and on the other at a doublet of acetylcholine" (succinylcholine).

Bovet (1951) classified the synthetic curare-like agents according to the nature of the structures separating the two quaternary ammonium groups:

1. Quinoline and isoquinoline series: The most active member of this series is 8′-8″-diquinolyloxy-1,5-pentane diiodoethylate, or compound 3381 R.P. (Fig. 4A). This was the first highly effective synthesized molecule taking the dTC molecule as a model (Bovet *et al.*, 1946).
2. Aromatic amines: A representative is bis-(dimethyl-amino-2,2′-phenoxy)-1,5-pentane diiodomethylate (3565 R.P.) (Fig. 4B).
3. Bis- and poly-quaternary derivatives of aromatic ethers and esters: An example is tri- (β-triethylammoniumethoxy)-1,2,3-benzene triiodide, a compound that became important in clinical and experimental applications under the names of gallamine and flaxedil (Fig. 4C).

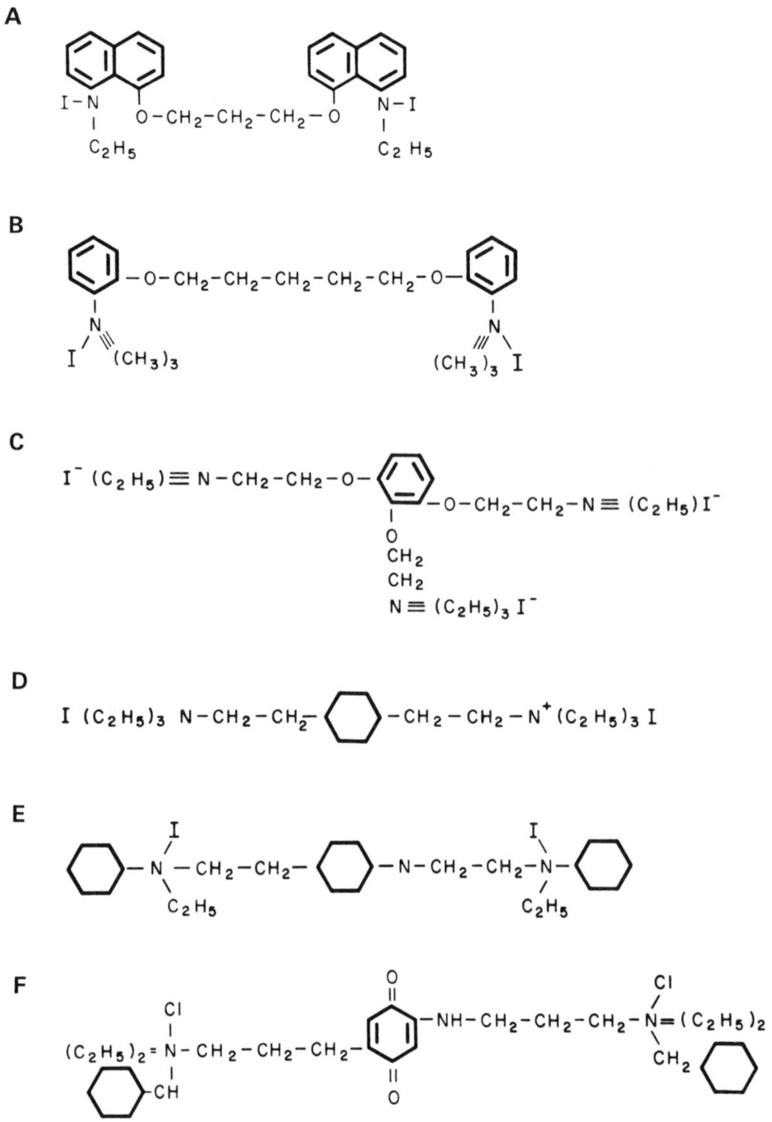

A

I−N O−CH2−CH2−CH2−O N−I
C2H5 C2H5

B

−O−CH2−CH2−CH2−CH2−CH2−O−
N N
I (CH3)3 (CH3)3 I

C

I⁻ (C2H5)≡N−CH2−CH2−O−
−O−CH2−CH2−N≡(C2H5)I⁻
O
CH2
CH2
N≡(C2H5)3 I⁻

D

I (C2H5)3 N−CH2−CH2− −CH2−CH2−N⁺(C2H5)3 I

E

I I
−N−CH2−CH2− −N−CH2−CH2−N−
C2H5 C2H5

F

O Cl
Cl
−NH−CH2−CH2−CH2−N=(C2H5)2
(C2H5)2=N−CH2−CH2−CH2−
CH2
CH
O

Fig. 4. Structures of 8′-8′′-diquinolyloxy-1,5-pentane diiodoethylate, or compound 3381 R.P. (A); bis-(dimethyl-amino-2,2′-phenoxy)-1,5-pentane diiodomethylate, or compound 3565 R.P. (B); tri-(β-triethylammoniumethoxy)1,2,3-benzene triiodide, known as gallamine or Flaxedil (C); 1-(β-diethyl-aminoethoxy)-4-(carboxy-β-diethyl-aminoethyl)-benzene diiodoethylate (D); bis-(β-piperidylethyl)piperazine diiodoethylate (E); and 2,5-bis-(3-diethyl-amino-propyl-amino)benzoquinone-bis-benzylchloride, known as mytolon or Win 2747 (F).

4. Arylaromatic amine series: An example is 1-(β-diethyl-amino-ethoxy)-4-(carboxy-β-diethyl-aminoethyl)-benzene diiodoethylate; this compound is of interest because it shows that the oxygen bridges present in dTC are not essential for curariform activity (Fig. 4D).
5. Piperidine series: The most active member of this group is bis-(β-piperidylethyl)piperazine diiodoethylate (Fig. 4E).
6. Alkylamino-benzoquinone series: 2,5-Bis-(3-diethyl-amino-propyl-amino)benzoquinone-bis-benzylchloride, known as mytolon (Win 2747) (Fig. 4F), is one of the most active molecules of this group and has been used clinically. The pharmacology of this compound was studied by Hoppe (1950).
7. Aliphatic series:
   a. Polymethylene series: Tetraethylammonium was long known to have paralyzing effects on muscle. Brieger (1886) and Willstaetter and Heubner (1907) investigated derivatives containing two quaternary ammonium groups and discovered the paralytic activity of tetramethylene-bis-trimethylammonium. In the late 1940s, Barlow and Ing (1948*a,b*) and Paton and Zaimis (1949) described independently the pharmacological properties of higher members of the polymethylene-bis-trimethylammonium series, of which decamethylene bis-trimethylammonium iodide, known as decamethonium, is the most active (Fig. 5A). Other compounds in this series, pentamethonium iodide and hexamethonium iodide have ganglionic blocking properties and also exert a marked antagonism against the effects of decamethonium on the motor end plate. Barlow and Zoller (1964) examined the effects of members of the same series with longer chains and discovered the presence of a second peak of activity in the compounds made of a chain of 16 carbon atoms.
   b. Ester series: The main representative of this group is bis-dimethylaminoethyl succinate diiodomethylate, known as succinylcholine, which is two acetylcholine (ACh) molecules linked by their acetyl ends (Fig. 5B). The pharmacology of succinylcholine was investigated as early as 1906 by Hunt and Taveau; however, because they employed curarized animals they failed to observe the neuromuscular blocking action of the drug. Succinylcholine is a powerful curarizing agent widely used in medicine; it has a duration of action shorter than that of curare, since it is easily hydrolyzed by acetylcholinesterase (AChE) (Glick, 1941; Bovet-Nitti, 1959; Castillo and de Beer, 1950). Succinylcholine does not have the muscarinic properties of ACh.

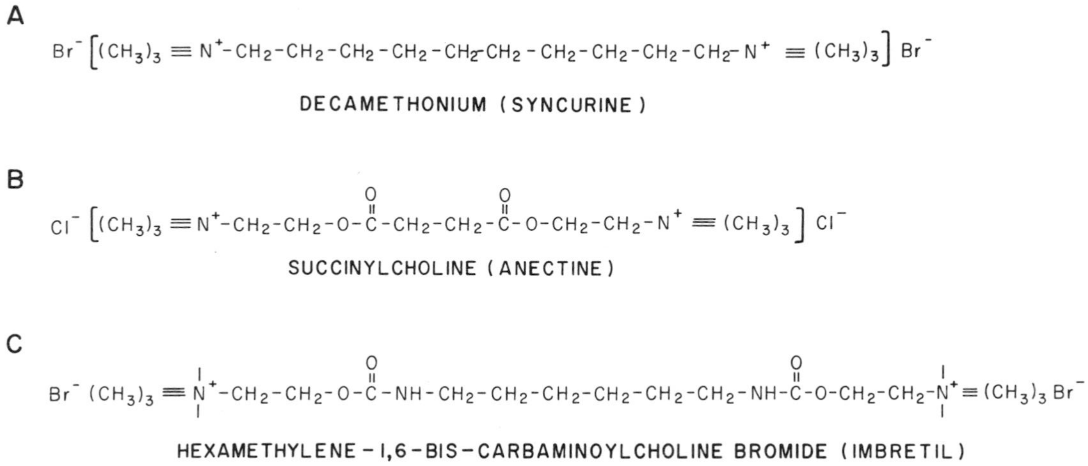

A

$$Br^- \left[(CH_3)_3 \equiv N^+ - CH_2 - CH_2 - CH_2 - CH_2 - CH_2 - CH_2 - CH_2 - CH_2 - CH_2 - CH_2 - N^+ \equiv (CH_3)_3\right] Br^-$$

DECAMETHONIUM (SYNCURINE)

B

$$Cl^- \left[(CH_3)_3 \equiv N^+ - CH_2 - CH_2 - O - \overset{O}{\overset{\|}{C}} - CH_2 - CH_2 - \overset{O}{\overset{\|}{C}} - O - CH_2 - CH_2 - N^+ \equiv (CH_3)_3\right] Cl^-$$

SUCCINYLCHOLINE (ANECTINE)

C

$$Br^- (CH_3)_3 \equiv N^+ - CH_2 - CH_2 - O - \overset{O}{\overset{\|}{C}} - NH - CH_2 - CH_2 - CH_2 - CH_2 - CH_2 - CH_2 - NH - \overset{O}{\overset{\|}{C}} - O - CH_2 - CH_2 - N^+ \equiv (CH_3)_3 Br^-$$

HEXAMETHYLENE – 1,6 – BIS – CARBAMINOYLCHOLINE BROMIDE (IMBRETIL)

Fig. 5. Structures of decamethylene-bis-trimethylammonium iodide, or decamethonium (A); bis-dimethylaminoethyl succinate diiodomethylate, or succinylcholine (B); and hexamethylene-1,6-bis-carbaminoylcholine, or Imbretil (C).

Many derivatives of succinylcholine have been prepared, but neither the monoester nor the tertiary diamine equivalent to succinylcholine has curarizing action. Also, the curarizing properties of succinylcholine are lost if the methyl groups attached to the nitrogen are replaced by other radicals.

The dicholinic esters of higher dicarboxylic acids have little curarizing activity under ordinary conditions, probably because of their rapid hydrolysis by AChE. By inhibiting AChE, eserine greatly potentiates the curare-like action of these compounds; however, the relationships between the length of the chain and curarizing potency in the presence of eserine are not clear, and all of the compounds having between 12 and 16 carbon atoms have approximately the same potency. These compounds also exert a prolonged stimulating action on amphibian and avian tonic muscles. In the absence of anticholinesterase agents, suberyldicholine, which has a chain of 14 carbons between the nitrogens, is the most potent stimulating compound; but in the presence of neostigmine, sebacinyldicholine, with a 16-carbon chain, is more potent than suberyldicholine (see references in Khromov-Borisov and Michelson, 1966). These observations have been interpreted as evidence that a peak of activity occurs both in compounds with a 10-atom and those with a 16-atom chain between the quaternary nitrogens.

c. Bis-carbaminoylcholine series: This series shows interesting structure–activity relationships. The molecule which represents a doublet of the carbaminoylcholine molecule, i.e., bis-carbaminoylcholine, has very little activity. This has been explained by the presence of a —N—N— bond in the central part of the molecule, which could lead to the formation of stable complexes in which the shape of the molecule would be completely distorted. The incorporation of one methylene group between the two carbaminic nitrogens increases the potency 50 times, and the potency continues to increase as the length of the chain between the two nitrogens is lengthened up to six methyl groups. This compound, hexamethylene-1,6-bis-carbaminoylcholine (Imbretil) (Fig. 5C), has a chain of 16 atoms between the two quaternary nitrogen groups. It has been suggested (de Beer, 1959) that the nitrogen atoms may introduce bends in the chain bringing the two cationic nitrogens to a distance similar to that of decamethonium (i.e., about 14 Å). However, this compound has also been used as proof that a second peak of curarizing activity occurs in compounds in which the two cationic nitrogens are separated by a distance of about 20 Å.

8. Other synthetic curarizing agents: New synthetic curarizing agents are pancuronium dimethobromide, a molecule unique among curarizing drugs because it has a steroid nucleus (Buckett *et al.*, 1968; Stovner and Lund, 1970; Karis and Gissen, 1971; see Speight and Avery, 1972, and Manani *et al.*, 1972, for clinical studies; see Dretchen *et al.*, 1972, and Galindo, 1972, for studies of mechanism of action), and 1,1′-azobis(3-methyl-2-phenyl-1*H*-imidazo[1,2-*a*]-pyridinium)dibromide (Brittain and Tyers, 1972). A number of curarizing compounds described in the Russian literature are mentioned by Khromov-Borisov and Michelson (1966).

In addition to the bis-quaternary neuromuscular blocking agents, a few monoquaternary molecules have proved to have curare-like action; among them are several monoquaternary derivatives of the alkylaminobenzoquinone series. Another is *p*-dimethylaminophenyl heptyl ketone semicarbazone ethiodide (Bamford *et al.*, 1972), which is a short-acting curare-like drug comparable to succinylcholine in the duration of its effects. Its block is reversed by anticholinesterases.

C. On the Size and Shape of the Curarizing Agents

Bovet (1951) proposed classifying all of the curarizing agents, both natural and synthetic, into two groups according to the size and shape of the region of the molecule between the two nitrogen atoms. In the *pachycurares*, which are fat or plump, the space between the cationic nitrogens is filled with structures such as cyclic rings and aromatic groups; the *leptocurares*, on the other hand, are long and slender molecules, such as decamethonium and succinylcholine.

D. Curarizing Agents of Animal Origin

A number of curare-like agents of animal origin have been described. These include insect poisons and snake venoms, e.g., bungarotoxin and cobrotoxin (See Volume 1 of *Neuropoisons*). Certain fractions of these snake venoms bind reasonably specifically and irreversibly with the cholinergic receptors, and they have become extremely useful tools for the biochemical isolation of the receptor substance.

III. GENERAL PHARMACOLOGICAL AND TOXIC EFFECTS OF CURARE

A. Peripheral Cholinergic Junctions

1. Skeletal Muscle

The intravenous injection of dTC into experimental animals causes muscle weakness, loss of muscle tonus, and, finally, complete flaccid paralysis. Muscle involvement follows a definite order: eye and ear muscles are the first to be affected; the neck muscles follow, then the limb muscles, the muscles of the trunk, and eventually the intercostal muscles and the diaphragm. Death is caused by anoxia due to respiratory failure. Artificial respiration prevents death, and, as the blood levels of the drug drop, muscle activity is reestablished in an order approximately the reverse of that occurring in paralysis, except that the facial muscles appear to recover at the same time as the diaphragm.

In man, the intravenous injection of the usual clinical paralyzing dose of dTC (10–15 mg) exerts very rapid effects. In less than 30 sec, strabismus and diplopia appear; palpebral ptosis, dysarthria, and dysphagia quickly follow. In about 2 min, paralysis of the facial and neck muscles sets in and then spreads to the limbs and abdomen. The intercostal muscles are affected in about 3 min. Respiration proceeds with difficulty and becomes purely diaphragmatic. As respiration becomes increasingly difficult, artificial respiration becomes necessary. After a period of paralysis with a duration depending on the dose (approximately 20–30 min with 10–15 mg), recuperation begins and becomes complete within 30–60 min.

2. Autonomic Effects

Curare acts not only on skeletal muscle but also at synapses of the autonomic ganglia, although its effect on ganglia is less intense than that at the motor end-plate. Blockage of autonomic ganglia is responsible in part for a drop in blood pressure and tachycardia (Sollman, 1957). Curarizing drugs have no conspicuous effects on the isolated heart–lung preparation (Dowdy *et al.*, 1971). In the heart *in situ*, in both experimental animals and man, the minute volume, venous pressure, and EKG are not altered, even if rather high doses are employed (Sollman, 1957). Sometimes, however, tachycardia can be observed due to vagal inhibition. Riker and Wescoe (1951) showed that dTC desensitizes the heart to epinephrine in subjects anesthetized with cyclopropane.

B. Central Nervous System

Because curare is a lipid-insoluble quaternary ammonium base, it does not penetrate the blood–brain barrier. Neither consciousness nor sensibility is affected following its intravenous injection, and neither sedation nor analgesia occurs. Smith *et al.*, (1947) injected a healthy, conscious subject with 2.5 times the dose of curare required for complete respiratory paralysis. The subject reported dizziness, sensation of warmth, difficulty in focusing, weakness of the jaw muscles, increasing difficulty in speech and in keeping the eyes open, diplopia, and dysphagia; his limbs felt heavy and difficult to move. When full paralysis occurred, shortness of breath was experienced in spite of artificially maintained respiration. The subject remained fully conscious throughout the experiment.

When injected directly into the cerebral ventricles, dTC behaves as a potent stimulant, similar to strychnine and picrotoxin, and gives rise to myoclonic contractions, convulsions which resemble epileptic seizures, and changes in the EEG similar to those observed during grand mal in man (See Section XI).

C. Histamine-Releasing Action

The slow intravenous injection of curare does not significantly modify the arterial blood pressure in animals and man, except at high doses which cause hypotension due to ganglionic block. However, the rapid intravenous injection of dTC can produce a sudden drop of blood pressure, leading to shock and death; this is the result of a sudden liberation of histamine, first demonstrated by Alam *et al.* (1939). These authors demonstrated that curare causes a release of histamine from skeletal muscle as well as from the heart, but not from the lung. Histamine release following the rapid injection of curare produces not only circulatory symptoms but also bronchospasm.

Other signs of histamine action have been reported following intraarterial injection of curare (Grob *et al.*, 1947), such as wheals, swelling of the limbs, local and generalized vasodilation, and increased secretion of gastric juice. These effects are prevented by tripelennamine, but not atropine.

The intradermal injection of dTC and toxiferines gives rise to the so-called triple response in the human skin (Paton and Perry, 1951).

IV. PHARMACODYNAMICS

A. Absorption and Distribution

Curares and curarines are not absorbed through the intact unbroken skin, and are hardly absorbed, if at all, from the gastrointestinal tract. As the South American Indians knew, curares are inactive if given orally. It is not clear, however, whether this lack of activity is due to the destruction of the curare or to failure of absorption.

Although absorption can be fast by subcutaneous and intramuscular injection, for clinical and experimental purposes curare is almost always introduced by intravenous injection. Following its injection, curare distributes itself widely throughout the body, although it crosses neither the blood–brain barrier nor the placenta (Marsh, 1951; Kalow, 1959). Paralysis occurs when the concentration of dTC in plasma rises above 2–4 μg/ml. After an initial peak concentration of the drug is reached, the concentration in the plasma decreases rapidly at first, and then more slowly until its complete disappearance from blood. There are no indications that curare either binds plasma proteins or penetrates the red cells.

The transient nature of the paralytic action following the usual clinical doses of curare is related to neither metabolism nor excretion, but to a rapid redistribution of the drug in the body. dTC is not concentrated at the neuromuscular junctions, but instead distributes itself uniformly throughout the body, and it has been estimated that only about one-thousandth of the clinical dose is actually needed to block the cholinergic receptor sites in skeletal muscle. The end of paralysis is reached when the curare molecules move from the blood and the cholinergic receptor sites to other acceptor sites or silent receptors.

B. Nonspecific Acceptors

The nature of the secondary acceptor sites is unknown, but studies on the distribution of curare in dogs during periods of full curarization show the existence of a rough correlation between the acidic mucopolysaccharide content of the tissues and the amount of curare fixed; also, more active binding appears to occur in tissues where neurovegetative synapses are abundant (Chagas, 1962). With large or repeated doses, the acceptor sites become saturated and the paralytic effects are prolonged considerably. Duration of paralysis thus becomes dependent on the rate of excretion.

Not all of the synthetic curarizing compounds seem to have the same degree of affinity for the nonspecific, or silent, acceptor sites. The short duration of action of some stable compounds (those not hydrolyzed by AChE) seems to depend on a vary rapid attachment to such acceptors. This occurs in particular with bis-(dimethyl-amino-butoxy)-1,4-benzene diiodomethylate and dodecamethylene-bis-(*N*-methyl)piperidinium iodide, which produce extremely short paralysis when given intravenously in dogs and rabbits. The rapid reversibility of their effects cannot be explained by either destruction or rapid elimination.

The hypothesis that the transient nature of the paralytic action of curare is linked to its attachment to nonspecific acceptors is supported by the observation that the effects of curare are potentiated by the administration of compounds that lack any cholinergic actions. Cheymol and Bourillet (1960) showed that many quaternary ammonium bases and other strong bases, which do not have biological activity on their own, potentiate the action of curare. It was suggested that this might be the result of a displacement of curare from the silent receptors or acceptors, resulting in an increase in the effective concentration of curare in blood. Bovet *et al.* (1956) have suggested an analogous mechanism for the potentiation of curariform drugs by the compound known as SKF 525-A. This compound, which by itself has no action on neuromuscular transmission, increases the intensity and duration of curarization in the rabbit and dog when injected immediately after the curarizing agent. This can be explained by a displacement of the curariform drug from the acceptor sites by competitive action. SKF 525-A particularly potentiates the effects of short-acting curariform compounds. Its effects are less apparent or even completely absent on long-lasting curares (see references in Bovet, 1951).

The action of curare can be antagonized, instead of potentiated, by the injection of heparine and other polysulfonates into the circulatory system (Cheymol *et al.*, 1955). This antagonism is probably due to a direct chemical interaction between the acidic polysulfonates and curare, i.e., a direct antagonism by extracellular chemical neutralization. Schueler (1960) synthesized a linear polymer containing anionic groups ($—SO_2O^-$) located at a distance of 14 Å from each other. This polymer, which may be considered a cholinergic receptor, competed with the curare-binding sites in the organism.

C. Elimination

Curare is poorly metabolized in the body, and most of it is excreted unchanged. Chagas and his coworkers have performed experiments to determine the fate of injected curariform drugs in various animals (For references to their extensive work, consult Chagas, 1962). Their experiments with ^{14}C-labeled dimethyl-dTC and gallamine in the dog showed that the urinary system is the principal pathway for the excretion of curares. From 50 to 70% of the drug was found in the urine from 3 to 6 hr after its injection. The total amount in the bile was no greater than 10%. Chromatography of dimethyl-dTC gave no indication of any molecular modifications of the eliminated drug. This, however, does not exclude the possibility of the elimination of the drug in the form of a complex, which might have dissociated during the assay. In experiments on the electric eel, the amount recovered from the urine plus that present in the blood added up to about 80% of the total injected dose. No traces of ^{14}C were found in the expired air (Chagas, 1962). Therefore, Chagas believed that the remainder of the drug remains attached to acceptor sites, from which it is liberated very slowly.

V. CHOLINERGIC RECEPTORS

With the exception of its histamine-releasing action, its desensitizing effects against epinephrine on the myocardium, and, perhaps, some other minor effects, the main toxicological and pharmacological actions of curare are believed to be due to its interaction with certain cholinergic receptors present on the surfaces of cells that are sensitive to ACh.

A. Classification

Long before the role of ACh in synaptic transmission was established, its pharmacological actions had been described as a combination of the effects elicited by the plant alkaloids nicotine and muscarine (see Dale, 1914–1915). The effects of these two alkaloids are believed to be mediated by two different types of cholinergic receptors, nicotinic and muscarinic receptors. As Dale (1914–1915) pointed out, the differences between the nicotinic and muscarinic receptors are apparent not only on the basis of the effects of activating or "agonist" drugs, but also on the basis of the "antagonist" or blocking drugs. The effects of muscarine are blocked by atropine, and the effects of nicotine by curare. The basic mechanism of action of curare appears to depend on its specific interaction with the nicotinic type of ACh receptors. The present ideas on such receptors are summarized below. We wish to emphasize, however, that a sharp distinction between nicotinic and muscarinic receptors derives from mammalian pharmacology.

Recent investigations on invertebrates have revealed new cholinergic receptors which cannot easily be fitted into either category (Kehoe, 1972).

B. Topography

In skeletal muscle fibers, cholinergic receptors are concentrated in the areas where the terminal arborizations of the motor nerve fiber establish functional contact with the muscle cell. This was first shown by the classical experiments of Kuffler (1942, 1943). He applied small droplets of ACh solution to a single nerve fiber–muscle fiber preparation and observed that the fiber would twitch only when the solution contacted the myoneural region.

The introduction of glass microelectrodes for recording (Ling and Gerard, 1949) and their subsequent use for the electrophoretic application of ACh (Nastuk, 1953; del Castillo and Katz, 1955) greatly increased the degree of resolution with which the ACh-sensitive areas could be mapped. It was possible to show that not all the surface of the fiber in the synaptic region was equally sensitive to ACh, but that chemical sensitivity was restricted to narrow regions corresponding presumably to the distribution of the terminal nerve filaments. Moving the tip of the micropipette away from these areas by as little as 10 μm caused the amplitude of the potential changes elicited by constant ACh pulses to decline to a fraction of their original value. At the same time, the rising phase of the ACh potential lengthened severalfold, showing that the diffusional pathways had increased considerably. del Castillo and Katz (1955) also showed that ACh and stable depolarizing agents such as carbaminoylcholine (CCh) are ineffective when injected inside the muscle fiber. This shows that the ACh-sensitive membrane is asymmetrical i.e., that the binding sites of the receptors are located only on the external surface of the membrane. More recently, a combination of microelectrophoresis and interference contrast (Nomarski) optics has permitted analysis of ACh sensitivity of postjunctional membranes in preparations in which nerve filaments could be clearly seen (Peper and McMahan, 1972). Such experiments have shown that peak ACh sensitivity is confined to an area of membrane within a few microns of the nerve terminal edge.

Interruption of the motor supply to the muscle fibers results, after a latent period, in change in the distribution of cholinergic sensitivity. As first demonstrated by Ginetsinsky and Shamarina (1942), the whole surface of the denervated muscle fiber becomes sensitive to ACh. This phenomenon was further studied with electrical techniques by Axelsson and Thesleff (1959) and Miledi (1960). Following denervation, the receptors spread out from the synaptic region. The opposite process takes place when the motor nerve is allowed to regenerate.

C. Receptor Activation

In the presence of ACh, the ionic permeability of the cholinoceptive areas of the muscle fiber membrane increases drastically, as shown by a great reduction in the fiber's electrical resistance (Fatt and Katz, 1951). This change in permeability is the result of a process known as *receptor activation*. It is generally accepted that the interaction between ACh and receptor sites at the external surface of the end-plate membranes causes the opening of ion-permeable channels which serve as pathways for small cations (del Castillo and Katz, 1955; Takeuchi and Takeuchi, 1960; Takeuchi; 1963). These pathways act as a shunt across the resting potential of the muscle membrane. As a consequence of receptor activation, the muscle membrane becomes depolarized and a muscle action potential is fired.

D. Desensitization

If the action of the transmitter on the cholinoceptive membrane is prolonged, the receptor molecules become refractory to activation. This is the phenomenon described as "desensitization" (Thesleff, 1955; Katz and Thesleff, 1957*a*). It has been assumed that desensitization involves the transformation of the drug-receptor complex from its active form, in which membrane permeability is increased, to an inactive form which fails to maintain or produce a high ionic permeability of the end-plate membrane (Thesleff, 1956). Whether desensitization is due to a conformational change in the receptor molecules or to a blockade of receptor sites is not clear (Thesleff, 1958). Although it is unlikely that desensitization plays a physiological role, it can be important in a number of pharmacological situations—for example, when ACh accumulates in large concentrations under the influence of anti-AChE agents, or when curare-like drugs, such as decamethonium and succinylcholine, are applied.

E. Binding Sites of the Nicotinic Receptor

The attachment of a drug to a receptor involves chemical interactions between pairs of complementary regions, or chemical functions, at one or more sites on the receptor surface and the drug molecule. The main

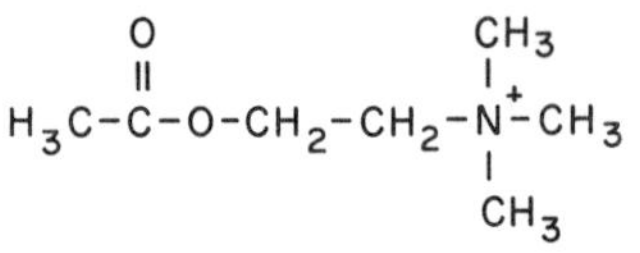

$$H_3C-\overset{\overset{\displaystyle O}{\|}}{C}-O-CH_2-CH_2-\overset{\overset{\displaystyle CH_3}{|}}{\underset{\underset{\displaystyle CH_3}{|}}{N^+}}-CH_3$$

Fig. 6. Structure of acetylcholine.

chemical features of the ACh molecule (Fig. 6) are its onium head (the quaternary nitrogen group) and its esteratic moiety, which includes an ether oxygen and a carbonyl group. The active center of AChE has been used, as suggested originally by Roepke (1937), as a convenient model for the cholinergic receptor. Accordingly, it is generally assumed that the ACh molecule interacts with the receptor in at least three separate sites (Barlow, 1964; Goldstein *et al.*, 1968):

1. A negative, or anionic, site, probably represented by a carboxyl (Edwards *et al.*, 1970) or phosphate (Hu, 1972) group, which attracts the positively charged quaternary nitrogen head of ACh and orients the molecule. Models of the ACh molecule show that its cationic nitrogen is free to rotate with reference to the carbon chain, and it has been suggested that the negative charge of the receptor is placed within a cavity that will accommodate two of the three methyl groups which would stabilize the transmitter–receptor complex through van der Waals forces.
2. An "esterophilic" or "carbonyl-binding" site that would interact with the ester moiety of the ACh molecule by involving either the carbonyl group alone or a dipole formed by the ether and carbonyl oxygens of ACh (Khromov-Borisov and Michelson, 1966).
3. Possible hydrophobic interactions of the carbon atoms between the nitrogen and the ether oxygen with a flat part of the receptor surface between the anionic and "esterophilic" sites.

Although receptor activation by ACh simultaneously involves these three sites and, perhaps, additional interactions (see Burgen, 1970), it is possible to activate the receptor with compounds that can act only at single sites. For instance, tetramethylammonium (TMA), a molecule that can interact only with the anionic site, is a strong activator of nicotinic receptors, both when injected (Burn and Dale, 1915) and when applied iontophoretically (del Castillo and Sobrino, 1973).

Recently, del Castillo and Sobrino (1973) have shown that drug–receptor interactions which exclude the participation of the anionic site also cause receptor activation. The microelectroosmotic application of methyl acetate, a compound which is equivalent to the esteratic moiety of the ACh molecule, gives rise to depolarizations similar to those elicited by pulses of ACh. Ethyl acetate has a similar effect. The activating action of methyl acetate and ethyl acetate on the cholinergic end-plate receptors appears to be due to the carbonyl group and not to the ester function of these compounds. In fact, diethyl ether, a molecule similar to ethyl acetate, in which the carbonyl oxygen has been replaced by two hydrogens, not only lacks a depolarizing action on the end-plate receptors but also has a curare-like action (Karis *et al.*, 1966). Acetone, on the other hand, which lacks an ether oxygen but possesses a carbonyl group, is an activator of the end-plate receptors (del Castillo and Sobrino, 1973).

F. Chemical Nature of the Cholinergic Receptors

1. The Protein Hypothesis

Proteins are particularly well suited to perform the dual function postulated for the synaptic receptors: (a) the recognition of transmitter molecules and (b) the conformational change needed to explain the sudden increase in the permeability of the postsynaptic membrane. Therefore, even in the absence of direct biochemical evidence, many authors followed Welsh's (1948) and Nachmansohn's (1955) suggestions that the synaptic receptors are protein molecules. Receptor activation has been envisaged as a change in the tertiary or quaternary configuration of these molecules resulting in the opening of ion-permeable channels.

2. Chemical Modification In Situ: The Nicotinic Receptor as a Sulfhydryl (SH) Protein

The experiments of Karlin and Bartels (1966) and Karlin and Winnik (1968) on isolated cells from the electric organ of *Electrophorus electricus* demonstrated that the receptors of the innervated surface of the electroplate possess a disulfide bond, situated at a distance of 9–10 Å away from the anionic subsite, whose degree of oxidation or reduction determines the sensitivity of the receptor to the depolarizing action of ACh and related drugs. These results were important not only because they confirmed that the receptor, or part of it, is a protein, but also because they showed that the conformational changes induced by the oxidation or reduction of such a disulfide bond were reflected in the efficacy of the drug–receptor interaction.

Del Castillo *et al.* (1971) and Sobrino and del Castillo (1972) studied the effects of microelectrophoretically applied SH reagents, and they found that end-plate receptors could be activated via their sulfhydryl groups. The most potent receptor activator among the various SH reagents tested proved to be *o*-iodosobenzoate (IB), which at a *p*H of 8.5 oxidizes highly specifically the —SH groups. The electroosmotic application of IB to the end-plate membrane results in phasic depolarizations or "IB-potentials" which are often faster than the ACh potentials elicited from the other barrel of double micropipettes. The effects of these reagents have been studied with the same techniques on the receptors of the electroplate preparation. The results obtained were essentially the same as those obtained in the motor end-plate (del Castillo *et al.*, 1972).

3. *Chemical Isolation*

Recently, several techniques have been developed to identify, isolate, and characterize the nicotinic receptor macromolecule. Agents that bind specifically and with high affinity have been used to label the receptor either reversibly or irreversibly. The report of a recent Neurosciences Research Program Work Session on the biophysics and biochemistry of receptors includes descriptions of several of the experimental approaches currently used in the study of various receptors, including the cholinergic receptor, and an extensive bibliography (Hammes *et al.*, 1973). The reader is directed to this source for references (see also Karlin, 1973).

G. Autoradiographic Studies

Molecules that possess high affinity for cholinergic receptor sites and combine with them with various degrees of reversibility can be used in tracer studies both to identify the binding sites and to obtain quantitative data on their number in a given tissue. Curares labeled with ^{14}C were first used by Chagas and collaborators. A complex formed by the injected curare and the bound macromolecule was isolated from homogenates of perfused curarized electric organs. Hassón and Chagas (1959, 1961) suggested that acidic mucopolysaccharides were responsible for curare fixation. Autoradiographic experiments showed that curare attaches to both the anterior and posterior surfaces of the electroplate and to the ground substance in the intracellular phase (Chagas, 1962).

Waser (1965, 1966, 1970) used autoradiographic techniques to explore the distribution, density, and specificity of binding sites in the end-plates of mouse diaphragm. Three different types of compounds were used: (1) the depolarizing agents decamethonium, muscarone, and carbachol; (2) an anti-AChE drug, diisopropylfluorophosphate (DFP); and (3) two calabash alkaloids (curarine and toxiferine) and dimethyl-dTC.

Of the depolarizing agents used, only radioactive decamethonium gave good radiographs: muscarone and carbachol gave only faintly detectable traces of radioactivity. With a minimal intravenous dose, 7.0×10^7 molecules of decamethonium were found in the end-plate region; about 1.9×10^9 molecules were found around the end-plate. The results obtained with both ^{32}P- and ^{14}C-labeled DFP showed that the binding sites in the active centers of AChE were saturated at a concentration of between 1.9 and 2.4×10^7 molecules per end-plate. Both calabash curare alkaloids accumulated in the end-plates, but curarine, the less active of the two, was found in the tendinous ends of muscle fibers. Toxiferine was fixed only in the end-plates. The number of radioactive curare molecules fixed per end-plate was 4×10^6 for both alkaloids.

As a result of these studies, Waser concluded that three different types of cholinergic binding sites are present in the end-plate region: (1) true ACh receptors, (2) active centers of AChE, and (3) curarine receptors. The possible significance of these findings will be discussed in Section XII.

Porter *et al.* (1973) used pure α-bungarotoxin, labeled by ^3H-acetylation, to study the distribution and numbers of ACh receptors in muscle fibers of mouse diaphragm. The grain counts obtained from electron micrographs of postjunctional membrane corresponded, after suitable corrections, to a surface density of 12,400 receptor molecules per square micron, or from 1.4 to 2.1×10^7 receptor molecules per end-plate. This number is lower, but of the same order of magnitude, as that obtained by Waser. It also agrees well with the value of $2\text{–}3 \times 10^7$ receptors per end-plate obtained by different autoradiographic methods using light microscopy (Barnard *et al.*, 1971).

In mouse, rat, monkey, and chicken muscles, the number of specific α-bungarotoxin sites per end-plate appears to equal the number of apparent active centers of AChE (Barnard *et al.*, 1971). The same equality or near equality was found by Kasai and Changeux (1971) for the electroplate membrane. It seems likely that there is some fundamental relationship between the two types of molecules, although there is good evidence that they are not identical.

The effects of saturating concentrations of dTC on the binding of α-bungarotoxin by mouse end-plate were studied by Porter *et al.* (1973). Their results confirmed a previous report by Miledi and Potter (1971) that showed that only 50% of the α-bungarotoxin-binding sites are protected by dTC. These results suggest that there are two different classes of receptor sites in the end-plates of vertebrate skeletal muscle. Both classes irreversibly bind α-bungarotoxin, but only one class binds dTC reversibly. The two types of sites number 1.2×10^4 per square micron, a figure which is approximately equal to the density of the active centers of AChE.

In frog muscle, Miledi and Potter (1971) reported that there are about 10^9 bungarotoxin-binding sites per end-plate (about 60 times the content of the mouse diaphragm end-plate) but that the cholinesterase-like sites in the frog muscle end-plate equal the number of receptors in the mouse end-plate. According to Porter *et al.* (1973), such a discrepancy is due to the presence of large numbers of extrajunctional receptors in the sarcoplasm inside the frog muscle fibers, and the specific end-plate ACh receptors number about 3×10^7 per end-plate.

VI. ACTIONS OF CURARE ON SKELETAL MUSCLE

A. Antagonism Between Curare and ACh

The theory that curare blocks neuromuscular transmission by changing the electrical excitability of muscle (Lapique, 1926) was disproved (Rushton, 1933), and, although curare may exert some presynaptic effects (see Sections VIII, IX, and X), the mass of experimental evidence indicates that, as Cowan first showed (1936), curare paralyzes skeletal muscle by antagonizing the depolarizing effect of ACh on the end-plate membrane. Even before the chemical nature of transmission at the neuromuscular junction was elucidated, Langley (1909) showed that curare greatly diminishes the stimulating action of nicotine on the sartorius and gastrocnemius muscles of the frog.

The antagonism between the curare and ACh on muscle has been demonstrated to be competitive by the determination of dose–response curves of ACh or other cholinergic agonists in the presence of increasing concentrations of dTC. Van Maanen (1950) studied the antagonism of dTC, curarine I, *C*-toxiferine II, and β-erythroidine on ACh-contracture of the frog rectus abdominis muscle. The effects of all of these alkaloids were essentially the same (Fig. 7). As the dTC concentration increases, the log concentration–response curves for ACh are shifted in a parallel fashion to the right. The amplitude of the maximal response is not reduced; muscles become less sensitive to ACh, but the maximal response can still be obtained and the slope of the curve is not significantly changed. These results suggest that there is a competitive antagonism between curare and ACh. Other experiments on the same preparation (Kirschner and Stone, 1951; Ariens *et al.*, 1956; Jenkinson, 1960) and on the sartorius and extensor digitorum longus of the frog (Jenkinson, 1960) have likewise demonstrated a competitive antagonism between cholinergic agonists and a number of synthetic curare-like agents.

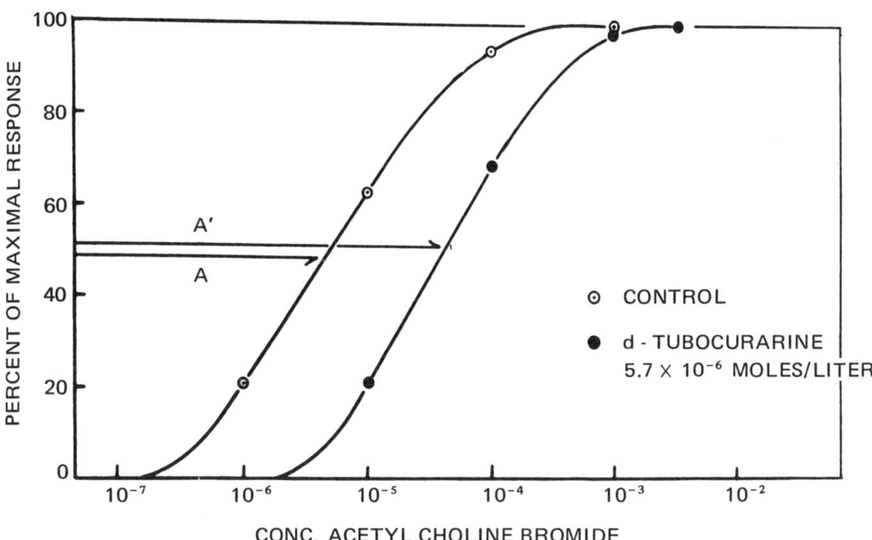

Fig. 7. Dose–response curve for acetylcholine, alone and in the presence of *d*-tubocurarine. A and A′ denote the concentrations of acetylcholine which produce 50% of the maximal contracture. Note that the presence of *d*-tubocurarine has shifted the dose–response curve for acetylcholine to the right. From van Maanen (1950).

B. End-Plate Potential in Curarized Muscle

Failure of neuromuscular transmission occurs in muscles exposed to curare when the motor nerve spike fails to trigger an action potential in the muscle fiber. When contraction ceases, however, the presynaptic action potential may still give rise to a potential change in the end-plate region. This potential is called the "end-plate potential" (e.p.p.). Although the e.p.p. was first described by Göpfert and Schaefer (1938) (see also Eccles and O'Connor, 1939), it had been known since the study of Adrian and Lucas (1912) that a nerve impulse which is partially blocked at the myoneural junction produces a transient excitatory effect in the muscle fiber that may help a second nerve impulse trigger an action potential in that muscle fiber. The time course of this local excitatory disturbance was studied by Katz (1939) in the curarized sciatic–sartorius preparation of the frog, and Eccles *et al.* (1941) thoroughly investigated the e.p.p. in both the curarized frog sartorius and the cat soleus. They showed that the e.p.p. is a local depolarization of the muscle fiber which behaves as a local, subthreshold catelectrotonic potential. Its amplitude decreases as the curare concentration increases; at 20°C the duration of its rising phase was 2.3 msec in the frog sartorius and 0.8 msec in the cat soleus, and the time constants of decay were 11 and 5 msec, respectively.

C. Curare Antagonists

When the amplitude of the e.p.p. elicited by nerve stimulation fails to reach the threshold for electrical stimulation of the muscle fiber (in the frog, a depolarization of about 30–35 mV from the resting potential) the junction becomes blocked. However, if the amplitude of the e.p.p. remains close to the threshold level, contraction will occur in the presence of curare if, by any means, the peak of the e.p.p. is made to cross the threshold level. The so-called curare antagonists help to make the amplitude of the e.p.p. exceed threshold: they exhibit four main mechanisms of action, discussed below.

1. *Increase in the Amount of Transmitter Released*

Calcium ions exert an anticurare effect (Eccles *et al.*, 1941) by increasing the amount of ACh liberated per nerve impulse (del Castillo and Stark, 1952). Guanidine, at a concentration of 10^{-4} to 10^{-3} M, has an effect similar to that of Ca^{2+} ions (Eccles *et al.*, 1941) and seems to increase the amount of ACh released per impulse (Otsuka and Endo, 1960).

2. *Block of the Hydrolysis of ACh*

Anticholinesterase agents such as physostigmine (eserine) and neostigmine inhibit AChE present in the junction, and thereby increase both the duration of action and the effective concentration of ACh released by a nerve impulse. The mechanism of the curare–eserine antagonism was analyzed by Eccles *et al.* (1942). With any concentration of curare, eserine, at a concentration of 10^{-5} (w/v), increased the amplitude and duration of the e.p.p, although the initial rate of rise was practically unaltered. These investigators concluded that the prolonged rising phase and increased amplitude of the e.p.p. showed that eserine had increased the duration of transmitter action about threefold, whereas the unaltered initial rate of rise indicated that there was no appreciable change of the intensity of transmitter action.

An anti-ChE agent that is often used in the clinic to combat muscle paralysis induced by curare is edrophonium bromide (Tensilon), a quaternary ammonium salt. The pharmacological actions and mechanism of action of edrophonium were investigated by Katz and Thesleff (1957*b*) and, more recently, Blaber (1972).

3. *Decrease in the Resting Potential of the Muscle Fiber*

When the muscle fiber membrane at the synaptic region is partially depolarized, the e.p.p. elicited by nerve stimulation will add to the depolarization so that threshold may be reached. This seems to be the main mechanism of the anticurare action of potassium ions following the intraarterial injection of KCl into the curarized cat gastrocnemius (Wilson and Wright, 1936). The same mechanism explains the "anticurare" effect of catelectrotonic potentials in curarized frog muscle fibers. When the nerve is stimulated during a local subthreshold depolarization produced by applied current, transmission is restored, as Katz (1939) demonstrated before the exact nature of the junctional potential changes was known.

4. Interaction with the Curare Molecule

Congo red and related dyes appear to antagonize the action of curare by combining with it chemically; congo red prevents dTC from inhibiting the response to ACh of the isolated rectus abdominis of the frog, but does not prevent erythroidic alkaloids from inhibiting the ACh response (Kensler, 1949). The action of the dye seems to be a direct chemical interaction with dTC, since, under suitable conditions, these two compounds form a precipitate.

Ferry and Marshall (1973) report that hexamethonium produces increased amplitude of e.p.p.'s in curarized rat phrenic nerve–diaphragm preparations. Since hexamethonium has no anti-ChE activity, and neither depolarizes muscle cells nor increases the quantity of transmitter released, Ferry and Marshall conclude that it exerts a "specific anticurare action."

D. Microelectrophoretic Studies

The interaction between dTC and ACh delivered from adjacent barrels of "twin" micropipettes was demonstrated by del Castillo and Katz (1957*a*). Pulses of dTC applied during both slow, steady depolarizations and trains of brief depolarizations produced by applied ACh cause a transient decrease in the amplitude of the ACh potentials. The overall course of dTC action has a relatively fast initial phase and is followed by a longer decay. In agreement with previous reports (Rushton, 1933; Kuffler, 1945; Fatt and Katz, 1951), del Castillo and Katz (1957*a*) confirmed with the electrophoretic method that dTC has no detectable effect on the electrical properties of the muscle membrane. Large dTC pulses have no influence on the electrotonic potentials produced by injection of current into the muscle fiber at spots where ACh or carbachol (CCh) potentials are fully blocked (del Castillo and Katz, 1957*a*).

It had been previously shown (del Castillo and Katz, 1955) that ACh is effective in eliciting a depolarization of the end-plate membrane only if applied to its external surface, and consistent results were obtained with curare (del Castillo and Katz, 1957*a*). Whereas extracellularly applied dTC almost completely blocked the depolarizing effect of ACh and CCh, intracellular injections of much larger amounts of dTC at the same sites failed to influence the size of the ACh and CCh potentials. These results provided further support for the view that ACh and dTC interact with the same or similar receptors attached to the same regions on the external surface of the end-plate membrane.

An interesting difference between ACh and dTC is the time course of their actions. The inhibitory effect of a given amount of dTC declined ($t_{1/2}$) in 1.4 sec, whereas the average $t_{1/2}$ of ACh and CCh potentials was 43 msec. Such a large difference can be attributed neither to differences in diffusion nor to enzymatic hydrolysis of ACh, since the half-decay time of the depolarizing potentials was not changed appreciably when CCh, which is not hydrolyzed by AChE, was used instead of ACh. Two alternative explanations for the slow rate of decay of the dTC inhibition were suggested by del Castillo and Katz (1957*a*). The first and more plausible is that the different rates of decay may be due to different dissociation rates of the drug–receptor complex. The second is the possible existence of a diffusion barrier for curare.

Curare not only antagonizes the action of ACh and its chemical analogues on the end-plate membrane, but also blocks the depolarizing action of electroosmotically applied iodosobenzoate (IB). Sobrino and del Castillo (1972) showed that the steady release of dTC from one of the barrels of a triple micropipette blocks to the same extent the potentials produced by pulses of CCh and IB applied with the other two barrels.

E. Depolarizing Curare-like Agents

Simple polymethylene-bis-quaternary derivatives possess curarizing properties which reach a peak potency when the chain separating the two nitrogen atoms is either 14 or 20 Å long. The 14 Å (C-10) compound is known as decamethonium. Although decamethonium is a "curare-like" agent, since it blocks transmission but affects neither nerve conduction nor twitch tension to direct stimulation, its mechanism of action on the end-plate membrane differs from that of curare. Decamethonium not only decreases the sensitivity of the end-plate membrane to ACh, but also exerts a depolarizing action (Brown *et al*., 1949; Castillo *et al*., 1949; Paton, 1951; Burns and Paton, 1951; Paton and Zaimis, 1952). This property of decamethonium is shared by other synthetic curare-like agents, especially the so-called leptocurares, in which the region between the two onium groups is slender and does not include cyclic groups. It is likely that the interaction of rings with the receptor surface is necessary to stabilize the receptor and prevent its activation. In the absence of cyclic groups, the simultaneous interaction of the two quaternary ammonium groups with receptors gives rise to a prolonged depolarization. As a consequence, these compounds block the myoneural junction both by competing with ACh and by causing densensitization of the receptor site (Thesleff, 1955, 1956). Bovet *et al.* (1951) examined the effects of lepto- and pachycurares on various preparations: On the frog rectus abdominis muscle, leptocurares (succinylcholine and decamethonium) elicited a contracture similar to that caused by ACh and nicotine, whereas dTC and Flaxedil produced a block without depolarization. On avian muscle, succinylcholine and decamethonium exerted purely nicotinic excitatory effects. In mammalian muscle, succinylcholine and decamethonium exerted a persistent depolarizing action which was antagonized by the pachycurares dTC and Flaxedil. Bovet *et al.* (1951) emphasize that the type of curarizing action depends not on the aliphatic or aromatic character of the molecule or on the presence or absence of methyl groups, but on the entire shape of the molecule.

del Castillo and Katz (1957*b*) found that decamethonium exerts at least three different types of actions at the frog neuromuscular junction. If a pulse of decamethonium is applied to the receptor surface just before a pulse of ACh, it depresses the initial part of the ACh potential, indicating a competitive action for the receptor sites; it potentiates the latter part of the ACh potential, an effect that can be attributed to an anti-AChE action since it is absent in preparations exposed to neostigmine; and when applied alone, it causes a small but prolonged depolarization.

F. Effects of Curare on Chronically Denervated Muscle

Curare increases the threshold for the depolarizing action of ACh on cholinergic receptors that proliferate and spread over the surface of muscle fibers during chronic denervation. However, denervated mammalian muscle responds to curare with an increase instead of a block of spontaneous electrical activity. This appears to be due to a depolarizing effect of curare outside the end-plate membrane (McIntyre *et al.*, 1945; McIntyre, 1947; Jarcho *et al.*, 1951; Bowman and Raper, 1965). β-Erythroidine also depolarizes chronically denervated muscle (Bowman and Raper, 1965).

Using iontophoretic application of ACh both to the end-plate and to regions of membrane distant from the end plate in muscle fibers of the rat diaphragm, Beránek and Vyskočil (1967) showed that sensitivity to ACh spreads from the end-plate region 15–25 days following denervation.

However, ACh receptors away from the end-plate were much less sensitive to the effects of applied dTC than were those at the end-plate. Bernánek and Vyskočil (1967) say that these results could suggest that the ACh receptors away from the end-plate are different from those at the end-plate.

Waser (1967) measured the changes in curare-binding sites of denervated mouse diaphragm using labeled curare. Soon after the phrenic nerve was cut, there was a 60–70% increase in the radioactivity within the end-plate region but not elsewhere which gradually diminished to the normal value after 40–60 days. The active centers of the esterase seemed to behave in the same way. However, in similar experiments, ^{14}C-labeled decamethonium spread over the surface of the muscle fiber. One would conclude from Waser's results that after denervation there is a dissociation between the ACh receptors on the one hand and the binding sites for curare and active centers for AChE on the other.

G. Other Effects of Curare on Skeletal Muscle

dTC has been shown to block the responses of intrafusal muscle fibers to stimulation of γ-fibers, and the therapeutic lissive effect attributed to curare may result from diminished spinal reflexes that govern muscle tonus (see Kuffler *et al.*, 1947; Hunt and Kuffler, 1950; Hunt, 1952; Hammond *et al.*, 1956).

H. Different Actions of dTC and Toxiferines on Skeletal Muscle

Paton and Perry (1951) compared the actions of toxiferines with those of dTC on skeletal muscle and found that, in general, they were similar. Therefore, all that we have discussed so far with regard to dTC can be inferred to apply to the toxiferines (see also van Maanen, 1950). Some minor differences were noticed, however (Paton and Perry, 1951): A muscle blocked with toxiferine often responds to tetanic stimulation with a sustained contraction. This is in marked contrast to the rapid decay in the amplitude of the e.p.p.'s seen in muscles blocked by dTC (Wedenski inhibition). The post-tetanic potentiation in muscles blocked by toxiferine is usually greater than in those blocked by dTC. In toxiferine-blocked muscles, neostigmine not only reverses the block but also potentiates the normal twitch tension. In addition, toxiferines have a negligible muscarinic action accompanied by a small atropinic action. In skeletal muscle, toxiferine is about 15 times as potent as dTC, but in ganglia it is less than four times as potent as dTC.

VII. EFFECTS OF CURARE ON OTHER POSTSYNAPTIC RECEPTORS

A. Autonomic Ganglion Cells

Although curare has more affinity for neuromuscular receptors than for autonomic ganglionic receptors, it does block ganglionic transmission (Langley, 1918). A transient phase of stimulation may precede paralysis. In this sense, curare resembles nicotine and differs from hexamethonium, which is exclusively a depressant. Curare prevents neither synthesis of ACh in the ganglia nor its release by preganglionic nerve impulses, but it blocks the depolarizing effect of ACh on ganglionic cells (Paton and Perry, 1953). After blockade, the cells do not respond to ACh, although they still discharge in response to high concentrations of K^+ ions. In autonomic ganglia, in contrast to skeletal muscle, dTC is more potent than dimethyl-dTC. Neostigmine and edrophonium can overcome to some extent the effect of curare on ganglion cells.

Different ganglia exhibit different sensitivities to curare. The ciliary and vagal ganglia are more sensitive than the ganglia that supply sympathetic fibers to the pupil, nictitating membrane, heart, and splanchnic blood vessels (Guyton and Reeder, 1950).

B. Electroplates

The electric organs of *Malapterurus, Torpedo,* and *Electrophorus* are blocked by curarization (Du Bois-Reymond, 1881; Albe-Fessard and Chagas, 1951; Chagas *et al.*, 1953; Chagas and Albe-Fessard, 1954). Chagas found in *Electrophorus* that the kinetics of the combination of curare with the receptors of muscle tissue and electric organ are different. Whereas a strong dose of curare induced muscle paralysis lasting up to 8 hr, the inhibition of the electric organ in the same eel continued up to 48 hr. Another effect of curare on the electric organ cells was to convert the all-or-nothing action potential into graded responses. Curare has also been reported to block spike production in these cells, but at doses much higher than those necessary to block neuroelectroplate transmission (Altamirano *et al.*, 1955).

C. Invertebrate Nerve and Muscle Cells

For references on the effects of curare on invertebrate nerve and muscle cells, the reader is referred to the recent and comprehensive review by Gerschenfeld (1973). Table I, which is based largely on that review, provides a summary of the effects of dTC and related drugs on cholinergic receptors of invertebrate organisms.

VIII. EFFECTS OF CURARE ON CHOLINERGIC RECEPTORS OF NERVE MEMBRANE

Armett and Ritchie (1960, 1961), using the sucrose gap technique, observed in the desheathed rabbit vagus and the cat hypogastric nerve that 1.7 mM ACh produces a rapid depolarization of about 3 mV, a reduction in the amplitude of the action potential to about 60% of its normal value, and a slowing in the speed of conduction. The receptors involved in these effects are nicotinic, since equimolar concentrations of nicotine, carbachol, and tetramethylammonium produce the same effects. Activation of these receptors seems to increase the resting permeability of the axonal membrane to Na^+ ions. Similar effects have been described by Dettbarn and Davis (1962, 1963) in crustacean nonmedullated nerve fibers.

The fact that the axonal membrane has cholinergic receptors similar to those present in postsynaptic membranes has been interpreted as support for the view that ionic permeability changes responsible for the action potential are due to release of ACh and its subsequent interaction with cholinergic receptors (see Nachmansohn, 1969). The effects of curare on impulse conduction are therefore important from the viewpoint of this hypothesis. Armett and Ritchie (1961) showed that low concentrations of dTC block the depolarizing action of ACh on C-fibers, and higher concentrations block the action potential altogether (Ritchie and Armett, 1963). However, the blocking effect of dTC on impulse conduction is not related to ACh antagonism. It seems to be the result of depolarization of the nerve membrane produced by dTC (30 mM of dTC causes a depolarization of about 10 mV in 20 min). Further, hexamethonium, which blocks the depolarizing action of ACh on nerve, does not affect the action potential even at concentrations as high as 50 mM. These observations oppose the view that cholinergic receptors in nerve are involved in impulse conduction.

Dettbarn and Davis (1963) observed that dTC depolarizes crustacean nerve fibers, but not sufficiently to block impulse conduction, when the nerve is immersed in normal seawater. After the calcium concentration was lowered by one tenth and magnesium removed entirely, dTC blocked conduction. The significance of this finding is questionable, however, since conduction is already impaired in this medium before dTC is added.

In contrast to nonmedullated fibers, medullated nerve fibers are generally insensitive to both ACh and curare. When applied to the whole

Table I. Cholinergic Transmission in Invertebrates

Animal	Effect of drug	Reference
1. Nematoda		
Ascaris	dTC blocks excitatory effects of ACh in myogenic somatic musculature	del Castillo *et al.* (1967)
2. Annelida		
Hirudo	Mechanism of neural excitation is very likely cholinergic	Gaskell (1914), Pantin (1935)
	dTC paralyzes voluntary muscle system	Gaskell (1914)
	dTC blocks effects of applied ACh	Bacq and Copée (1937), Flacke and Yeoh (1968)
Pheretima	dTC blocks e.p.s.p.'s in muscle	Ito *et al.* (1969)
Brachioma vesiculosum (Montagu)	dTC does not block contractions induced by ACh	Nicol (1952)
Sabellastarte	dTC does not block but seems to increase contractions induced by ACh	Alvarez *et al.* (1969)
3. Crustacea		
Homarus	dTC and atropine partially block e.p.s.p.'s at synapses between sensory fibers and central neurons	Barker *et al.* (1972)
Procambarus	dTC blocks excitatory postsynaptic activity of tonic postural flexor muscles	Futamachi (1972)
Procambarus and *Atya*	dTC does not block excitatory postsynaptic activity	Evoy and del Castillo (unpublished)
Various crayfish	dTC and dihydro-β-erythroidine block the neuromuscular system, but are not antagonized by neostigmine	Wright (1949)
	Stretch receptor organs contain AChE and may be cholinergic	Maynard and Maynard (1960)
	Stretch receptor organs are excited by both muscarinic and nicotinic cholinergic agonists; such effects are blocked by atropine, hexamethonium, and β-erythroidine	McLennan and York (1966)
4. Insecta		
Periplaneta	dTC and gallamine block e.p.s.p.'s in neurons, and gallamine reversibly blocks responses elicited by applied ACh	Callec and Boistel (1967), Pitman and Kerkut (1970)
	At concentrations as high as 10^{-2} M, dTC has a complete lack of action in ganglia	Roeder (1948)
	dTC has a synaptic blocking effect in ganglia	Kerkut *et al.* (1969), Shankland *et al.* (1971), Suga and Katsuki (1961)

Table I.—Continued

Animal	Effect of drug	Reference
Various insects	ACh does not participate in neuromuscular transmission	Colhoun (1963)
	dTC injected intraabdominally produces flaccid paralysis and blockade of synaptic activity in leg muscles[a]	Larsen *et al.* (1966), McCann (1966), McCann and Reece (1967)
5. Mollusca	Central ganglia of *Aplysia* and brain of *Octopus* contain high concentrations of ACh	Bacq (1935, 1947), Bacq and Copée (1937)
Aplysia and *Helix*	Low concentrations of perfused ACh cause excitatory depolarizations in some neurons (D-response mediated by D-receptors) and two types of inhibitory hyperpolarizations [H-responses mediated by H-receptors; one type (fast) due to increased conductance to Cl^- ions; the other (slow) due to conductance of K^+ ions]	Tauc and Gerschenfeld (1961, 1962), see also Tauc (1967), Gerschenfeld (1970)
	Iontophoretic application of ACh produces responses similar to those obtained by perfusion	Kandel *et al.* (1967), Kehoe (1967, 1972), Tauc and Gerschenfeld (1961)
	dTC and atropine block D-receptors and fast H-receptors; hexamethonium blocks D-receptors but not fast H-receptors	Kehoe (1972), Tauc and Gerschenfeld (1961, 1962)
Aplysia	Slow H-receptors are not affected by dTC, atropine, or hexamethonium but are selectively blocked by TEA and methylxylocholine	Kehoe (1969, 1972)
Aplysia and *Helix*	Depolarizations elicited by dopamine are blocked by dTC and strychnine	Ascher (1968, 1972)
	dTC blocks both A (depolarizing response) and C (inhibitory response) types of serotonin receptors	Gerschenfeld (1971), Gerschenfeld and Paupardin, cited by Gerschenfeld (1973)
Mytilus	ACh-elicited depolarizations and contractions of anterior byssus retractor muscle are blocked by dTC	Hidaka and Twarog, cited by Gerschenfeld (1973)
Venus	dTC slightly potentiates the responses of muscarinic receptors at concentrations of 10^{-5} to 10^{-6} M; blocking action occurs at 10^{-3} M and higher; decamethonium is also a poor ACh antagonist; mytolon[b] (Win 2747) at 10^{-6} M completely blocks a dose of ACh that would by itself produce an inhibition of cardiac activity of from 20 to 80%	Welsh and Taub (1953)

(*Footnotes on p. 133*)

sciatic nerve, dTC does not affect electrical excitability. This has been attributed by Dettbarn (1967) to the low solubility of dTC in lipids. The same author, however, reported a reversible block of conduction by dTC applied to single nodes of Ranvier, where the conducting membrane is less protected (Dettbarn, 1960). Hubbard *et al.* (1965) also concluded that both ACh and dTC depolarize the membrane of the nodes of Ranvier adjacent to nerve terminals. This is discussed further in the next section.

IX. EFFECTS OF CURARE ON CHOLINERGIC SENSITIVITY OF MOTOR AXON TERMINALS

After intravenous injection of eserine to cats, Masland and Wigton (1940) observed repetitive discharges in motor nerve fibers. These discharges did not originate in the motoneurons. They apparently originated in motor nerve terminals, were conducted antidromically, and were associated with twitching and fasciculations of muscle. Similar observations were reported by Feng and Li (1941) following the direct application of anticholinesterase agents to muscle. These observations were confirmed by Eccles *et al.* (1942); they established, however, that some nerve discharges were independent from and occurred prior to muscle action potentials.

Langley and Kato (1915) observed that the twitching and fasciculations produced by eserine were abolished by curare in doses much lower than those needed to block neuromuscular transmission. Masland and Wigton (1940) showed that dTC at low doses blocked antidromic nerve discharges in eserinized preparations, and they concluded that cholinergic receptors are present not only in postsynaptic membranes but also in motor nerve endings; these receptors would be depolarized and electrically excited by ACh accumulated in the presence of a cholinesterase inhibitor. The depolarization of nerve endings following application of ACh was confirmed by Werner (1961). However, none of these experiments fully excluded the possibility that ACh might depolarize nerve filaments indirectly as a consequence of the release of K^+ ions from the muscle fiber during de-

---

[a] It has been suggested that this effect is due to the direct action of curare on conduction of impulses in the motor nerves (Faeder *et al.*, 1970; Friedman and Carlson, 1970).

[b] Such a marked contrast between dTC and mytolon can probably be explained by the important role that the carbonyl group of ACh plays in the interaction between the transmitter and the receptor. Both dTC and decamethonium lack carbonyl groups, and their interactions are thus limited to the coulombic forces at each end of their molecules; the effectiveness of mytolon is, however, likely to be due to the two carbonyl groups in its molecules. (Other compounds that have carbonyl groups, such as barbiturates, also block the effects of ACh on the *Venus* heart.)

polarization of the end-plate membrane. For this reason, the effects of ACh and dTC on the nerve terminals of diaphragm were reinvestigated by Hubbard *et al.* (1965), who confirmed the presence of presynaptic ACh receptors. ACh and dTC both reduced the quantal content of the e.p.p.'s and decreased the threshold for the direct electrical stimulation of nerve terminals. In preparations blocked by high Mg^{2+}, dTC was also found to lower the threshold. These observations indicate that both ACh and dTC depolarize the nerve membrane. However, since the application of ACh or dTC had no effect on the frequency of release of miniature end-plate potentials (m.e.p.p.'s), a process which is very sensitive to membrane potential changes, Hubbard *et al.* (1965) concluded that the membrane that is depolarized by both ACh and dTC cannot be that surrounding motor terminals. They suggested that depolarization occurs at adjacent nodes of Ranvier. In their opinion, these nodes, instead of the terminals themselves, are the sites of the initiation of the antidromic spikes recorded from preparations treated with eserine or neostigmine.

If there are ACh receptors in the membrane of motor terminals, the consequences would be very interesting. First, there would be the possibility of a feedback process following transmitter release. Second, the properties of the presynaptic terminals might be influenced by drugs acting on such receptors. The first possibility led Koelle (1962) to the hypothesis that in all synapses, both cholinergic and noncholinergic, the arrival of a nerve impulse would release a small number of ACh quanta; the released ACh would act on the presynaptic membrane to trigger or increase the liberation of additional transmitter.

X. EFFECTS OF CURARE ON ACH RELEASE

Certain investigators have asserted that the proposed presynaptic action of dTC is more important in producing neuromuscular blockade than its postsynaptic action. Standaert (1964) noted that post-tetanic repetitive activity, which is a purely neural phenomenon, was abolished by dTC. This occurred at a concentration of dTC which had no appreciable effect on isometric twitch tension of the indirectly stimulated muscle. These observations led Standaert to conclude that the principal site of action of dTC at the neuromuscular junction is presynaptic. Riker and his collaborators (see Riker and Okamoto, 1969, for references) cite experiments showing that the intraarterial injection of ACh in the cat excites motor nerve terminals and causes them to fire antidromically, and they propose that this evidence strongly implies that the competition between ACh and curare is not a postsynaptic event, but is instead presynaptic.

Galindo (1971, 1972) also proposes that the main action of curare used in surgical applications is to cause prejunctional failure. In the phrenic nerve–hemidiaphragm preparation of the rat, Galindo (1971) reported that dTC added to the bath at a concentration of 1×10^{-8} g/ml reduced the frequency of m.e.p.p.'s by about 44% without appreciably altering their size, and that the sensitivity of the postsynaptic membrane to applied ACh was reduced only in the presence of concentrations of dTC greater than 10^{-6} g/ml. In contrast to these results, other investigators have found in the same preparation that dTC has no effect on the release of m.e.p.p.'s (Hubbard *et al.*, 1965) and that postsynaptic effects are observed at lower concentrations of dTC than presynaptic effects (Hubbard and Wilson, 1973).

Other workers have noted that dTC has a synaptic action in addition to its postsynaptic action. Gergis *et al.* (1971), using a bioassay technique, observed that dTC (0.1–1.0 μg/ml) reduces the amount of ACh released from the motor nerve terminals in the frog gastrocnemius nerve–muscle preparation, in addition to decreasing the indirectly evoked twitch contractions of the muscle. Auerbach and Betz (1971), however, using similar concentrations of dTC (0.5–0.9 μg/ml) on the frog sartorius, reached opposite conclusions. They found that the amplitudes of spontaneous m.e.p.p.'s and end-plate currrents (measured under voltage clamp conditions) were reduced to the same extent. They interpreted these results to mean that dTC did not change the number of transmitter quanta released, and they concluded that dTC had no presynaptic effects at these concentrations. With higher concentrations of dTC, Auerbach and Betz (1971) observed some increase in the coefficient of variation of the end-plate currents, which could imply a presynaptic effect of the drug.

Lilleheil and Naess (1961) used the isolated phrenic nerve diaphragm preparation of the rat to study the effects of tetanic stimulation during various stages of curarization. They noted that the work of Dale *et al.* (1936) showed that dTC competes with ACh for the postsynaptic receptor at frequencies of stimulation ranging from 5 to 15 stimuli/sec, but that Dale *et al.* had not investigated the effects of higher frequencies of stimulation. Lilleheil and Naess were interested in determining the mechanism of the so-called Wedensky inhibition (Wedensky, 1903), a rapid depression of muscular contractions that occurs during high frequencies of stimulation and is particularly pronounced in curarized preparations. They showed that during prolonged stimulation of curarized preparations, several minutes after the disappearance of the contraction, the e.p.p. declines in amplitude and finally disappears. This process is reversible, and the e.p.p. reappears when dTC is washed out. Since Hutter (1952) showed that the sensitivity of the end-plate to ACh does not change during Wedensky inhibition, Lilleheil and Naess (1961) concluded that the decrease in amplitude of the e.p.p. was a result of presynaptic changes produced by the dTC. They suggested that the dTC reinforces the tendency of tetanic impulses to block propagation in the terminal arborizations of the nerve fiber.

Hubbard and Wilson (1973), using cut and uncut muscle preparations of the rat diaphragm, recorded e.p.p.'s intracellularly and estimated their quantum content in the presence of dTC. Frequencies of stimulation ranged from 50 to 150 Hz. They found that dTC, at a concentration of 4×10^{-8}, had no effect on quantal content, but a postsynaptic effect was noticeable. At higher concentrations (8×10^{-8} g/ml to 4×10^{-7} g/ml), dTC caused a dose-related decrease in quantal content, which indicates a presynaptic action of the drug.

Beani *et al.* (1964) found that dTC, at 5×10^{-6} g/ml, reduces the release of ACh (assayed against standards on guinea pig ileum) from stimulated phrenic nerve–diaphragm preparations of guinea pig. In these preparations, dTC had no effect on release at rest or during stimulation at 6 Hz, but it had a marked effect at 50 Hz. The inhibition of release is present at 38°C and is more marked at 33 and 28°C.

Blaber (1970), using the isolated tenuissimus muscle of the cat, reported that dTC at a concentration of 5.0×10^{-7} g/ml not only had a postsynaptic blocking effect but also increased the quantum content of the e.p.p.'s. Higher (unspecified) concentrations decreased the presynaptic quantal release.

Beránek and Vyskočil (1967) used the phrenic nerve–diaphragm preparation of the rat, but they found no change in the quantum content of the evoked e.p.p.'s in the presence of dTC at concentrations of $1\text{–}4 \times 10^{-8}$ g/ml. Such concentrations are, according to Hubbard and Wilson (1973), too low to produce a presynaptic effect in this preparation.

Hubbard and Wilson (1973) found, as did Lilleheil and Naess (1961), that the presynaptic and postsynaptic effects of dTC occur with different time courses. Quantal size decreased within 4 min of application of dTC, whereas quantal content began to decline within this time but continued to do so for 10–15 min more.

Hubbard and Wilson (1973) note that many investigators have found that noncurarized muscle preparations *in situ* contract reliably throughout a period of prolonged stimulation at frequencies of 5–15 Hz, whereas *in vitro* curarized muscle preparations show a rapid decline in transmitter release and even failure of transmission at similar frequencies. They suggest that this difference can be explained by the presynaptic action of dTC, and that, since the postsynaptic effect of dTC appears at a lower concentration than the presynaptic effect, consideration of the doses used experimentally is important.

XI. CENTRAL EFFECTS OF CURARE

At the level of the central nervous system (CNS), the pharmacological interactions between ACh, nicotine, and curare are different from those in the periphery. Nicotine, which can cross the blood–brain barrier, behaves as a powerful stimulant of the CNS. ACh, which cannot cross the blood–brain barrier, produces predominantly inhibitory effects when applied directly to the CNS (Dikshit, 1934). Effects similar to those of ACh result from intraventricular injection of anti-AChE agents (Feldberg and Sherwood, 1954). Curare, which cannot pass the blood–brain barrier, exerts excitatory effects resembling those of strychnine and picrotoxin when applied directly to the CNS. An apparent exception to this seems to be the amphibian CNS. Pick and Unna (1945) showed that both dTC and dihydro-β-erythroidine suppressed electrical activity of the frog brain.

When topically applied to the mammalian brain cortex, dTC has from five to ten times the convulsivant potency of strychnine (Banerjee *et al.*, 1970); Bhargava and Meldrum, 1969). Injected in small doses into the brain ventricles of the cat, dTC produces tremor, myoclonic contractions, and calling. Larger doses cause general convulsions which are associated with a variety of autonomic effects (for a detailed discussion, see Feldberg, 1963). As Wright (1955) first showed, intraventricular injection of dTC gives rise to EEG alterations typical of epilepsy. The profound changes in electrical activity of the brain induced by dTC are not restricted to the cerebral cortex, but extend to the hippocampus, amygdala, cerebellar cortex, and thalamus as well. The electrical changes are more pronounced ipsilateral to the injection, suggesting a local action of the drug in areas in the vicinity of the lateral ventricles. The injection of dTC into the cisterna magna is not followed by excitatory effects. This indicates that dTC acts on deep structures.

The excitatory effects of dTC on the central nervous system appear to be related to a direct and specific stimulating action on nerve cells. Cholinergic blockade is unlikely, since other curarizing agents such as gallamine, decamethonium, and dihydro-β-erythroidine do not have convulsant effects. Moreoever, it has been shown by Krnjević and Phillis (1963) and Anderson and Curtis (1964) that cells in the cerebral cortex and the thalamus are excited by dTC applied electrophoretically. Hill *et al.* (1972) studied the effects of iontophoretic application of dTC on cortical inhibition and on the actions of applied γ-aminobutyric acid (GABA), other amino acids, and drugs delivered from multiple-barrel pipettes. They showed that dTC consistently antagonized the depressant effects of GABA, and they suggest that the convulsant action of dTC is due, at least in part, to an antagonism of the inhibitory influence of endogenous GABA.

dTC given intravenously is ineffective in blocking cholinergic transmission from motor axon collaterals to Renshaw cells in the ventral horn of the spinal cord. However, dihydro-β-erythroidine, in doses as low as 0.1 mg/kg, has a powerful depressant action on Renshaw cells. Gallamine and dimethyl-dTC are as ineffective as dTC, even at large doses, and atropine is only slightly effective (Eccles *et al.*, 1954, 1956).

β-Erythroidine and the related compound dihydro-β-erythroidine are known to exert a gradual and complete relaxing action on the enhanced muscle tonus of the decerebrate cat preparation. However, this lissive action cannot be attributed to a peripheral neuromuscular block, since after rigidity has disappeared the tendon reflexes are present and apparently normal (Smith, 1947). This effect was further investigated by Smith *et al.* (1949), who concluded that the decreased muscle tonus is due to blockade of interneurons of the spinal cord. In this sense, these curare-like alkaloids act in a manner similar to that of centrally acting muscle relaxant agents such as mephenesin (see del Castillo-Nicolau, 1948).

Sauvage *et al.* (1949) confirmed the selective depressive effect of *Erythrina* alkaloids on spinal interneurons and showed that apo-β-erythroidine produces in the cat, at a dose of 150 mg/kg, a flaccid paralysis with loss of postural tonus. This compound, however, lacks any peripheral curarizing actions.

XII. INTERACTION OF CURARE WITH CHOLINERGIC RECEPTORS

A. Sites and Modes of Action of Curare

The question of whether the sites that bind curare to cholinoceptive membranes are identical to ACh receptors has been raised several times in the literature. Shanes (1958) has interpreted the action of curare as being a nonspecific stabilizing influence, probably of a physical nature, on the surface membrane of the cell. As he pointed out, the idea of such a general, nonspecific antagonism is not inconsistent with quantitative formulations based on the assumption of competitive inhibition as applied to final effector response. The idea that curare and ACh may act on different membrane sites was supported by the autoradiographic observations of Waser (1970). The results of Miledi and Potter (1971), Lester (1972), and Porter *et al.* (1973) also suggested a duality of receptor sites. All the ACh receptor sites would irreversibly bind α-bungarotoxin, but only some of them would reversibly bind curare and thereby be protected against α-bungarotoxin.

The excitatory actions of curare must also be considered. Curare is not exclusively a depressant drug, but instead exerts excitatory and/or depolarizing effects at a number of sites: in the central nervous system, on nonmedullated nerve fibers, possibly at some nodes of Ranvier of medullated fibers, and on chronically denervated mammalian muscle.

B. Minimal Requirements for Curarizing Action

To compete with ACh for the active surface of the receptor and antagonize its activating effect, a molecule should have sufficiently high affinity for any or all of the interaction subsites discussed in Section V. The simplest molecules that act in such a manner are TMA and tetraethylammonium (TEA), which can interact only with the anionic site of the receptor. Crum-Brown and Fraser (1868, 1869) observed that compounds with this general structure exerted a curare-like action on skeletal muscle. Some of these substances also have a muscarinic effect, since they can slow the heart.

The receptor-activating action of TMA can be accounted for by its interaction with the anionic site. When the methyl groups are replaced with ethyl groups, the density of charge of the molecule will decrease and its diameter will increase. Such a combination could explain the curarizing activity of TEA, which would be attracted to the negative site of the receptor without fitting into it well enough to cause activation. Although this explanation appears plausible, TEA could also prevent activation by combining with other anionic sites of the receptor molecule that are not normally involved in the activation process. This might prevent activation by allosteric inhibition.

Perhaps the simplest curarizing alkaloids are those derived from *Erythrina* plants. It is likely that the tertiary nitrogen has an affinity for the anionic site of the ACh receptor and that the ring system interacts with the receptor molecule forming a stable complex that prevents activation. However, a quaternary nitrogen and a ring system are not by themselves sufficient for curarizing action. The quaternary derivatives of coclaurine, which esterically represent one-half of the dTC molecule, have been shown to have very low curarizing activity.

C. Waser's Model of Curare Action

Waser (1962, 1966, 1970), mainly on the basis of his autoradiographic observations on the mammalian end plate, concludes that the cholinergic receptors are different from the active centers of AChE. Furthermore, they differ in quantity and distribution from the curare-receptive sites of the postsynaptic membrane. Waser thinks that these different binding sites might be uniformly distributed on the membrane, but he prefers his model first proposed in 1962 in which these different receptive sites might be arranged around the membrane pores or channels through which the depolarizing ionic currents flow. Because of the close agreement between the number of receptors and AChE molecules, Waser (1970) assumes a number of 5×10^6 receptor complexes working as units in the postsynaptic membrane of one end plate. The pore permitting the ion flux would be surrounded by two molecules of AChE with four active centers. ACh or decamethonium would interact with the many cholinergic receptor molecules located near the cholinesterase, perhaps in close association with its protein outside the active center. An allosteric action would change the structure of the membrane and open the pores. The open pores would be blocked by the large curare molecules, whose cationic nitrogens would react with the anionic center sites of the receptor or the AChE.

D. Bis-quaternary Compounds and the C-10 and C-16 Patterns

The possibilities of interaction between the receptor surface and the curarizing molecules increase in the case of bis-quaternary compounds, since these can combine simultaneously with two anionic sites of the same or adjacent receptors. Such double binding seems very likely since the distance between the two cationic nitrogens is one of the critical features of curare-like molecules. Moreover, this suggests that the anionic groups in the receptor surface are not distributed at random, but instead form patterns or arrays with preferred average distances between them.

The anionic sites of cholinergic receptors of the motor end plate appear to form an array in which two distances equivalent to the length of ten (C-10) and sixteen (C-16) carbon atom chains predominate, i.e., of about 14 and 20 Å. The existence of the C-10 pattern was established by the pioneer work of Barlow and Ing (1948*a,b*) and Paton and Zaimis (1949) on the neuromuscular blocking action of the polymethylene-bis-quaternary series. If the relative pharmacological potency of the different compounds is plotted against the number of atoms in the interquaternary polymethylene chain, peak activity is shown by deca compound. That such a distance is significant from the viewpoint of structure–activity relationships is supported by the fact that the equivalent distance in the bis-quaternary curare alkaloids is also close to 14 Å. It should be emphasized, however, that curare alkaloids also block ganglionic transmission, although in autonomic ganglia the most active polymethylene-bis-quaternary compounds are those with five or six carbons between the cationic nitrogens (Gill, 1959).

The C-16 pattern was suspected when the biological actions of longer members of several series of cholinergic agonists and antagonists were examined. Bovet *et al.* (1951) studied the stimulating effects of a number of dicholinic esters of dicarboxyl acids on the tonic muscles of frog and chicken. In the presence of neostigmine, used to prevent the fast hydrolysis of these compounds, sebacyldicholine (with a 16-atom chain) was the most potent.

Similar results favoring C-10 and C-16 patterns were found with the bis-carbaminoyl series (Brücke, 1956; Cheymol *et al.*, 1954) and also with the higher members of the polymethylene-bis-quaternary series (Barlow and Zoller, 1964).

E. Distribution of Anionic Sites on the Receptor Surface

The presence of two peaks of activity for the C-10 and C-16 compounds strongly suggests that the cholinergic receptors are arranged in such a way that the average values of the interanionic distances are predominantly 14 and 20 Å.

1. Barlow's Model

Barlow (1964) suggested that the anionic sites of adjacent receptors are located at the angles of rectangles or squares. In the case of the rectangle, one side would measure 14 Å and the other 20 Å. A square could be equally likely, since the ratio of 14 to 20 is also the ratio of the side of a square to its diagonal.

2. Rybolovlev's Model

Rybolovlev (for references, see Khromov-Borisov and Michelson, 1966) suggested that a linear sequence of ACh-binding sites arranged in a "head-to-head and tail-to-tail" fashion could also explain the peak activities of the C-10 and C-16 compounds while taking into account the esterophilic sites of the receptor. The C-10 compounds would bind simultaneously to two anionic groups with no carbonyl-binding sites interposed between them. On the other hand, the C-16 compounds would bridge a distance of 20 Å to interact with two anionic groups, but in this case two carbonyl-binding sites would be interposed between them.

This hypothesis would predict that the activity of thin C-10 compounds should not be greatly influenced by the presence of ester functions at any point on the chain, since these would not come into contact with esterophilic sites. However, the activity of these compounds would be markedly altered by the removal of one of the quaternary groups, since the stability of the drug–receptor complex would be due predominantly to the two simultaneous interactions with the anionic groups at each end of the chain. Conversely, the activity of thin C-16 compounds should be greatly influenced by the presence and the position of ester functions in the chain, but should not depend critically on the presence of both quaternary groups since additional interactions should be expected to occur at the esterophilic sites. All of these predictions appear to be corroborated by experimental data (see Khromov-Borisov and Michelson, 1966, for details).

3. The Khromov-Borisov and Michelson Model

Rybolovlev's model was modified by Khromov-Borisov and Michelson (1966), who suggested a tetrameric arrangement of the cholinergic receptors. According to this scheme, the C-10 compounds would form bridges between adjacent protein molecules, whereas the C-16 compounds would bridge the tetramers diagonally.

In suggesting the tetrameric structure of the receptor, Kromov-Borisov and Michelson (1966) took into consideration the properties of self-regulating proteins, such as enzymes and hemoglobin, which are arranged in oligomeric structures. Moreover, they suggested that allosteric interactions between adjacent protein molecules might play a significant role in the interaction of ACh with the tetrameric receptor. The polymeric arrangement of receptor macromolecules is strongly supported by Changeux *et al.* (1967), who believe that the receptors can be organized not only in oligomeric structures but even in infinite lattices.

F. Bis-atropinic Character of the Curare Molecule

Kimura *et al.* (1948) were intrigued by the similarity between each of the two halves of the dTC molecule and the structure of muscarinic drugs. Each cationic end of the dTC molecule, they point out, resembles atropine in both the "umbrella structure" and the spatial arrangements of the three oxygens with regard to the nitrogen. These authors synthesized new molecules by joining two quaternary atropine molecules through an amyl chain, and these new compounds proved to have a powerful curarizing action. Also, a bis-Benadryl derivative proved to have a marked curarizing action. The synthesis of this molecule was suggested by the atropine-like properties of Benadryl (or diphenhydramine), an antihistaminic compound.

Kimura *et al.* (1948) suggest a hypothesis to account for fact that atropine by itself has no demonstrable blocking action. Since they see no reason why an atropine molecule could not interact with a nicotinic receptor and antagonize ACh, they propose that the attachment of an atropine molecule to a receptor, through interactions with the three oxygen prosthetic groups, would prevent by an allosteric mechanism the interaction of other atropine molecules on neighboring receptors. As a consequence, the potential blocking actions of atropine on nicotinic receptors would be autoinhibitory. It is interesting to note in this regard that for muscarinic receptors there are indications that small amounts of atropine will not block but instead sensitize the receptor to ACh (Hazard *et al.*, 1959).

G. Curare Action as a Function of Receptor Density

The notion that ACh receptors may form aggregates of various degrees of complexity can help one to understand some puzzling aspects of curare action. We have already described how ACh-sensitivity of the end-plate membrane decreases sharply as the tip of the exploring ACh-micropipette moves away from the synaptic groove. The simplest way to explain this observation is to assume that receptor density is not uniform. Only in the synaptic groove is the density high enough to allow most receptors to be organized in oligomeric or polymeric structures.

Taking the Khromov-Borisov and Michelson model as an example of an oligomeric structure, one can visualize the dTC–receptor interaction as the formation of a complex involving at least one drug molecule and two receptor molecules. The dTC molecule, attracted to the receptor surface by the ionic forces between the nitrogens and the anionic sites (which would serve as "anchoring sites"; Gill and Ing, 1958), and oriented by the same forces, would form a bridge between two adjacent receptor molecules. As the distance between the drug and the receptor protein decreased, multiple interactions involving short-range forces would take place between the macromolecules and the ring system of the curare molecule. As a result, a stable complex would be formed by what Burgen (1970) has called the "chelate effect," which would not only prevent ACh from reaching the receptor but would also hinder its activation.

Cavallito (1962, 1967) has emphasized that, in addition to coulombic-bonding properties represented by the charge and size of the onium groups of the curare molecules, steric factors and the hydrophilic–lipophilic balance of the molecule are important for the formation of a complex.

Steric factors determine not only the closeness of the approach between drug and receptor, and as a consequence the intervention of close-range secondary binding forces, but also the very nature and type of these forces. The hydrophilic–lipophilic balance of the molecule will determine the bonding between the bulky part of the curariform molecule and the receptor protein. In the case of the thin curare molecules, such as decamethonium and succinylcholine, the interaction between the polymethylene or ester chain and the macromolecules will influence the kinetics of the drug–receptor interaction, but will not be strong enough to fully stabilize the receptors. The receptors will thus be activated by the coulombic interactions taking place at each end of the chain where the trimethylammonium groups fit into the anionic cavities.

For the ganglionic blocking agents, Gill (1959) distinguishes between two types of bis-quaternary compounds: (1) those in which the blocking activity depends on the length of the carbon chain separating the two cationic nitrogens and (2) those in which blocking activity is independent of the length of the chain. The cationic groups of the first type of blocking compounds fit closely into the anionic cavities of the receptors, separated by a distance of 6–7.8 Å, and lock the receptor protein in its resting configuration. This will prevent the reversible rearrangement of the protein which would lead to the permeability change. The compounds of the second type are not able to approach the receptor sufficiently to induce or prevent the molecular rearrangement for activation, but they hinder the approach of ACh. As a result, they compete with ACh without actually locking the receptor structure in its resting configuration.

If the density of the receptor molecules is low, the probability of oligomeric arrangements will be decreased. Most of the receptor molecules will be separated by distances greater than 14 or 20 Å. As a consequence, the curare molecules will react with the receptors in a one-to-one fashion. This will lead to weaker and more easily reversible drug–receptor complexes. We have already mentioned that molecules which are equivalent to one-half of the dTC molecule have only a weak curarizing action.

Waser's (1970) autoradiographic observations could be explained on the basis of these arguments. Only at the end-plate region, where receptor density is highest, will the curarine- or toxiferine–receptor complex be stable enough for the labeled drugs to expose the photographic emulsion. In the extrajunctional areas of chronically denervated muscle, the receptor density will be low, most receptor molecules will be isolated, and drug–receptor complexes will be weak and easily reversible. The same argument can be used to explain why only a fraction of the end-plate receptors are protected by dTC against α-bungarotoxin. We may assume that only dTC–receptor complexes involving two receptor macromolecules would be stable enough to prevent the α-bungarotoxin from irreversibly binding the receptor.

H. Curare as a Receptor Activator

Whether a curare-like molecule will act as a blocking nondepolarizing drug (such as dTC), as a depolarizing competitive drug (decamethonium), or as an activating agonist drug (CCh) appears to depend on three factors:

1. Characteristics of the drug molecule (coulombic-bonding properties, steric factors, and hydrophilic–lipophilic character): High charge density and a good fit into the anionic cavity will favor activation; slender and flexible interquaternary structures leading to the formation of weak or flexible complexes will similarly allow some degree of activation.
2. Receptor density: Oligomeric or polymeric arrangements making it possible for a single curare molecule to interact with more than one receptor macromolecule will favor the stability of the drug–receptor complex and prevention of activation.
3. Relationship between the receptor macromolecule and the membrane matrix surrounding it: If a relatively large area of the receptor macromolecule, including its active site, is exposed to an aqueous environment, the formation of an extensive stabilizing complex will be facilitated. If only the active site is exposed, the interaction of one of the onium groups of the curare molecule with the anionic site may lead to activation.

In view of these possibilities, it is not surprising that dTC may act as a receptor activator in certain systems, such as the brain.

Acknowledgments

This work was supported in part by USPHS Grants No. KGN-14938 and N5-07464 to Jose del Castillo. This is contribution No. 52 of the Laboratory of Neurobiology.

XIII. REFERENCES

Adrian, E. D., and Lucas, K., 1912, On the summation of propagated disturbances in nerve and muscle, *J. Physiol.* (*Lond.*) **44**:68.

Alam, M., Anrep, G. V., Barsoum, G. S., Talaat, M., and Wieninger, E., 1939, Liberation of histamine from skeletal muscle by curare, *J. Physiol.* (*Lond.*) **95**:148.

Albe-Fessard, D., and Chagas, C., 1951, Action d'une substance curarisante sur la décharge électrique de l'*Electrophorus electricus* L., *Compt. Rend. Seanc. Soc. Biol.* (*Paris*) **145**:248.

Altamirano, M., Schleyer, W., Coates, C. W., and Nachmansohn, D., 1955, Electrical activity in electric tissue. I. The difference between tertiary and quaternary nitrogen compounds in relation to their chemical and electrical activities, *Biochem. Biophys. Acta* **16**:268.

Alvarez, M. C., del Castilo, J., and Sanchez, V., 1969, Pharmacological responses of the dorsal longitudinal muscle of *Sabellastarte magnifica, Comp. Biochem. Physiol.* **29**:931.

Anderson, P., and Curtis, D. R., 1964, The pharmacology of the synaptic and acetylcholine-induced excitation of ventrobasal thalamic neurones, *Acta Physiol. Scand.* **61**:100.

Arïens, E. J., van Rossum, J. M., and Simonis, A. M., 1956, A theoretical basis of molecular pharmacology, Part I: Interactions of one or two compounds with one receptor system, *Arzneim. Forsch.* **6**:282.

Armett, C. J., and Ritchie, J. M., 1960, The action of acetylcholine on conduction in mammalian non-myelinated fibres and its prevention by an anticholinesterase, *J. Physiol.* (*Lond.*) **152**:141.

Armett, C. J., and Ritchie, J. M., 1961, The action of acetylcholine and some related substances on conduction in mammalian non-myelinated nerve fibres, *J. Physiol.* (*Lond.*) **155**:372.

Ascher, P., 1968, Electrophoretic injections of dopamine on *Aplysia* neurones, *J. Physiol.* (*Lond.*) **198**:48 P.

Ascher, P., 1972, Inhibitory and excitatory effects of dopamine on *Aplysia* neurones, *J. Physiol.* (*Lond.*) **255**:173.

Auerbach, A., and Betz, W., 1971, Does curare effect transmitter release? *J. Physiol.* (*Lond.*) **213**:691.

Axelsson, J., and Thesleff, S., 1959, A study of supersensitivity in denervated mammalian skeletal muscle, *J. Physiol.* (*Lond.*) **147**:178.

Bacq, Z., 1935, Recherches sur la physiologie et la pharmacologie du système nerveux autonome. XVII. Les esters de la choline dans les extraits de tissu des Invertébrés, *Arch. Internat. Physiol.* **42**:24.

Bacq, Z., 1947, L'acétylcholine et l'adrénaline chez les Invertébrés, *Biol. Rev.* **22**:73.

Bacq, Z., and Copée, G., 1937, Réaction des Vers et des Mollusques à l'ésérine: Existence de nerfs cholinergiques chez les Vers, *Arch. Internat. Physiol.* **45**:310.

Bamford, D. G., Biggs, D. F., Chaplen, P., Davis, M., and Maconochie, J., 1972, A novel monoquaternary neuromuscular blocking agent, *Experientia* **28**:1069.

Banerjee, U., Feldberg, W., and Georgiev, V. P., 1970, Microinjections of tubocurarine, leptazol, strychnine and picrotoxin into the cerebral cortex of anaesthetized cats, *Brit. J. Pharmacol.* **40**:6.

Barker, D. L., Herbert, E., Hildebrand, J. G., and Kravitz, E. A., 1972, Acetylcholine and lobster sensory neurones, *J. Physiol.* (*Lond.*) **226**:205.

Barlow, R. B., 1964, *Introduction to Chemical Pharmacology*, Methuen, London.

Barlow, R. B., and Ing, H. R., 1948*a*, Curare-like action of polymethylene bis-quaternary ammonium salts, *Nature* (*Lond.*) **161**:718.

Barlow, R. B., and Ing, H. R., 1948*b*, Curare-like action of polymethylene bis-quaternary ammonium salts, *Brit. J. Pharmacol.* **3**:298.

Barlow, R. B., and Zoller, A., 1964, Some effects of long chain polymethylene bis-onium salts on junctional transmission in the peripheral nervous system, *Brit. J. Pharmacol.* **23**:131.

Barnard, E. A., Wieckowski, J., and Chiu, T. H., 1971, Cholinergic receptor molecules and cholinesterase molecules at mouse skeletal muscle junctions, *Nature* (*Lond.*) **234**:207.

Barneby, R. C., and Krukoff, B. A., 1971, Supplementary notes on American Menispermaceae: VIII. A generic survey of the American Triclisieae and Anomospermeae, *Mem. N.Y. Bot. Gard.* **22**:1.

Beani, L., Bianchi, C., and Ledda, F., 1964, The effect of tubocurarine on acetylcholine release from motor nerve terminals, *J. Physiol.* (*Lond.*) **174**:172.

Beránek, R., and Vyskočil, F., 1967, The action of tubocurarine and atropine on the normal and denervated rat diaphragm, *J. Physiol.* (*Lond.*) **188**:53.

Bernard, C., 1857, *Leçons sur les Effets des Substances Toxiques et Medicamenteuses*, J.-B. Baillière et Fils, Paris.

Bhargava, V. K., and Meldrum, B. S., 1969, The strychnine-like action of curare and related compounds on the somatosensory evoked response of the rat cortex, *Brit. J. Pharmacol.* **37**:112.

Blaber, L. C., 1970, The effect of facilitatory concentrations of decamethonium on the storage and release of transmitter at the neuromuscular junction of the cat, *J. Pharmacol. Exptl. Therap.* **175**:664.

Blaber, L. C., 1972, The mechanism of the facilitatory action of edrophonium in cat skeletal muscle, *Brit. J. Pharmacol.* **46**:498.

Boehm, R., 1920, Curare und Curarealkaloide, in: *Hefter's Handbuch der experimentelle Pharmakologie*, Vol. 2, pp. 179–248, Springer, Berlin.

Bovet, D., 1951, Some aspects of the relationship between chemical constitution and curare-like activity, *Ann. N.Y. Acad. Sci.* **54**:407.

Bovet, D., Courvoiser, S., Ducrot, R., and Horclois, R., 1946, Proprietes curarisantes du di-iodoethylate de bis (quinoleyloxy-8′)-1,5-pentane, *Compt. Rend. Acad. Sci.* (*Paris*) **223**:597.

Bovet, D., Bovet-Nitti, F., Guarino, S., Longo, V. G., and Fusco, R,. 1951, Recherches sur les poisons curarisants du synthèse. III Partie: Succinylcholine et dérivés aliphatiques, *Arch. Int. Pharmacodyn. Therap.* **88**:1.

Bovet, D., Bovet-Nitti, F., Bettschart, S., and Scognamiglio, W., 1956, Mécanisme de la potentialisation par la chlorhydrate de diethylamino-ethyldiphénylpropylacétate des effets de quelques agents curarisants, *Helv. Physiol. Acta* **14**:430.

Bovet, D., Bovett-Nitti, F., and Marini-Bettòlo, G. B., eds., 1959, *Curare and Curare-like Agents*, Elsevier, Amsterdam.

Bovet-Nitti, F., 1959, Les curares à brève durée d'action, in: *Curare and Curare-like Agents* (D. Bovet, F., Bovet-Nitti, and G. B. Marini-Bettòlo, eds.) pp. 230–244, Elsevier, Amsterdam.

Bowman, W. C., and Raper, C., 1965, The effects of sympathomimetic amines on chronically denervated skeletal muscles, *Brit. J. Pharmacol.* **24**:98.

Brieger, L., 1886, *Untersuchüngen über Ptomaine*, Vol. III, A. Hirschwald, Berlin.

Brittain, R. T., and Tyers, M. B., 1972, AH 8165: A new short-acting, competitive neuromuscular blocking drug, *Brit. J. Pharmacol.* **45**:158 P.

Brown, G. L., Paton, W. D. M., and Vianna Dias, M., 1949, The depression of the demarcation potential of cat's tibialis by bistrimethylammonium decane diiodide (C_{10}). *J. Physiol.* (*Long.*) **109**:15P.

Brücke, F., 1956, Dicholinesters of α,ω-dicarboxylic acids and related substances, *Pharmacol. Rev.* **8**:265.

Buckett, W. R., Marjorbanks, C. E., and Morton, M. B., 1968, The pharmacology of pancuronium bromide (Org. NA97), a new potent steroid neuromuscular blocking agent, *Brit. J. Pharmacol.* **32**:671.

Burgen, A. V. S., 1970, The nature of complex formation, in: *Molecular Properties of Drug Receptors*, A Ciba Foundation Symposium (R. Porter and M. O'Connor, eds.) pp. 263–269, J. & A. Churchill, London.

Burn, J., and Dale, H. H., 1915, The action of certain quaternary ammonium bases, *J. Pharmacol. Exptl. Therap.* **6**:417.

Burns, B. D., and Paton, W. D. M., 1951, Depolarization of the motor end-plate by decamethonium and acetylcholine, *J. Physiol.* (*Lond.*) **115**:41.

Callec, J. J., and Boistel, J., 1967, Les effets de l'acétylcholine aux niveaux synaptique et somatique dans le cas du dernier ganglion abdominal de la blatte *Periplaneta americana, Compt. Rend. Seanc. Soc. Biol.* (*Paris*) **161**:442;

Castillo, J. C., and de Beer, E. J., 1950, The neuromuscular blocking action of succinylcholine (diacetylcholine), *J. Pharmacol. Exptl. Therap.* **99**:458.

Castillo, J. C., Phillips, A. P., and De Beer, E. J., 1949, Curariform action of decamethylene-1,10-bis-trimethylammonium bromide, *J. Pharmacol. Exptl. Therap.* **97**:150.

Cavillito, C. J., 1962, Structure–action relations throwing light on the receptor, in: *Curare and Curare-like Agents*, Ciba Foundation Study Group No. 12 (A. V. S. de Reuck, ed.) pp. 55–74, Little, Brown, Boston.

Cavillito, C. J., 1967, Bonding characteristics of acetylcholine simulants and antagonists and cholinergic receptors, *Ann. N.Y. Acad. Sci.* **144**:900.

Chagas, C., 1962, The fate of curare during curarization, in: *Curare and Curare-like Agents*, Ciba Foundation Study Group No. 12 (A. V. S. de Reuck, ed.) pp. 2–20, Little, Brown, Boston.

Chagas, C., and Albe-Fessard, D., 1954, Action de divers curarisants sur l'organe électrique de l'*Electrophorus electricus* (Linnaeus), *Acta Physiol. Latinoam.* **4**:49.

Chagas, C,, Bovet, D., and Sollero, L., 1953, Curarisation musculaire et curarisation electrique chez le poisson *Electrophorus electricus, Compt. Rend. Acad. Sci.* (*Paris*) **236**:1997.

Changeux, J.-P., 1969, Remarks on the symmetry and cooperative properties of biological membranes, in: *Symmetry and Function of Biological Membranes at the Macromolecular Level*, (A. Engström and B. Strandberg, eds.) pp. 235–256, Wiley, New York.

Changeux, J.-P., and Podleski, T. R., 1968, On the excitability and cooperativity of the electroplax membrane. *Proc. Natl. Acad. Sci.* **59**:944.

Changeux, J.-P., Thiéry, J., Tung, Y., and Kittel, C., 1967, On the cooperativity of biological membranes, *Proc. Natl. Acad. Sci.* **57**:335.

Cheymol, J., 1949, Curares naturels et curares de synthese, in: *Actualites Pharmacologiques*, Vol. 1 (R. Hazard, ed.) Masson et Cie, Paris.

Cheymol. J., and Bourillet, F., 1960. Curarizing substances and those modifying curarization, *Actual. Pharmacol.* **13**:63.

Cheymol, J., Delaby, R., Chabrier, P., Najer, H., and Bourillet, F., 1954, Activité acetylcholinomimètique de quelques dèrivés de la carbaminoylcholine, *Arch. Int. Pharmacodyn. Therap.* **98**:161.

Cheymol, J., Bourillet, F., and Lavassort, C., 1955, Action anti-curarimimétique de l'héparine et d'héparinöides de synthèse chez le lapin, *J. Physiol.* (*Paris*) **47**:132.

Colhoun, E. H., 1963, The physiological significance of acetylcholine in insects and observations upon other pharmacologically active substances, *Advan. Insect Physiol.* **1**:1.

Cowan, S. L., 1936, The initiation of all-or-none responses in muscle by acetylcholine, *J. Physiol.* (*Lond.*) **88**:3 P.

Craig, L. E., 1955, Curare-like effects, in: *The Alkaloids: Chemistry and Physiology*, Vol. V (R. H. F. Manske, ed.) Chap. 46, pp. 265–293, Academic Press, New York.

Crum-Brown, A., and Fraser, T. R., 1868, On the connection between chemical constitution and physiological action. Part I. On the physiological action of the salts of ammonium bases derived from strychnia, brucia, thebaia, codeia, morphia, and nicotia, *Trans. Roy. Soc. Edinb.* **25:**151.

Crum-Brown, A., and Fraser, T. R., 1869, On the connection between chemical constitution and physiological action. Part II. On the physiological action of the ammonium bases derived from atropia and conia, *Trans. Roy. Soc. Edinb.* **25:**693.

Dale, H. H., 1914–1915, The action of certain esters and ethers of choline and their relation to muscarone, *J. Pharmacol. Exptl. Therap.* **6:**147.

Dale, H. H., Feldberg, W., and Vogt, M., 1936, Release of acetylcholine at voluntary motor nerve endings, *J. Physiol.* (*Lond.*) **86:**353.

de Beer, E. J., 1959, The chemistry of the muscle relaxants, *Anesthesiology* **20:**416.

del Castillo, J., and Katz, B., 1955, On the localization of acetylcholine receptors, *J. Physiol.* (*Lond.*) **128:**157.

del Castillo, J., and Katz, B., 1957*a*, A study of curare action with an electrical micromethod, *Proc. Roy. Soc. Lond. Ser. B* **146:**339.

del Castillo, J., and Katz, B., 1957*b*, Interaction at end-plate receptors between different choline derivatives, *Proc. Roy. Soc. Lond. Ser. B* **146:**369.

del Castillo, J., and Sobrino, J. A., 1973, Carbonyl binding sites in the cholinergic receptors of the motor-end-plate. *Internat. J. Neurosci.* **6:**67.

del Castillo, J., and Stark, L., 1952, The effect of calcium ions on the motor end-plate potentials, *J. Physiol.* (*Lond.*) **116:**507.

del Castillo, J., de Mello, W. C., and Morales, T., 1967, The initiation of action potentials in the somatic musculature of *Ascaris lumbricoides*, *J. Exptl. Biol.* **46:**263.

del Castillo, J., Escobar, I., and Gijon, E., 1971, Effects of the electrophoretic application of sulfhydryl reagents to the end-plate receptors, *Internat. J. Neurosci.* **1:**199.

del Castillo, J., Bartels, E., and Sobrino, J. A., 1972, Microelectrophoretic application of cholinergic compounds, protein oxidizing agents, and mercurials to the chemically excitable membrane of the electroplax, *Proc. Natl. Acad. Sci.* **69:**2081.

del Castillo-Nicolau, J., 1948, Acciones centrales de la myanesina, *Trab. Inst. Nac. Cien. Med.* **12:**363.

de Reuck, A. V. S., ed., 1962, *Curare and Curare-like Agents,* Ciba Foundation Study Group No. 12, Little, Brown, Boston.

Dettbarn, W. D., 1960, Effect of curare on conduction in myelinated, isolated nerve fibers of the frog, *Nature* (*Lond.*) **186:**891.

Dettbarn, W. D., 1967, The acetylcholine system in peripheral nerve, *Ann. N.Y. Acad. Sci.* **144:**483.

Dettbarn, W. D., and Davis, F. A., 1962, Effect of acetylcholine on the electrical activity of somatic nerves of the lobster, *Science* **136:**716.

Dettbarn, W. D., and Davis, F. A., 1963, Effects of acetylcholine on axonal conduction of lobster nerve, *Biochim. Biophys. Acta* **66:**397.

Dikshit, B. B., 1934, The production of cardiac irregularities by excitation of the hypothalamic centres, *J. Physiol.* (*Lond.*) **81:**382.

Dowdy, E. G., Holland, W. C., Yamanaka, I., and Kaya, K., 1971, Cardioactive properties of *d*-tubocurarine with and without preservatives, *Anesthesiology* **34:**257.

Dretchen, K. L., Sokoll, M. D., Gergis, S. D., and Long, J. P., 1972, Effects of pancuronium on the motor nerve terminal, *Europ. J. Pharmacol.* **20:**46.

Du Bois-Reymond, E., 1881, *Dr. Carl Sachs: Untersuchungen am Zitteraal Gymnotus electricus*, Veit, Leipzig.

Eccles, J. C., and O'Connor, W. J., 1939, Responses which nerve impulses evoke in mammalian striated muscles, *J. Physiol.* (*Lond.*) **97:**44.

Eccles, J. C., Katz, B., and Kuffler, S. W., 1941, Nature of the "end-plate potential" in curarized muscle, *J. Neurophysiol.* **4**:362.

Eccles, J. C., Katz, B., and Kuffler, S. W., 1942, Effect of eserine on neuromuscular transmission, *J. Neurophysiol.* **5**:211.

Eccles, J. C., Fatt, P., and Koketsu, K., 1954, Cholinergic and inhibitory synapses in a pathway from motor–axon collaterals to motoneurones, *J. Physiol.* (*Lond.*) **126**:524.

Eccles, J. C., Eccles, R. M., and Fatt, P., 1956, Pharmacological investigations on a central synapse operated by acetylcholine, *J. Physiol.* (*Lond.*) **131**:154.

Edwards, C., Bunch, W., Marfey, P., Marois, R., and Van Meter, D., 1970, Studies on the chemical properties of the acetylcholine receptor site of the frog neuromuscular junction, *J. Membrane Biol.* **2**:119.

Faeder, I. R., O'Brien, R. D., and Salpeter, M. M., 1970, A re-investigation of evidence for cholinergic neuromuscular transmission in insects, *J. Exptl. Zool.* **173**:187.

Fänge, R., 1962, Pharmacology of poikilothermic vertebrates and invertebrates, *Pharmacol. Rev.* **4**:281.

Fatt, P., and Katz, B., 1951, An analysis of the end-plate potential recorded with an intracellular electrode, *J. Physiol.* (*Lond.*) **115**:320.

Feldberg, W., 1963, *A Pharmacological Approach to the Brain from Its Inner and Outer Surface*, Williams and Wilkins, Baltimore.

Feldberg, W., and Sherwood, S. L., 1954, Behaviour of cats after intraventricular injections of eserine and DFP, *J. Physiol.* (*Lond.*) **125**:488.

Feng, T. P., and Li, T. H., 1941, Studies on the neuromuscular junction, XXIII. A new aspect of the phenomena of eserine potentiation and posttetanic facilitation in mammalian muscles, *Chin. J. Physiol.* **16**:37.

Ferry, C. B., and Marshall, A. R., 1973, An anti-curare effect of hexamethonium at the mammalian neuromuscular junction, *Brit. J. Pharmacol.* **47**:353.

Flacke, W., and Yeoh, T. S., 1968, Differentiation of acetylcholine and succinylcholine receptors in leech muscle, *Brit. J. Pharmacol.* **33**:154.

Friedman, K. J., and Carlson, A. D., 1970, The effects of curare in the cockroach. II. Blockage of nerve impulses by dTC, *J. Exptl. Biol.* **52**:593.

Futamachi, K. J., 1972, Acetylcholine: Possible neuromuscular transmitter in crustacea, *Science* **175**:1373.

Galindo, A., 1971, Prejunctional effect of curare: Its relative importance, *J. Neurophysiol.* **34**:289.

Galindo, A., 1972, Curare and pancuronium compared: Effects on previously undepressed mammalian myoneural junctions, *Science* **178**:753.

Gaskell, J. F., 1914, The chromaffin system of annelids and the relation of this system to the contractile vascular system in the leech, *Hirudo medicinalis, Phil. Trans. Roy. Soc. Lond. Ser. B.* **205**:153.

Gergis, S. D., Dretchen, K. L., Sokoll, M. D., and Long, J. P., 1971, The effect of neuromuscular blocking agents on acetylcholine release, *Proc. Soc. Exptl. Biol. Med.* **138**:693.

Gerschenfeld, H. M., 1970, Acetylcholine transmission at central synapses of Mollusca, a survey, in: *Structure and Function of Synapses* (G. D. Pappas and D. Purpura, eds.) Chap. 9, Raven Press, New York.

Gerschenfeld, H. M., 1971, Serotonin: Two different inhibitory actions on snail neurones, *Science* **171**:1252.

Gerschenfeld, H. M., 1973, Chemical transmission in invertebrate central nervous systems and neuromuscular junctions, *Physiol. Rev.* **53**:1.

Gill, E. W., 1959, Inter-quaternary distance and ganglion-blocking activity in bis-quaternary compounds, *Proc. Roy. Soc. Lond. Ser. B* **150**:381.

Gill, E. W., and Ing, H. R., 1958, The problem of hexamethonium, *Il Farmaco* (*Sci. Ed.*) **13**:244.

Gill, R. C., 1940, *White Water and Black Magic*, Holt, New York.

Ginetsinsky, A. G., and Shamarina, N. M., 1942, The tonomotor phenomenon in denervated muscle (D. S. I. R. Translation RTS 1710), *Advan. Mod. Biol.* (*USSR*) **15**:283.

Glick, D., 1941, Some additional observations on the specificity of cholinesterase, *J. Biol. Chem.* **137**:357.

Goldstein, A., Aronow, L., and Kalman, S. M., 1968, *Principles of Drug Action: The Basis of Pharmacology*, Hoeber Medical Division, Harper and Row, New York.

Göpfert, H., and Schaefer, H., 1938, Ueber den direkt und indirekt erregten Aktionstrom und die Funktion der motorischen Endplatte, *Pflüger's Arch. Ges. Physiol.* **239**:597.

Granier-Doyeux, M., 1951, *Contribution al Estudio Historico, Geografico y Etnografico de los Curares*, Caracas.

Grob, D., Lilienthal, J. L., Jr., and Harvey, A. M., 1947, On certain vascular effects of curare in man: The "histamine" reaction, *Bull. Johns Hopkins Hosp.* **80**:299.

Guyton, A. C., and Reeder, R. C., 1950, Quantitative studies on the autonomic actions of curare, *J. Pharmacol. Exptl. Therap.* **98**:188.

Hammes, G. G., Molinoff, P. B., and Bloom, F. E., eds., 1973, Receptor biophysics and biochemistry, *Neurosci. Res. Prog. Bull.* **11**:159.

Hammond, P. H., Merton, P. A., and Sutton, G. G., 1956, Nervous gradation of muscular contraction, *Brit. Med. Bull.* **12**:214.

Harvey, A. M., 1939, The actions of quinine on skeletal muscle, *J. Physiol.* (*Lond.*) **95**:45.

Harvey, A. M., 1940, The action of quinine methochloride on neuromuscular transmission, *Bull. Johns Hopkins Hosp.* **66**:52.

Hassón, A., and Chagas, C., 1959, Selective capacity of components of the aqueous extract of the electric organ to bind curarizing quaternary ammonium derivatives, *Biochim. Biophys. Acta.* **36**:301.

Hassón, A., and Chagas, C., 1961, Purification of macromolecular components of the aqueous extract of electric organ [*E. electricus* (L.)] with binding capacity *in vitro* for quaternary ammonium bases, in: *Bioelectrogenesis* (C. Chagas and A. Paes de Carvalho, eds.) pp. 362–378, Elsevier, Amsterdam.

Hazard, R., Savini, E., and Renier-Cornec, A., 1959, Augmentation par des doses minimes d'atropine de la sensibilité de l'intestin isolé a l'acétylcholine, *Arch. Int. Pharmacodyn. Therap.* **120**:369.

Hill, R. G., Simmonds, M. A., and Straughan, D. W., 1972, Convulsive properties of *d*-tubocurarine and cortical inhibition, *Nature* (*Lond.*) **240**:51.

Hoppe, J. O., 1950, A pharmacological investigation of 2,5-bis(3-diethylaminopropylamino)benzoquinone-bis-benzyl chloride (Win 2747): A new curarimimetic drug, *J. Pharmacol. Exptl. Therap.* **100**:333.

Hu, J. H., 1972, Nature of postjunctional receptors, *Am. J. Physiol.* **223**:882.

Hubbard, J. I., and Wilson, D. F., 1973, Neuromuscular transmission in a mammalian preparation in the absence of blocking drugs and the effect of *d*-tubocurarine, *J. Physiol.* (*Lond.*) **228**:307.

Hubbard, J. I., Schmidt, R. F., and Yokota, T., 1965, The effect of acetylcholine upon mammalian motor nerve terminals, *J. Physiol.* (*Lond.*) **181**:810.

Hunt, C. C., 1952, Drug effects on mammalian muscle spindles, *Fed. Proc.* **11**:75.

Hunt, C. C., and Kuffler, S. W., 1950, Pharmacology of the neuromuscular junction, *J. Pharmacol. Exptl. Therap.* **98**:96.

Hunt, R., and Taveau, R. de M., 1906, On the physiological action of certain choline derivatives and new methods for detecting choline, *Brit. Med. J.* **2**:1788.

Hutter, O. F., 1952, Post-tetanic restoration of neuromuscular transmission blocked by *d*-tubocurarine, *J. Physiol.* (*Lond.*) **118**:216.

Ito, Y., Kuriyama, H., and Tashiro, N., 1969, Miniature excitatory junction potentials in the somatic muscle of the earthworm, *Pheretima communissima,* in sodium free solution, *J. Exptl. Biol.* **51**:107.

Jarcho, L. W., Berman, B., Eyzaguirre, C., and Lilienthal, J. L., Jr., 1951, Curarization of denervated muscle, *Ann. N.Y. Acad. Sci.* **54**:337.

Jenkinson, D. H., 1960, The antagonism between tubocurarine and substances which depolarize the motor end-plate, *J. Physiol.* (*Lond.*) **152**:309.

Kalow, W., 1959, The distribution, destruction and elimination of muscle relaxants, *Anesthesiology* **20**:505.

Kandel, E. R., Frazier, W. T., Waziri, R., and Coggeshall, R. E., 1967, Direct and common connections among the identified neurones in the abdominal ganglion of *Aplysia, J. Neurophysiol.* **30**:1352.

Karis, J., Gissen, A. J., and Nastuk, W. L., 1966, Mode of action of diethyl-ether in blocking neuromuscular transmission, *Anesthesiology* **27**:42.

Karis, J., Gissen, A. J., and Nastuk, W. L., 1966, Mode of action of deithyl-ether in blocking neuromuscular transmission, *Anesthesiology* **27**:42.

Karlin, A., 1973, Molecular interactions of the acetylcholine receptor, *Fed. Proc.*32:1847.

Karlin, A., and Bartels, E., 1966, Effects of blocking sulfhydryl groups and of reducing disulfide bonds on the acetylcholine-activated permeability system of the electroplax, *Biochim. Biophys. Acta* **126**:525.

Karlin, A., and Winnik, M., 1968, Reduction and specific alkylation of the receptor for acetylcholine, *Proc. Natl. Acad. Sci.* **60**:668.

Kasai, M., and Changeux, J.-P., 1971, *In vitro* excitation of purified membrane fragments by cholinergic agonists. III. Comparison of the dose–response curves to decamethonium with the corresponding binding curves of decamethonium to the cholinergic receptor, *J. Membrane Biol.* **6**:58.

Katz, B., 1939, The "anti-curare" action of a subthreshold catelectrotonus, *J. Physiol.* (*Lond.*) **95**:286.

Katz, B., and Thesleff, S., 1957*a*, A study of the "desensitization" produced by acetylcholine at the motor end-plate, *J. Physiol.* (*Lond.*) **138**:63.

Katz, B,. and Thesleff, S., 1957*b*, The interaction between edrophonium (Tensilon) and acetylcholine at the motor end-plate, *Brit. J. Pharmacol.* **12**:260.

Kehoe, J. S., 1967, Pharmacological characteristics and ionic bases of a two component synaptic inhibition, *Nature* (*Lond.*) **215**:1503.

Kehoe, J. S., 1969, Single presynaptic neurone mediates a two component postsynaptic inhibition, *Nature* (*Lond.*) **221**:866.

Kehoe, J. S., 1972, Three acetylcholine receptors in *Aplysia* neurones, *J. Physiol.* (*Lond.*) **225**:115.

Kensler, C. J., 1949, The antagonism of curare by congo red and related compounds, *J. Pharmacol. Exptl. Therap.* **95**:28.

Kerkut, G. A., Pitman, R. M., and Walker, R. J., 1969, Sensitivity of neurones of the insect central nervous system to iontophoretically applied acetylcholine or GABA, *Nature* (*Lond.*) **222**:1075.

Khromov-Borisov, N. Y., and Michelson, M. J., 1966, The mutual disposition of cholinoreceptors of locomotor muscles and the changes in their disposition in the course of evolution, *Pharmacol. Rev.* **18**:1051.

Kimura, K. K., Unna, K., and Pfeiffer, C. C., 1948, Diatropine derivatives as proof that *d*-tubocurarine is a blocking moiety containing twin atropine–acetylcholine prosthetic groups, *J. Pharmacol. Exptl. Therap.* **95**:149.

King, H., 1935, Curare alkaloids. I. Tubocurarine, *J. Chem. Soc.* **1935**:1381.

Kirschner, L. B., and Stone, W. E., 1951, Action of inhibitors at the myoneural junction, *J. Gen. Physiol.* **34**:821.

Koelle, G. B., 1962, A new general concept of the neurohumoral functions of acetylcholine and acetylcholinesterase, *J. Pharm. Pharmacol.* **14**:65.

Koelle, G. B., 1970, Neuromuscular blocking agents, in: *The Pharmacological Basis of Therapeutics,* 4th ed. (L. S. Goodman and A. Gilman, eds.) pp. 601–619, Macmillan, New York.

Kreig, M. B., 1964, *Green Medicine*, Rand McNally, Chicago.

Krnjević, K., and Phillis, J. W., 1963, Pharmacological properties of acetylcholine-sensitive cells in the cerebral cortex, *J. Physiol.* (*Lond.*) **166**:328.

Krukoff, B. A., and Moldenke, H. N., 1938, Studies of American Menispermaceae with special reference to species used in the preparation of arrow poisons, *Brittonia* **3**:1.

Kuffler, S. W., 1942, Electrical potential changes at an isolated nerve–muscle junction, *J. Neurophysiol.* **5**:18.

Kuffler, S. W., 1943, Specific excitability of the endplate region in normal and denervated muscle, *J. Neurophysiol.* **6**:99.

Kuffler, S. W., 1945, Electric excitability of nerve–muscle fibre preparations, *J. Neurophysiol.* **8**:77.

Kuffler, S. W., Laporte, Y., and Ransmeier, R. E., 1947, The function of the frog's small-nerve motor system, *J. Neurophysiol.* **10**:395.

Langley, J. N., 1909, On the contraction of muscle, chiefly in relation to the presence of "receptive" substances. Part IV. The effect of curari and of some other substances on the nicotine response of the sartorius and gastrocnemius muscles of the frog, *J. Physiol.* (*Lond.*) **39**:235.

Langley, J. N., 1918, On the stimulation and paralysis of nerve cells and nerve endings. Part II. Paralysis by curari, strychnine and brucine and its antagonism by nicotine, *J. Physiol.* (*Lond.*) **52**:247.

Langley, J. N., and Kato, T., 1915, The physiological action of physostigmine and its action on denervated skeletal muscle, *J. Physiol.* (*Lond.*) **49**:410.

Lapique, L., 1926, *L'Excitabilité en Fonction du Temp; la Cronaxie, sa Signification et sa Mesure*, Presses Universitaires de France, Paris.

Larsen, J. R., Miller, D. M., and Yamamoto, T., 1966, *d*-Tubocurarine chloride: Effect on insects, *Science* **152**:225.

Lehman, A. J., 1935–1936, Curare actions of erythrina alkaloids, *Proc. Soc. Exptl. Biol. Med.* **33**:501.

Lester, H. A., 1972, Vulnerability of desensitized or curare-treated acetylcholine receptors to irreversible blockade by cobra toxin, *Mol. Pharmacol.* **8**:632.

Lilleheil, G., and Naess, K., 1961, A presynaptic effect of *d*-tubocurarine in the neuromuscular junction, *Acta Physiol. Scand.* **52**:120.

Ling, G., and Gerard, R. W., 1949, The normal membrane potential of frog sartorius fibers, *J. Cell. Comp. Physiol.* **34**:383.

MacNutt, F. A., 1912, Translation of P. M. D'Anghera's *De Orbe Novo*, G. P. Putnam's Sons, New York.

Manani, G., Galzigna, L., Mammona, S., and Gasparetto, A., 1972, Experimental and clinical study of the effects of pancuronium bromide, a neuromuscular blocking agent, *Arzneim. Forsch.* **22**:1528.

Marsh, D. F., 1951, The pharmacology of calabash curare. *Ann. N.Y. Acad. Sci.* **54**:307.

Masland, R. L., and Wigton, R. S., 1940, Nerve activity accompanying fasciculation produced by prostigmin, *J. Neurophysiol.* **3**:269.

Mats, M. N., 1972, Study of new curare-like agents of plant origin, *Rastit. Resur.* **8**:249.

Maynard, E. A., and Maynard, D. M., 1960, Cholinesterase in the crustacean muscle receptor organ, *J. Histochem. Cytochem.* **8**:376.

McCann, F. V., 1966, Curare as a neuromuscular blocking agent in insects, *Science* **154**:1023.

McCann, F. V., and Reece, R. W., 1967, Neuromuscular transmission in insects: Effect of injected chemical agents, *Comp. Biochem. Physiol.* **21**:115.

McIntyre, A. R., 1947, *Curare: Its History, Nature, and Clinical Use*, University of Chicago Press, Chicago.

McIntyre, A. R., King, R. E., and Dunn, A. L., 1945, Electrical activity of denervated mammalian skeletal muscle as influenced by *d*-tubocurarine, *J. Neurophysiol.* **8**:297.

McLennan, H., and York, D. H., 1966, Cholinoceptive receptors of crayfish stretch receptor neurones, *Comp. Biochem. Physiol.* **17**:327.

Miguel, J., and Vela, R., 1953, Contribución española a la historia del curare, *Hypnos* (Official Bull. Spanish Ass. Anesthesiol.), 1.

Miledi, R., 1960, The acetylcholine sensitivity of frog muscle fibres after complete and partial denervation, *J. Physiol.* (*Long.*) **151**:1.

Miledi, R., and Potter, L. T., 1971, Acetylcholine receptors in muscle fibers, *Nature* (*Lond.*) **233**:599.

Miner, R. W., Henegan, B. J., and Aeschlimann, J. A., eds., 1951, Curare and anti-curare agents, *Ann. N.Y. Acad. Sci.* **54**:297.

Nachmansohn, D., 1955, Metabolism and function of the nerve cell, in: *Harvey Lectures 1953/1954,* Vol. 49, pp. 57–99, Academic Press, New York.

Nachmansohn, D., 1969, Proteins of excitable membranes, *J. Gen. Physiol.* **54**:187.

Nastuk, W. L., 1953, Membrane potential changes at a single muscle end-plate produced by transitory application of acetylcholine with an electrically controlled microjet, *Fed. Proc.* **12**:102.

Nicol, J. A. C., 1952, Muscle activity and drug action in the body wall of the sabellid worm *Branchioma vesiculosum* (Montagu), *Physiol. Comp. Oecol.* **2**:339.

Otsuka, M., and Endo, M., 1960, The effect of guanidine on neuromuscular transmission, *J. Pharmacol. Exptl. Therap.* **128**:273.

Pantin, C. F. A., 1935, Response of the leech to acetylcholine, *Nature* (*Lond.*) **135**:875.

Paton, W. D. M., 1949, The pharmacology of curare and curarizing substances, *J. Pharm. Pharmacol.* **1**:273.

Paton, W. D. M., 1951, The pharmacology of decamethonium, *Ann. N.Y. Acad. Sci.* **54**:347.

Paton, W. D. M., and Perry, W. L. M., 1951, The pharmacology of the toxiferines, *Brit. J. Pharmacol.* **6**:299.

Paton, W. D. M., and Perry, W. L. M., 1953, The relationship between depolarization and block in the cat's superior cervical ganglion, *J. Physiol.* (*Lond.*) **119**:43.

Paton, W. D. M., and Zaimis, E. J., 1948, Curare-like action of polymethylene bis-quaternary ammonium salts, *Nature* (*Lond.*) **161**:718.

Paton, W. D. M., and Zaimis, E. J., 1949, The pharmacological actions of polymethylene bistrimethylammonium salts, *Brit. J. Pharmacol.* **4**:381.

Paton, W. D. M., and Zaimis, E. J., 1952, The methonium compounds, *Pharmacol. Rev.* **4**:219.

Peper, K., and McMahan, U. J., 1972, Distribution of acetylcholine receptors in the vicinity of nerve terminals on skeletal muscle of the frog, *Proc. Roy. Soc. Lond. Ser. B.* **181**:431.

Pick, E. P., and Unna, K., 1945, The effect of curare and curare-like substances on the central nervous system, *J. Pharmacol. Exptl. Therap.* **83**:59.

Pitman, R. M., and Kerkut, G. A., 1970, Comparison of the actions of iontophoretically applied acetylcholine and gamma-aminobutyric acid in cockroach central neurons, *Comp. Gen. Pharmacol.* **1**:221.

Porter, C. W., Chiu, T. H., Wieckowski, J., and Barnard, E. A., 1973, Types and locations of cholinergic receptor–like molecules in muscle fibers, *Nature New Biology* **241**:3.

Riker, W. F., Jr., and Okamoto, M., 1969, Pharmacology of motor nerve terminals, *Ann. Rev. Pharmacol.* **9**:173.

Riker, W. F., Jr., and Wescoe, W. C., 1951, The pharmacology of Flaxedil, with observations on certain analogs, *Ann. N.Y. Acad. Sci.* **54**:373.

Ritchie, J. M., and Armett, C. J., 1963, On the role of acetylcholine in conduction in mammalian nonmyelinated nerve fibres, *J. Pharmacol. Exptl. Therap.* **139**:201.

Roeder, K. D., 1948, The effect of anticholinesterases and related substances on nervous activity of the cockroach, *Bull. Johns Hopkins Hosp.* **83**:587.

Roepke, M. H., 1937, A study of choline esterase, *J. Pharmacol. Exptl. Therap.* **59**:264.

Rushton, W. A. H., 1933, Lapique's theory of curarization, *J. Physiol.* (*Lond.*) **77**:337.

Sauvage, G. L., Berger, F. M., and Boekelheide, V., 1949, The conversion of β-erythroidine to derivatives of the desmethoxy series and some pharmacological properties of apo-β-erythroidine, *Science* **109**:627.

Schueler, F. W., 1960, *Chemobiodynamics and Drug Design*, p. 484, McGraw-Hill, New York.

Shanes, A. M., 1958, Electrochemical aspects of physiological and pharmacological action in excitable cells. Part I. The resting cells and its alteration by extrinsic factors, *Pharmacol. Rev.* **10**:59.

Shankland, D. L., Rose, J. A., and Donniger, C., 1971, The cholinergic nature of the cercal nerve–giant fiber synapse in the sixth abdominal ganglion of the American cockroach *Periplaneta americana L., J. Neurobiol.* **2**:247.

Smith, S. M., Brown, H. O., Toman, J. E. P., and Goodman, L. S., 1947, The lack of cerebral effects of *d*-tubocurarine, *Anesthesiology* **8**:1.

Smith, W. K., 1947, The differential action of erythroidine in the normal and in the decerebrate animal, *Fed. Proc.* **6**:205.

Smith, W. K., Dodge, P., Luttrell, C., and Feldmahn, A., 1949, The site of action of some chemical agents in diminishing normal and excessive muscle tension, *Science* **110**:96.

Sobrino, J. A., and del Castillo, J., 1972, Activation of the cholinergic end-plate receptors by oxidizing reagents, *Internat. J. Neurosci.* **3**:251.

Sollman, T., 1957, *A Manual of Pharmacology and Its Applications to Therapeutics and Toxicology*, Saunders, Philadelphia.

Speight, T. M., and Avery, G. S., 1972, Pancuronium bromide: A review of its pharmacological properties and clinical application, *Drugs* (Australasian Drug Inform. Serv., Auckland), 4.

Standaert, F. G., 1964, The action of *d*-tubocurarine on the motor nerve terminal, *J. Pharmacol. Exptl. Therap.* **143**:181.

Stovner, J., and Lund, I., 1970, The muscle relaxants and their antagonists, *Brit. J. Anesth.* **42**:235.

Suga, N., and Katsuki, Y., 1961, Pharmacological studies on the auditory synapses in a grasshopper, *J. Exptl. Biol.* **38**:759.

Takeuchi, A., and Takeuchi, N., 1960, On the permeability of end-plate membrane during the action of transmitter, *J. Physiol.* (*Lond.*) **154**:52.

Takeuchi, N., 1963, Some properties of conductance changes at the end-plate membrane during the action of acetylcholine, *J. Physiol.* (*Lond.*) **167**:128.

Tauc, L., 1967, Transmission in vertebrate and invertebrate ganglia, *Physiol. Rev.* **47**521.

Tauc, L., and Gerschenfeld, H. M., 1961, Cholinergic transmission mechanisms for both excitation and inhibition in molluscan central synapses, *Nature* (*Lond.*) **192**:366.

Tauc, L., and Gershenfeld, H. M., 1962, A cholinergic mechanism of inhibitory synaptic transmission in a molluscan nervous system, *J. Neurophysiol.* **25**:236.

Taylor, D. B., and Nedergaard, O. A., 1965, Relation between structure and action of quaternary ammonium neuromuscular blocking agents, *Physiol. Rev.* **45**:523.

Thesleff, S., 1955, The mode of neuromuscular block caused by acetylcholine, nicotine, decamethonium and succinylcholine, *Acta Physiol. Scand.* **34**:218.

Thesleff, S., 1956, A further analysis of the neuromuscular block caused by acetylcholine, *Acta Physiol. Scand.* **37**:330.

Thesleff, S., 1958, A study of the interaction between neuromuscular blocking agents and acetylcholine at the mammalian motor end-plate, *Acta Anaesthesiol. Scand.* **2**:69.

van Maanen, E. F., 1948, A comparison of curare alkaloids, *Fed. Proc.* **7**:261.

van Maanen, E. F., 1950, The antagonism between acetylcholine and the curare alkaloids, *d*-tubocurarine, *c*-curarine-I, *c*-toxiferine-II and β-erythroidine in the rectus abdominis of the frog, *J. Pharmacol. Exptl. Therap.* **99**:255.

Waser, P. G., 1953, Calebassen-Curare, *Helv. Physiol. Pharmacol. Acta Suppl.* **8**:II.

Waser, P. G., 1962, Relation between enzymes and cholinergic receptors, in: *Enzymes and Drug Action*, A Ciba Foundation Symposium (A. V. S. de Reuck, ed.) pp. 206–219, Little, Brown, Boston.

Waser, P. G., 1965, The molecular distribution of ^{14}C-decamethonium in and around the motor end plate and its metabolism in cats and mice, in: *Pharmacology of Cholinergic and Adrenergic Transmission*, pp. 129–136, Pergamon Press, Oxford.

Waser, P. G., 1966, Autoradiographic investigations of cholinergic and other receptors in the motor endplate, in: *Advances in Drug Research* (N. J. Harper and A. B. Simmonds, eds.) pp. 81–120, Academic Press, New York.

Waser, P. G., 1967, Receptor localization by autoradiographic techniques, *Ann. N.Y. Acad. Sci.* **144**:737.

Waser, P. G., 1970, On receptors in the postsynaptic membrane of the motor endplate, in: *Molecular Properties of Drug Receptors*, A Ciba Foundation Symposium (R. Porter and M. O'Connor, eds.) pp. 59–74, J. & A. Churchill, London.

Wedensky, N. E., 1903, Die Erregung, Hemmung und Narkose, *Pflüger's Arch. Ges. Physiol.* **10**:1.

Welsh, J. H., 1948, Concerning the mode of action of acetylcholine, *Bull. Johns Hopkins Hosp.* **83**:568.

Welsch, J. H., and Taub, R., 1953, The action of acetylcholine antagonists on the heart of *Venus mercenaria, Brit. J. Pharmacol.* **8**:327.

Werner, G., 1961, Antidromic activity in motor nerves and its relation to a generator event in nerve terminals, *J. Neurophysiol.* **24**:401.

Willstaetter, R., and W. Heubner, 1907, Über eine neue Solanaceenbase, *Ber. Deutsch. Chem. Ges.* **40**:3869.

Wilson, A. T., and Wright, S., 1936, Anti-curare action of potassium and other substances, *Quart. J. Exptl. Physiol.* **26**:127.

Wintersteiner, O., and Dutcher, J. D., 1943, Curare alkaloids from *Chondodendron tomentosum, Science* **97**:467.

Wright, E. B., 1949, The action of erythroidine, curare and chlorobutanol in the crayfish, *J. Cell. Comp. Physiol.* **33**:301.

Wright, S., 1955, Electroencephalographic patterns following intraventricular injection of tubocurarine in the cat, *J. Physiol.* (*Lond.*) **130**:35P.

Chapter 4

Atropine

R. D. O'Brien

Section of Neurobiology and Behavior
Cornell University
Ithaca, New York, U.S.A.

I. INTRODUCTION

Atropine is one of the oldest known poisons, with references to plant extracts that contain it going back to the Ebers papyrus of 1550 B.C. Its name derives from the plant which produces it, *Atropa belladonna*, or deadly nightshade. *Atropos* was the Greek Fate whose business was to cut the thread of life (spun by her kindlier sister), without regard to sex, age, or quality; her name means "unmovable." This etymology is a reflection of its long history of use as a poison, having been referred to as such by authors from Pliny to Shakespeare. By contrast, the *belladonna* ("beautiful woman") term refers to its use by women, up to the nineteenth century, to dilate their pupils and thus enhance their beauty (the catastrophic effects on vision being presumably of lesser importance). Thus the toxic and the parasympatholytic properties have long been entwined in the plant's name, which was given by Linnaeus in 1753. Atropine itself was discovered in 1809 by Vacquelin, and isolated in 1831 by Mein.

It has been known since 1867 that atropine caused the heart rate to quicken (tachycardia) by blocking vagal stimulation, and by the later part of the nineteenth century it was recognized that muscarine's ability to slow the heart was antagonized by atropine (e.g., Pickering, 1896). When Loewi (1921) showed that heart slowing was caused by a chemical released by the vagus nerve [called *Vagusstoff*; subsequently identified as acetylcholine by Loewi and Navratil (1926)], he was quick to note that its action was blocked by atropine. Even before this, Dale (1914) had noted that injected acetylcholine had two kinds of effects: One kind was mimicked by muscarine and blocked by atropine; he called these "muscarinic" (examples are the response of the pupil and the heart). The other kind was mimicked by nicotine and was insensitive to atropine; he called them "nicotinic" (an example is the effect on neuromuscular junctions of skeletal muscles). Once the work of Loewi, and of others who followed him, had shown that acetylcholine was the transmitter at numerous chemically mediated junctions, the Dale categorization achieved major importance, and atropine became an essential tool in establishing the character of any particular junction.

Because of the long history and unusual importance of atropine, a full review of its use is not possible in a few pages. Fortunately, its pharmacology, chemistry, metabolism, and clinical use were reviewed at length several years ago (Cullumbine, 1967; Innes and Nickerson, 1965; Triggle, 1965). Consequently, I have attempted to give an account which, although fairly complete in itself, stresses the value of atropine as a tool in studying the nervous system and makes reference principally to experiments published during the last decade.

II. MODE OF ACTION

A. Postsynaptic Actions

All nerves act either on nerves or on effectors, such as muscles or glands. In most cases, they act by releasing a chemical mediator called a "transmitter," which combines with a receptor macromolecule in the receiving cell and, by modifying the ionic permeability of that cell, either excites it or reduces its excitability. Acetylcholine is one such transmitter, and the various acetylcholine receptors in the *periphery* were classified by Dale (see above); atropine blocks the category he called "muscarinic." This blockade can be shown as an interruption of the response normally provoked neurally or as a block of response to exogenously applied transmitters (such as acetylcholine) or agonistic drugs (such as muscarine).

The principal muscarinic receptors include the cholinergic receptors of most smooth muscles (such as trachea, bronchi, gastrointestinal tract, iris and ciliary muscles of the eye), which are therefore relaxed or prevented from contraction if enough atropine is given. Atropine also blocks the inhibitory or slowing action of the vagus nerve on the heart and consequently causes cardiac acceleration. Furthermore, it has central actions, which in normal animals and man can lead to quite complex effects, including effects on mood and electroencephalogram. As we shall see, these central effects are of paramount importance in the antidotal action of atropine against poisoning by anticholinesterases. However, these findings do not permit us to classify the corresponding central receptors as muscarinic, for the situation may be much more complex. Thus the Renshaw cells of the spinal cord appear to have three kinds of receptors: an excitatory nicotinic receptor, an excitatory muscarinic receptor, and an unspecified inhibitory cholinergic receptor (Curtis and Ryall, 1966). Some deep pyramidal cells of the cortex are classically muscarinic, but other central cells have a mixed nicotinic–muscarinic character (Phillis, 1970).

The postsynaptic effects described above represent the "classical" action of atropine. But in recent years some additional, quite different actions have been reliably reported. Obviously, they complicate the relatively simple interpretation of atropine's action and need to be taken into account if one attempts to use atropine as a tool in studying the nervous system.

B. Presynaptic Actions

In recent years, it has become apparent that in addition to the well-known effects of atropine on the postsynaptic receptor, it is active presynaptically even at very low concentrations. Acetylcholine release is enhanced by atropine, as can be shown in preparations whose acetylcholinesterase has been blocked by a suitable inhibitor. This was shown 10 years ago with the intact exposed cerebral cortex of the cat, rabbit, and sheep (Mitchell, 1963; Szerb, 1964). More recent studies (Molenaar and Polak, 1970; Polak, 1971) have made use of cortical slices from rat brain, in which the concentrations of added agents can be more precisely controlled. In this preparation, a base level of acetylcholine release was obtained by incubating in high concentrations (25 mM) of K^+. Atropine at 0.3 μM increased the acetylcholine release from the slices by three-fold to about 13 μg/g. The increase was not affected by 10 μg/ml of tetrodotoxin (a gigantic concentration), in contrast to the effect of the toxin in reducing acetylcholine release from the intact cat cortex (Dudar and Szerb, 1969). But botulinum toxin, which is known to block acetylcholine release, antagonized the atropine effect. In this set of experiments, the acetylcholine release from slices, which was normally 6 μg/g, was increased by 0.3 μM atropine to 13 and decreased by botulinum toxin alone (20,000 mouse LD_{50}/ml) to 3; with both atropine and toxin, the release was 5.

Atropine increases the total as well as the released acetylcholine in cortical slices and therefore must enhance acetylcholine synthesis. Thus the extractable (i.e., not released) acetylcholine was increased about 30% (from

9.8 to 13 μg/g) by 0.7 μM atropine. This finding raised the question of whether the increase in released acetylcholine was caused by greater synthesis or whether increased synthesis was the result of more extensive acetylcholine loss from the presynapse. Because botulium toxin, which is believed to act only on acetylcholine release, had the effect of abolishing atropine's effect on extractable acetylcholine, it seems likely that atropine directly affected release, not synthesis. And indeed atropine was ineffectual on acetylcholine synthesis in a cell-free system (Giarman and Pepeu, 1964). Other antimuscarinic drugs such as hyoscyamine were highly effective in promoting acetylcholine release from slices (Bertels-Meeuws and Polak, 1968).

Although most of the work on atropine with cortical slices has employed high K^+ as the primary acetylcholine releaser, precisely comparable results were obtained when square-wave stimulation was employed. Atropine at 3×10^{-7} M had no effect on the resting output of acetylcholine (18.4 ng/g/min), but a peak-effect stimulation rate of 16/sec led to an output of 50 ng in the control and 127 ng in the atropinized preparation (Bourdois *et al.*, 1971). This effect is illustrated in Fig. 1.

The most satisfactory resolution of these presynaptic effects may come from the demonstration by Schuberth and Sundwall (1967) that atropine shares with hemicholinium, eserine, oxotremorine, and morphine the ability to block acetylcholine uptake. The uptake was demonstrated in slices of mouse brain cortex, but there was evidence that the nerve-ending fraction was involved, so that it is tempting to conclude that an uptake into end bulbs is implied. The drug concentrations were of the order of 10^{-5} M, and K_i values for the various drugs ranged from 5 to 30 μM, that for atropine being 16 μM. A comparable block by atropine or carbamylcholine uptake into a similar preparation had been shown earlier by Creese and Taylor (1965). A tentative hypothesis is, therefore, that net acetylcholine release reflects the differential between total release from end bulbs and total uptake back into them; atropine increases net release by blocking reuptake, and promotes new synthesis by depleting the end bulbs of their acetylcholine content.

A quite different presynaptic mechanism was postulated by Polak (1971). He suggested that normally the released acetylcholine inhibits further release and this inhibition is blocked by atropine. If this "disinhibition" mechanism were true, one should be able to overcome it by adding extra acetylcholine. Although this was not experimentally feasible, Polak was able to add oxotremorine or acetyl-β-methylcholine and block atropine's action, and he felt that this supported his proposal. But very high concentrations were needed: the effect of 0.3 μM atropine was abolished only by 300 μM acetyl-β-methylcholine and was not fully abolished by 100

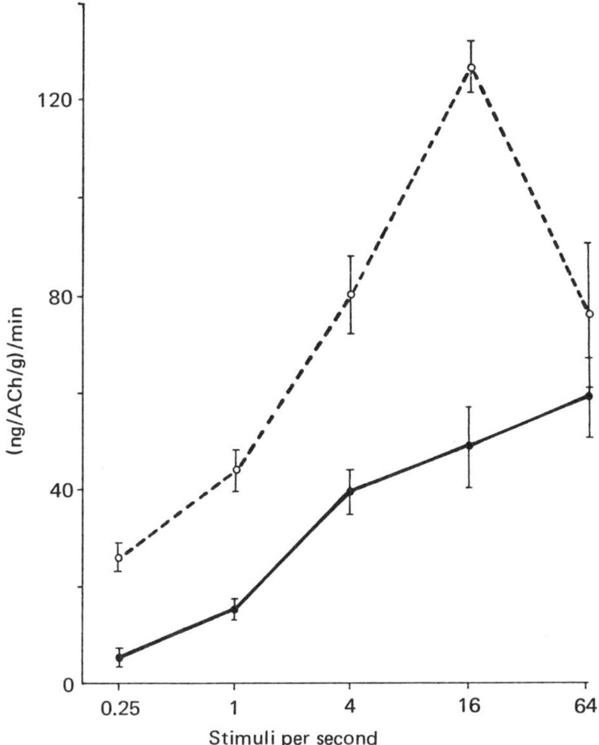

Fig. 1. Release of acetylcholine from rat cortex slices stimulated electrically. Values are for acetylcholine release in excess of that in prestimulation period. ●——●, Without atropine. ○---○, With 3×10^{-7} M atropine. From Bourdois *et al.* (1971).

μM oxotremorine. Such concentrations profoundly reduce acetylcholine uptake in the absence of atropine (see above), and the only counter to this consideration by Polak was that 100 μM eserine, which can also block acetylcholine uptake, did not interfere with atropine's releasing action. However, the puzzling feature is surely eserine's inability to antagonize atropine's action; the concentration of acetyl-β-methylcholine or oxotremorine was about 100 times greater than the acetylcholine in the medium and 100 times greater than the atropine concentration, suggesting that their action was not simply to reverse atropine's disinhibition by competing with the hypothetical disinhibition site.

A completely different approach to accounting for atropine's enhancement of acetylcholine release is that of Dudar and Szerb (1969) in support of an earlier proposal by MacIntosh (1963). They propose that the neurons whose acetylcholine release is affected are normally inhibited by a customary postsynaptic blockade of secondary cholinergic neurons. Working with cats, they showed that atropine applied to the right cortex enhanced acetylcholine release from the left cortex, thus demonstrating action-at-a-distance. Several other experiments showed that neural activity was a precondition for atropine's effect; for instance, its effect was lost if tetrodotoxin was applied or if mesencephalic lesions were made to turn off the neural input into the cortex. If depolarization was induced by high (45 μM) potassium rather than neurally, atropine had no effect. This study, which used approximately 3 μM atropine (about ten times more concentrated than in the *in vitro* studies), raises difficult questions. Certainly atropine's action-at-a-distance implies that one of its effects *in vivo* may well be block of an inhibitory pathway (if one can readily exclude diffusional leakage of atropine from the site of application). Some of the findings simply confirm those made in the less complex *in vitro* preparations, i.e., the fact that atropine has no action on resting release of acetylcholine. But some of the findings are quite unlike those described above for *in vitro* preparations: the sensitivity to tetrodotoxin and the failure of effect on high K^+–treated preparations. At the moment, one can say little more than that with 3 μM atropine in the intact cat cortex the evidence implies that at least a part of atropine's action on acetylcholine release involves a blockade of neural inhibition through a postsynaptic action, but with 0.3 μM atropine in rat cortical slices a direct presynaptic effect is probable.

Using a frog sartorius muscle preparation, Beránek and Vyskočil (1968) also proposed presynaptic actions of atropine but argued that acetylcholine release was not affected, since the quantum content of the neurally evoked junctional potentials was unaffected. The quantum content is defined as the mean amplitude of the junctional potential divided by the mean amplitude of the miniature end-plate potentials (m.e.p.p.'s); each was about halved by 60 μM atropine. Since this concentration also profoundly reduced the depolarization caused by electrophoretically added acetylcholine, there must surely be a large receptor blockade under these conditions, in addition to the effect on the m.e.p.p.'s. As to the presynaptic actions, the authors argue that acetylcholine release must be unimpaired, because the quantum content was unaltered, and one assumes that the size of each quantum of acetylcholine is not subject to change. Therefore, it is the effectiveness of that fixed acetylcholine release which is modified. Although the authors point to the possibility of promoted acetylcholine reuptake, I feel that all the effects seen in this preparation on both junctional potentials and m.e.p.p.'s can be readily accounted for by a simple receptor blockade by atropine. These same authors, using similar techniques, earlier concluded that the actions of low concentrations of atropine on the rat diaphragm were entirely postsynaptic, primarily because the quantum content was unaffected (Beránek and Vyskočil, 1967).

It has been hypothesized by Burn and Rand (see review by Burn and Rand, 1965) that in sympathetic nerve endings the release of norepinephrine is caused by the prior release of acetylcholine. A part of their evidence is that several agents affect both cholinergic and adrenergic systems; examples are botulinum toxin, bretylium, and guanidium. If the hypothesis is correct, there must be a presynaptic cholinergic "receptor" with which the released acetylcholine reacts. But in view of the fact (Burn *et al.*, 1963) that one can evoke these "cholinergic sympathetic" responses (e.g., in the nictitating membrane) even when 1 mg/kg of atropine is injected, it presumably follows that atropine does not block this particular presynaptic receptor.

C. Noncholinergic Effects

Atropine has classically been used to block gastric secretion, presumably by blockade of the receptors of the parasympathetic innervation of the stomach. However, it also has direct effects which can be seen in denervated preparations and in isolated mucosa preparations. In the vagally denervated dog's stomach, it was shown that H^+ movement across the fundic mucosa was approximately doubled by intravenous atropine, 0.05 mg/kg. The method involved studying loss from solutions introduced into a pouch formed in the fundus or the antrum (Rudick *et al.*, 1970). The effects of atropine on other ion fluxes were subsequently studied under a variety of conditions in this same preparation, and it was found that the effects on H^+ and K^+ were always closely correlated, whereas those on H^+ and Na^+ were not, thus suggesting a coupling mechanism for H^+ and K^+ movement (Berkowitz *et al.*, 1970).

No information is available on the mechanism of these noncholinergic effects. They confirm earlier reports on atropine block of water flux in rat erythrocytes (Hirschowitz *et al.*, 1960) and Na^+ flux in frog skin (Kirschner, 1955). Recently it has been shown that 10^{-6} M atropine reduced by 21% the fragility of erythrocytes (presumably human) as judged by hemolysis, but the effect was rather small compared with that of a classical "membrane stabilizer," chlorpromazine, which reduced fragility 83% at 10^{-6} M (Mikikits, 1970).

As with so many drugs, the high specificity of atropine which is typical at low drug concentrations is lost when high concentrations are employed. For instance, it can reduce the effect of epinephrine or of sympathetic stimulation on arterial beds (Bussell, 1940) and can block the lethal action of epinephrine in rats (Luduena and Branin, 1966). High concentrations have some nerve-blocking action, similar to that of local anesthetics. Thus 60 mM atropine sulfate caused 50% block of frog sciatic nerve in 15 min. This was one-sixteenth of the effectiveness of procaine on this preparation (Sheu *et al.*, 1969). A local anesthetic-like effect on single brain neurons can also be seen occasionally when atropine is applied to them electrophoretically; it is of a few minutes' duration and acts indiscriminately on cells sensitive or insensitive to acetylcholine (Curtis and Phillis, 1960; Spehlmann, 1969). Similarly, in the so-called CILDA cells of the mollusk *Aplysia* it was found that iontophoretic atropine depressed nonspecifically the curare-sensitive cholinergic receptors, the curare-insensitive receptors, and the serotonin receptors (Gerschenfeld *et al.*, 1967).

D. Intracellular Effects

Most of the effects of atropine discussed in this chapter involve reactions with membrane-bound receptors whose normal response is a change in plasma membrane permeability, especially to cations. In at least one instance, the pancreas, it has been postulated that there is a cholinergic receptor whose stimulation produces "an increase of an intracellular substance which enhances synthesis at the ribosomal level." The evidence is that administration of atropine *in vivo* in pigeons had effects *in vitro* on the pancreas which in most cases were the opposite of applying acetyl-β-methylcholine or urecholine. The doses were rather high, e.g., 3 mg/kg intramuscularly. The effects included up to twofold increases in the amylase content of the pancreas, a 35% reduction in phenylalanine incorporation, and small reductions in O_2 uptake and glucose and palmitate oxidation (Morisset and Webster, 1970). Subsequently, reductions up to 35% in uridine incorporation into soluble RNA were observed, without effect on nuclear RNA (Webster and Morisset, 1971).

E. Atropine Binding and Transport

Many drugs in the bloodstream are bound to plasma proteins. Such binding can have important effects by (1) increasing the amount of drug carried in the blood, (2) promoting the uptake into the blood by decreasing the free drug level of the blood, which is the factor of importance in establishing a concentration gradient with respect to the locus of application, and (3) decreasing the availability of the drug in the blood to the tissues, including target tissues. This decrease can be caused simply because the level of free drug is reduced by any kind of binding; if the binding is not rapidly reversible, the availability of the drug is even further reduced.

Orozlau and Maengweyn-Davies (1962*a*) explored atropine binding to purified bovine serum albumin. The binding was highly *p*H-dependent, being absent at the isoelectric point of the protein (*p*H 5) and increasing sharply at higher or lower *p*H. Increasing *p*H increased the number of binding sites per molecule of albumin, from 20 at *p*H 6 to 100 at 7. This fivefold increase was partially offset by a four-fold decrease in affinity, the dissociation constant, K_d, increasing from 8.6 mM at *p*H 6 to 38.2 mM at *p*H 8 (this affinity effect would not be apparent if saturating concentrations of atropine were always used). It should be noted that these affinities are extremely low, so that the influence of such binding under physiological conditions would be correspondingly small. Thus the large dose of 100 mg/kg of atropine, if evenly distributed throughout the body, would be only 0.3 mM, a value so far from the K_d that little of the potential binding would be realized. Thus if the K_d at blood *p*H were about 30 mM, only 1.3% of the total binding sites would actually bind. The percent binding is given by $100/[(K_d/L) + 1]$, where L is the ligand concentration.

N-Acetylated bovine serum albumin did not bind atropine, suggesting that the binding involves the amino group (and perhaps histidine nitrogens) of the protein. This observation, added to the large number of binding sites per protein molecule and the very low affinity, implies that the binding is highly nonspecific, and not due to anything that could be called a true "atropine-binding site."

These authors then showed (Orozlau and Maengweyn-Davies, 1962*b*) that acetylcholine and choline could affect the atropine binding of bovine serum albumin in very different ways, dependent on the *p*H, the atropine–acetylcholine or atropine–choline ratio, and the buffer. Effects varying from substantial (sixfold) activation of binding to about 50% inhibition were seen. The unexpected activation was due to a change in the affinity rather than in the number of binding sites. The authors correctly point to the inappropriateness of carrying over these observations to true receptor effects, but the possibility of such complex interactions occurring in receptors has to be seriously considered, especially since the effects were seen with acetylcholine at only half the concentration of atropine. However, the concentrations were quite high, in the millimolar range.

F. Tachyphylaxis

Tachyphylaxis, also called "acute tolerance," consists of the development of a decreased response to repeated applications of a drug.

Atropine was shown to have such an effect on the intestine of man (Quigley, 1973) and dog (Gray and Seevers, 1955). Recently, Goldenberg (1969) showed for rat ileum that tachyphylaxis in atropine blockade developed when the stimulation was by nicotine, but not when it was acetylcholine. Since nicotine is presumed to act in this preparation by causing acetylcholine release from nerve terminals, Goldenberg proposed that the tachyphylaxis involved presynaptic release rather than postsynaptic receptor. Tachyphylaxis is by no means universally found with atropine. Working with the frog sartorius muscle, Beránek and Vyskočil (1968) found that *d*-tubocurarine, on repeated applications, lost its effect on neurally evoked end-plate potentials, but atropine did not.

III. TOXICOLOGY

A. Toxicity

The acute toxicities of atropine are listed by Spector (1956). The average oral LD_{50} values in mg/kg are 948 for the mouse, 875 for the rat, 1100 for the guinea pig, and 1450 for the rabbit, a surprisingly narrow range. As usual, the intravenous and intraperitoneal routes yield higher toxicities, by about two- to tenfold in most cases; thus the averaged intraperitoneal LD_{50} values are 250 for the mouse, 440 for the rat, and 400 for the guinea pig. These values make it surprising that atropine was well known as a poison, for if the lethal dose for a human is (let us guess) 800 mg/kg orally, then it would take 56 g of pure alkaloid to kill a 70-kg man. Presumably, the poisoners used chronic doses.

The use of atropine in control of respiratory infections of infants requires caution. A 2-month-old boy who received 0.4 mg of the methyl nitrate (well within the therapeutic dose) with each feeding developed high fever (107°F, rectal), dilated pupils, and abdominal distension, all symptomatic of atropine poisoning (Purcell, 1966).

Eyedrops can cause toxic effects systemically. An 82-year-old woman with partial renal dysfunction received an unspecified number of drops, each drop with 0.75 mg of atropine. After 3 days of such treatment, signs of severe atropine poisoning developed, which subsided on discontinuation of the atropine. It seems likely that impaired excretion of the drug was involved (German and Siddigrie, 1970).

Psychotic symptoms have also been noted at common therapeutic doses such as the 4 mg per day used in the treatment of myocardial infarction. Erikssen (1969) observed, within a 6-month period, 30 cases of "serious mental aberrations," ranging all the way from inattention and paranoid ideas to auditory and visual hallucinations.

B. Antidotal Use in Poisoning by Anticholinesterase

The primary effect of poisonous organophosphates and carbamates is to block the acetylcholinesterase in nerve junctions, so that the pulse of acetylcholine generated in the synapse is sustained instead of being rapidly destroyed. Atropine can block the muscarinic acetylcholine receptor and thus compensate for the sustained acetylcholine. Atropine was one of the first agents studied for this purpose and is still the commonest antidote. The early literature has been reviewed extensively elsewhere (Koelle, 1963; O'Brien, 1960; Karczmar, 1970).

The military and commercial anticholinesterases are almost exclusively nonionic and consequently have both central and peripheral effects. The damaging central effects are on the respiratory center, and the peripheral ones include bronchial constriction, excessive respiratory tract secretions, paralysis of respiratory muscles, and cardiovascular effects. The relative contributions of these various factors to poisoning vary with animal species and with the anticholinesterase. Atropine is particularly valuable against the central effects, although the course of its effectiveness and the need for its continued application can be conveniently followed by observing its reversal of such peripheral symptoms of poisoning by anticholinesterase as myosis (contraction of the pupil) and salivation. Atropine alone is often used, in doses of 1–4 mg for an adult, repeated at intervals of from 5 to 60 min depending on the severity of poisoning. It is common to use an additional agent to control the neuromuscular effects. In the early work, a variety of oximes were tested, but now there is only one in common civilian use, known variously as pralidoxime chloride, 2-PAM chloride, or pyridoxime-2-aldoxime chloride, used in a dose of about 1 g intravenously. There is a useful brief review of the use of atropine plus pralidoxime for parathion poisoning, which is by far the commonest problem (Hayes, 1965).

Madill *et al.* (1968) have shown that for a series of drugs including atropine the ability to antagonize sarin poisoning in the guinea pig was correlated with the relative central anticholinergic potency (as judged by ability to antagonize seizures induced by intracerebral carbachol) and not with the relative peripheral anticholinergic potency (as judged by such tests as the abilty to cause mydriasis or to block slowing of the heart by acetyl-β-methylcholine). This was evidence that sarin poisoning was primarily due to a central effect on the respiratory center, and not to effects on such peripheral junctions as those of the neuromuscular junctions or the cardiovascular system. An incidental feature of the study was that of the ten drugs examined, atropine was the least effective against sarin. The best was scopolamine, which was 16 times more potent. Yet atropine remains the most popular drug for this purpose.

IV. ATROPINE AS A TOOL FOR STUDYING THE NERVOUS SYSTEM

A. Presence or Absence of Muscarinic Pathways

When atropine is found to have blocking activity, the conclusion is commonly drawn that a muscarinic pathway is involved, as in the following diverse recent examples.

The salivation induced in dogs by prostaglandin $F_{2\alpha}$ was augmented by the anticholinesterase eserine and blocked by atropine (Hahn and Patil, 1972). Single neurons in the cat's visual cortex were excited by acetylcholine and depressed by atropine, both applied iontophoretically (Spehlmann, 1969). Nerve transmission in the mammalian stellate ganglion is classically considered to be nicotinic, but it was shown in the dog (Flacke and Gillis, 1960) that high doses of nicotinic blockers failed to produce total blockade, yet this nonnicotinic residue could be fully blocked by 0.03 mg/kg of atropine. Consequently, there is a muscarinic pathway in this ganglion. Predatory aggression in rats (an aggressive response to specific prey, and not a reflection of generalized aggression) was suppressed when atropine was applied to certain highly localized sites in the lateral hypothalamus. These findings, along with the extensive related studies with other drugs, supported a hypothesis of cholinergic involvement in this specific behavioral pattern (Bandler, 1970). Atropine (0.1 mg/kg) abolished the ability of the centrally acting agent 2-deoxy-D-glucose to promote secretion of gastric pepsin, suggesting that the vagal nerve is the major pathway for the sugar's action (Johansson *et al.*, 1971). Atropine implanted at 1 mg/kg in the hypothalamus of rats reduced by 92% the growth of the ovary, implying the involvement of a cholinergic pathway in release of folliculotrophic hormones (Monti *et al.*, 1970).

The turnover of cerebral dopamine in rats has a cholinergic involvement, as judged by the effect of atropine on the production of dopamine's breakdown product, homovanillic acid. When given intraperitoneally, 5 mg/kg diminished production by 40%, without changing the dopamine level. But intraventricular atropine (200 μg) had the opposite effect, giving a doubling of production, again without changing the dopamine level (Bartholini and Pletscher, 1971).

Cholinergic mechanisms are implicated in the states of sleep and wakefulness. Atropine is known to inhibit the alerting response in rabbits which is produced either by external stimulation or by stimulating the midbrain reticular formation, the neural source of the alerting response; excitatory cholinergic drugs have the opposite effect (Rinaldi and Himwich, 1955). However, this effect of atropine is due only in part to atropine-sensitive synapses in the reticular formation. In addition, the cortex itself is a site of action of atropine, as can be shown by applying it via the cortical artery and stimulating via the untreated reticular formation (Rinaldi, 1965).

A study was made of the ability of muscarinic and nicotinic antagonists to block the arousal (measured by electroencephalogram activation) caused by muscarinic and nicotinic agonists (Domino *et al.*, 1968). Both kinds of agonists were highly effective, but atropine strongly blocked muscarinic agonists yet not nicotinic agonists. The reverse was true when atropine was replaced by nicotinic antagonists. It follows that the cholinergic pathways involved in arousal are not of some kind of mixed nicotinic–muscarinic character but contain separate nicotinic and muscarinic synapses.

The presence in cat jejunum of an inhibitory neural network with at least some muscarinic synapses was indicated when it was shown that atropine, tetrodotoxin (a specific axonic blocker), and xylocaine all caused excitation of the circular muscles of the excised gut. Several lines of evidence suggested that the effect was not a direct one on the muscle cells but involved inhibitory neurons in an enteric system (Wood, 1972).

Within the adrenal medulla, there appear to be separate muscarinic and nicotinic pathways, the former leading to the secretion of epinephrine only, the latter to a mixture of epinephrine and norepinephrine. Thus stimulation of the denervated cat adrenal gland with pilocarpine or muscarine produced only epinephrine, and the effect was blocked by atropine. The classical nicotinic pathway could be evoked by neural stimulation or acetylcholine or nicotine, and was blocked by hexamethonium. The authors pointed to the danger of confusing "nicotinic sites," in the sense of sites whose innervation had nicotinic character, with "nicotinic receptors": clearly, in the adrenal medulla the innervation is nicotinic, but the receptors include both nicotinic and muscarinic varieties (Douglas and Poisner, 1965).

The high specificity of the postsynaptic action of atropine has made the drug a favorite tool for showing the absence of muscarinic cholinergic involvement in various processes or for showing a nonmuscarinic component. A few diverse examples are as follows. Changes in ATP-induced mitochondrial swelling properties are caused by norepinephrine or vagal stimulation but not by atropine (Rosenblum and Rosenblum, 1969). The excitatory innervation of the urinary bladder of vertebrates is largely atropine resistant; the neurally evoked excitation differs in drug response from the acetylcholine-induced excitation; because ATP and other pyrophosphate purine nucleotides mimic the neural excitation, a possible mediation by such a nucleotide transmitter was postulated (Burnstock *et al.*, 1972). The innervation of the mammalian colon appears to have an atropine-resistant component when studied by a techique using an intraluminal balloon in cats or dogs which measures effects on the circular musculature (Fulgraff *et al.*, 1964; Gray *et al.*, 1955). But when the muscles of the longitudinal coat of the colon of the guinea pig were examined by a direct method, atropine at 0.03 mg/kg blocked all responses (Soldani *et al.*, 1970).

B. Measurement and Properties of the Muscarinic Receptor

It is axiomatic that if atropine affects a physiological system, it must affect a target macromolecule within that system such as an enzyme, a receptor, a nucleic acid, or a structural protein. And if atropine affects a macromolecule, it must bind to that macromolecule at least transiently. The binding could in principle be reversible or irreversible; since the postsynaptic action of atropine is reversible, it is likely that the binding to the target is reversible. "Reversibility" in this context is operationally defined, and includes not only true reversibility but also pseudoreversibility, in which the target could recover fully from its attack, whereas the atropine could be hydrolyzed or otherwise altered in the process. A classical case of pseudoreversibility is the reaction between carbamates and acetylcholinesterase; if one inhibits the enzyme, it becomes carbamylated, and if one removes residual inhibitor, the enzyme recovers by spontaneous decarbamylation, to yield unaltered enzyme (so it is reversible in that sense) and the hydrolysis products of the carbamate. Since atropine is an ester, the parallel possibility exists in its "reversible" action.

In the last 10 years, there has been a great interest in the use of radioactive drugs to bind directly to receptors in three kinds of studies. First, one should in principle be able to measure directly how many receptors there are in a tissue, and what their affinity is for the drug, in those cases (which are a majority) where binding is fully reversible. Second, one should be able to use the ability to bind the drug as an index of receptor activity in attempts to purify and characterize receptors. Third, it may be possible to visualize the location of binding of labeled drugs by radioautographic techniques.

Atropine was the original radioactive drug to be studied in the first way. A classical study by Paton and Rang (1966) involved both physiological and radioactive techniques. In physiological work, they first measured the rates of onset and recovery of the antagonistic effect against acetylcholine, and from the ratio of these rates computed a dissociation constant (which we shall call K_d) of 1.02 nM. They then measured K_d by equilibrium studies of antagonism and found a value of 1.11 nM. Labeled atropine uptake was next studied by an equilibrium technique: Pieces of muscle were equilibrated with ^{3}H-atropine at 37°C, then the muscle was removed and incubated with a solution of high concentration of nonradioactive atropine in ethanol. This incubation displaced over 95% of the radioactivity from the muscle into the solution, which was then counted. Three uptake phenomena were found: one binding that saturated with a high affinity (K_d = 1.11 nM), another with a low affinity (K_d = 450 nM), and a partitioning process which did not saturate and whose partition coefficient was 4.67 in favor of the muscle. The values of B_m (binding at saturation, expressed in pmol/g) were 180 for the high affinity and 974 for the low. It would seem likely that the high-affinity binding is to the true acetylcholine receptor, since the K_d values from physiological and radioactive studies are literally identical. By contrast, the low-affinity site is presumably unrelated to the muscarinic receptor and represents either nonspecific binding or possibly low-affinity binding to other more prolific receptors such as that for histamine (Table I).

In our laboratory, we have studied extensively the binding of reversible cholinergic ligands to electroplax preparations, a particularly rich source of nicotinic receptors (O'Brien *et al.*, 1971, 1972, 1973, 1974). Recently, we

Table I. Binding to Possible Receptors

		High affinity		Low affinity	
Tissue	Authors	K_d (nM)	B_m (pmol/g)	K_d (nM)	B_m (pmol/g)
	Radioactive Assay				
Guinea pig ileum muscle	Paton and Rang (1966)	1.11	180	450	974
Rat brain synaptosome membranes	Farrow and O'Brien (1973)	0.6	6.6	900	86
Mouse brain crude mitochondrial fraction	Schleifer and Eldefrawi (1973)	2.6	39	1000	250
	Physiological Assay				
Guinea pig ileum	Paton and Rang (1966)	1.11	—	—	—
Guinea pig ileum (for histamine)	Arunlakshana and Schild (1959)	—	—	2400	—

extended this technique to rat brain and examined the usefulness of binding of radioactive atropine as an index of muscarinic receptor sites (Farrow and O'Brien, 1973). We used equilibrium dialysis at 4°C overnight, and by performing studies at various concentrations of atropine from 40 pM to 5 μM were able to titrate the sites and so measure their quantity and affinity. We found (Fig. 2) that the synaptic membrane fraction contained two binding sites with dissociation constants of 0.6 nM (high affinity) and 0.9 μM (low affinity) present in that fraction to the respective extents of 6.6 and 0.86 pmol/g of whole brain. With 10 nM atropine (under which condition virtually all the binding is high affinity), the binding was shown to be reversible by addition of sufficient nonradioactive atropine, and little atropine hydrolysis was found. Study of the various subcellular fractions showed that the high-affinity binding was richest in synaptosomes, both on a total-

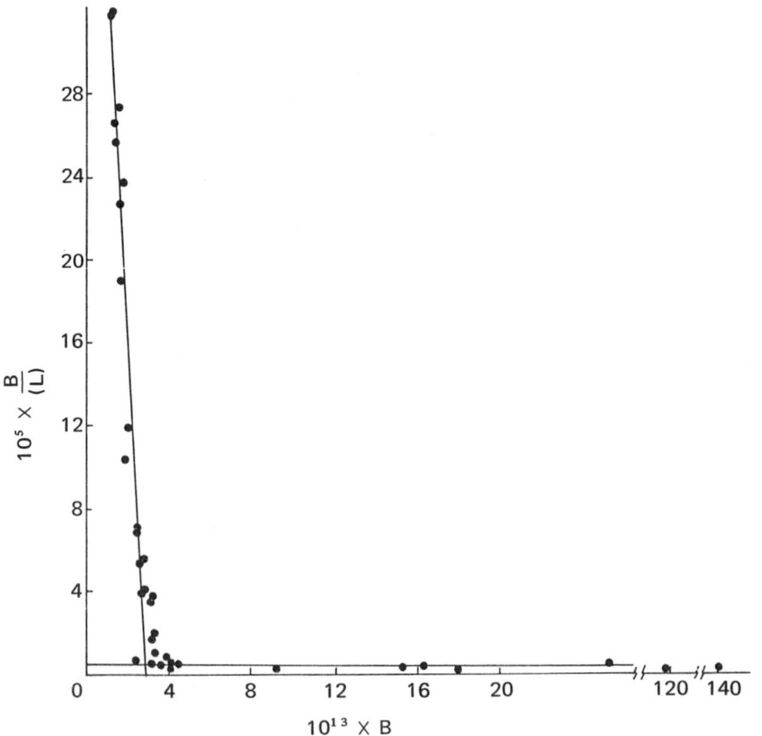

Fig. 2. Scatchard plot of binding of atropine to synaptic membranes from whole rat brains. *B*, Moles bound per 100 μg protein. *L*, Final free atropine concentration (molar). The concentration range is 40 pM to 5 μM. From Farrow and O'Brien (1973).

amount basis and a per-milligram-protein basis. However, a good deal of binding (60%) was distributed among the nonsynaptosomal fractions, primarily in membrane fractions of uncertain origin. Of 16 drugs tested at 50 nM against binding of 5 nM atropine, only scopolamine gave significant blockade, of 92%. Agents such as nicotine, hexamethonium, and decamethonium were entirely inactive, suggesting that the high-affinity receptor is a "pure" muscarinic type. By contrast, the receptor from electroplax is a "pure" nicotinic type, for its binding of radioactive acetylcholine is little affected by atropine (Eldefrawi *et al.*, 1972), and that from housefly brain appears to be "mixed," for it is sensitive to both nicotinic and muscarinic agents, including atropine (Eldefrawi and O'Brien, 1970). Supporting evidence that atropine binding was to a neural receptor was the fact that no binding occurred to kidney or lung homogenates. A little binding was found to liver mitochondria, a fact tentatively attributed to their content of atropinesterase, an enzyme lacking in brain.

Recently, Schleifer and Eldefrawi (1973) used an identical technique to study atropine binding to the lysed mitochondrial fraction from whole mouse brain; this fraction contains synaptosomes as well as mitochondria and myelin. Their findings (Table I) were in quite good agreement with the data on rat brain synaptosomes: they found for the mouse a low-affinity binding of almost the same affinity as that in rat brain but of three times the amount and a high-affinity binding of fourfold less affinity and six times the amount. However, the amounts of high-affinity atropine sites (39 pmol/g) were well in excess of the 5.6 pmol/g of acetylcholine-binding sites which they found. Unfortunately, atropine binding was measured with a crude mitochondrial fraction, whereas the acetylcholine binding was measured with the synaptosomal membrane fraction. Consequently, one must have reservations about the authors' assertion that the discrepancy between the amounts of atropine and acetylcholine binding means that atropine binds to numerous sites in addition to the acetylcholine sites.

An indirect approach to labeling atropine sites was taken by Takagi and Takahashi (1968). The nitrogen mustard derivative dibenamine (Fig. 3)

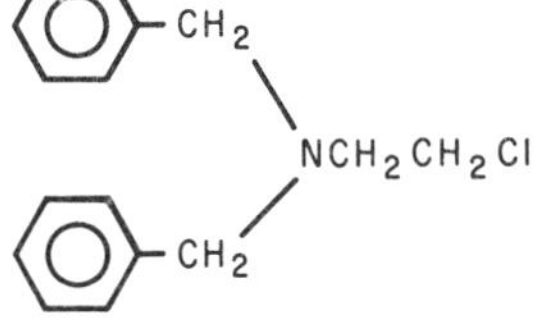

$$(C_6H_5CH_2)_2NCH_2CH_2Cl$$

Fig. 3. Structure of dibenamine.

reacts irreversibly with acetylcholine receptors as well as with numerous other molecules. They protected the atropine-binding sites in smooth muscle of dog intestine by incubating with nonradioactive atropine while reacting the other dibenamine-binding sites with nonradioactive dibenamine. Then they washed the preparation and treated it with ^{3}H-dibenamine to react with the now-exposed atropine sites. Some preliminary results were obtained which suggested the proteinaceous character of the atropine-binding macromolecules, but control experiments showed that most dibenamine (73%) bound to atropine-insensitive sites, so the potential errors were very high.

A quite different experimental approach to binding has been used by the De Robertis group (Gonzalez-Rodriguez *et al.*, 1970). They have used chloroform–methanol extracts of bovine cerebral cortex, subfractionated by elution from a Sephadex LH20 column with organic solvent mixes whose polarity is increased in a stepwise fashion. One such subfraction showed changes in lightscattering and polarized fluorescence which increased with increasing atropine concentration up to 10^{-5} M. The effect of 10^{-5} M atropine was reduced about 36% by 1 mM acetylcholine and 57% by 1 mM homatropine.

This whole approach has been questioned on several grounds. First, Levinson and Keynes (1972) have reported that the elution technique employed simply creates solvent fronts that dissociate ligands from binding to the column; they were able to repeat the experiments with protein-free preparations. Second, the same technique, using labeled acetylcholine, gives identical results with nonneural as with neural tissues (Eldefrawi, unpublished). Third, the binding of acetylcholine to electroplax extracts, when conducted in a chloroform–methanol medium (in this case employing equilibrium dialysis), has been shown to be blocked only by high concentrations of polar drugs, without any specificity (O'Brien *et al.*, 1973). Such nonspecificity echoes that reported by De Robertis *et al.* (1969), who found that the effect of atropine sulfate on light scattering in chloroform–methanol extracts could be mimicked by a variety of sulfates, such as dibenzylamine and eserine. By contrast, high specificity of receptor properties is retained in all the other isolation approaches described above. Fourth, the number of apparent binding sites found in *Torpedo* electroplax by this procedure is over 100 times larger than has been reported from two other laboratories using aqueous preparations (O'Brien *et al.*, 1972). Fifth, the acetylcholine receptor, judged by muscarone binding, is destroyed by organic solvents such as cold toluene (O'Brien *et al.*, 1970). Similarly, Molinoff and Potter (1972) reported that the receptor–α-bungarotoxin complex could not be extracted into chloroform–methanol nor could chloroform–methanol extracts of receptor bind to α-bungarotoxin (a toxin with very high and specific affinity for acetylcholine receptor).

The tentative conclusion is that in chloroform–methanol, polar drugs such as acetycholine partition into the polar regions of macromolecules in a nonspecific way and are displaced only by high concentrations of polar agents acting in nonstereospecific way. If this conclusion is correct, the events are entirely unrelated to cholinergic receptors.

V. REFERENCES

Arunlakshana, O., and Schild, H. O., 1959, Some quantitative uses of drug antagonists, *Brit. J. Pharmacol.* **14**:48.

Bandler, R. J., 1970, Cholinergic synapses in the lateral hypothalamus for the control of predatory aggression in the rat, *Brain Res.* **20**:409.

Bartholini, G., and Pletscher, A., 1971, Atropine-induced changes of cerebral dopamine turnover, *Experimentia* **27**:1302.

Beránek, R., and Vyskočil, F., 1967, The action of tubocurarine and atropine on the normal and denervated rat diaphragm, *J. Physiol.* (*Lond.*) **188**:53.

Beránek, R. B., and Vyskočil, F., 1968, The effect of atropine on the frog sartorius neuromuscular junction, *J. Physiol.* (*Lond.*) **195**:493.

Berkowitz, J. M., Warner, R. P., Janowitz, H. D., and Miller, I. F., 1970, Effects of some pharmacologic agents on gastric cation secretion: Ratio of hydrogen to potassium ions, *Proc. Soc. Exptl. Biol. Med.* **135**:804.

Bertels-Meeuws, M. M., and Polak, R. L., 1968, Influence of antimuscarinic substances on *in vitro* synthesis of acetylcholine by rat cerebral cortex, *Brit. J. Pharmacol.* **33**:368.

Bourdois, P. S., Mitchell, J. F., and Szerb, J. C., 1971, Effect of atropine on acetylcholine release from cerebral cortical slices stimulated at different frequencies, *Brit. J. Pharmacol.* **42**:640P.

Burn, J. H., and Rand, M. J., 1965, Acetylcholine in adrenergic transmission, *Ann. Rev. Pharmacol.* **5**:163.

Burn, J. H., Rand, M. J., and Wien, R., 1963, The adrenergic mechanism in the nictitating membrane, *Brit. J. Pharmacol.* **20**:83.

Burnstock, G., Dumsday, B., and Smythe, A., 1972, Atropine resistant excitation of the urinary bladder: The possibility of transmission via nerves releasing a purine nucleotide, *Brit. J. Pharmacol.* **44**:451.

Bussell, L. J., 1940, Relation of atropine to adrenaline and sympathetic system, *J. Pharmacol. Exptl. Therap.* **69**:128.

Creese, R. C., and Taylor, D. B. T., 1965, Effect of atropine on the uptake of labeled carbachol by rat brain slices, *Life Sci.* **4**:1545.

Cullumbine, H., 1967, Muscarinic blocking drugs, in: *Physiological Pharmacology* (W. S. Root and F. G. Hofmann, eds.) Vol. 3C, pp. 324–357, Academic Press, New York.

Curtis, D. R., and Phillis, J. W., 1960, The action of procaine and atropine in spinal neurones, *J. Physiol.* (*Lond.*) **153**:17.

Curtis, D. R., and Ryall, R. W., 1966, The excitation of Renshaw cells by cholinomimetics, *Exptl. Brain Res.* **2**:66.

Dale, H. H., 1914, The action of certain esthers and esthers of choline and their relation to muscarine, *J. Pharmacol. Exptl. Therap.* **6**:147.

De Robertis, E., Gonzalez-Rodriguez, J., and Teller, D. N., 1969, The interaction between atropine sulphate and a proteolipid from cerebral cortex studied by light scattering, *FEBS Letters*, **4**:4.

Domino, E. F., Yamamoto, K., and Dren, A. T., 1968, Role of cholinergic mechanisms in states of wakefulness and sleep, *Prog. Brain. Res.* **28**:113.

Douglas, W. W., and Poisner, A. M., 1965, Preferential release of adrenaline from the adrenal medulla by muscarine and pilocarpine, *Nature* (*Lond.*) **208**:1102.

Dudar, J. D., and Szerb, J. C., 1969, The effect of topically applied atropine on resting and evoked cortical acetylcholine release, *J. Physiol* (*Lond.*) **203**:741.

Eldefrawi, A. T., and O'Brien, R. D., 1970, Binding of muscarone by extracts of housefly brain: Relationship to receptors for acetylcholine, *J. Neurochem.* **17**:1287.

Eldefrawi, M. E., Eldefrawi, A. T., Seifert, S., and O'Brien, R. D., 1972, Properties of lubrol-solubilized acetylcholine receptor from *Torpedo* electroplax, *Arch. Biochem. Biophys.* **150**:210.

Erikssen, J., 1969, Atropine psychosis, *Lancet*, p. 53 (Jan.).

Farrow, J. T., and O'Brien, R. D., 1973, Binding of atropine and muscarone to rat brain fractions and its relation to acetylcholine receptor, *Mol. Pharmacol.* **9**:33.

Flacke, W., and Gillis, R. A., 1960, Dual transmission in the stellate ganglion of the dog, *Naunyn-Schmiedeberg's Arch. Pharmakol.* **259**:165.

Fulgraff, G., Schmidt, L., and Azokwu, P., 1964, Über die Atropin resistente neuromuskulare Übertragung am Pelvicus-Colon-Praparat der Katze, *Arch. Int. Pharmacodyn. Therap.* **149**:537.

German, E., and Siddigrie, N., 1970, Atropine toxicity from eyedrops, *New Engl. J. Med.* **282**:689.

Gerschenfeld, H. M., Ascher, P., and Tauc, L., 1967, Two different excitatory transmitters acting on a single molluscan neurone, *Nature* (*Lond.*) **28**:358.

Giarman, N. J., and Pepeu, G., 1964, The influence of centrally acting cholinolytic drugs on brain acetylcholine levels, *Brit. J. Pharmacol. Chemotherap.* **23**:123.

Goldenberg, M. M., 1969, Tachyphylaxis to the inhibitory action of atropine on the cholinergic response to nicotine *in vitro*, *Arch. Int. Pharmacodyn. Therap.* **180**:264.

Gonzalez-Rodriguez, J., La Torre, J. L., and De Robertis, E., 1970, The interaction between atropine sulfate and a proteolipid from cerebral cortex studied by polarization of fluorescence, *Mol. Pharmacol.* **6**:122.

Gray, G. W., and Seevers, M. H., 1955, *In vivo* observations on the nature of atropine tachyphylaxis exhibited by intestinal smooth muscle, *J. Pharmacol.* **113**:319.

Gray, G. W., Hendershot, L. C., Whitrock, R. M., and Seevers, M. H., 1955, Influence of the parasympathetic nerves and their relation to the action of atropine in the ileum and colon of the dog, *Am. J. Physiol.* **181**:679.

Hahn, R. A., and Patil, P. N., 1972, Salivation induced by prostaglandin $F_{2\alpha}$ and modification of the response by atropine and physostigmine, *Brit. J. Pharmacol.* **44**:527.

Hayes, W. J., 1965, Parathion poisoning and its treatment, *J. Am. Med. Ass.* **192**:135.

Hirschowitz, B. I., O'Leary, D. K., and Marks, I. N., 1960, Effects of atropine on synthesis and secretion of pepsinogen in the rat, *Am. J. Physiol.* **198**:108.

Innes, I. R., and Nickerson, M., 1965, Drugs inhibiting the action of acetylcholine on structures innervated by postganglionic parasympathetic nerves (antimuscarinic or atropinic drugs), in: *The Pharmacological Basis of Therapeutics*, 3rd ed. (L. S. Goodman and A. Gilman, eds.), pp. 521–545, Macmillan, New York.

Johansson, I., Lundell, L., and Svensson, S. E., 1971, Inhibition of gastric secretion by atropine in conscious rats, *J. Physiol.* (*Lond.*) **217**:723.

Karczmar, A. G., ed., 1970, *Anticholinesterase Agents*, Vol. 1, Pergamon Press, New York.

Kirschner, L. B., 1955, The effect of atropine and the curares on the active transport of sodium by the skin of *Rana esculenta, J. Cell. Comp. Physiol.* **45**:89.

Koelle, G. B., ed., 1963, *Cholinesterases and Anticholinsterase Agents,* Springer, Berlin.

Levinson, S. R., and Keynes, R. D., 1972, Isolation of acetylcholine receptors by chloroform–methanol extraction: Artifacts arising in use of Sephadex LH-20 columns, *Biochim. Biophys. Acta* **288**:241.

Loewi, O., 1921, Über humorale Übertragbarkeit der Herznervenwirkung, *Pflüger's Arch. Ges. Physiol.* **189**:239.

Loewi, O., and Navratil, E., 1926, Über humorale Übertragbarkeit der Herznervenwirkung. X. Uber das Schicksal des Vagusstoffes, *Pflüger's Arch. Ges. Physiol.* **214**:678.

Luduena, F. P., and Branin, M. J., 1966, Adrenolytic activity of atropine, (+)-hyoscyamine, atroscine, homatropine and related compounds, *J. Pharm. Sci.* **55**:280.

MacIntosh, F. C., 1963, Synthesis and storage of acetylcholine in nervous tissue, *Can. J. Biochem. Physiol.* **41**:2555.

Madill, H. D., Stewart, W. C., and Savoie, M. L., 1968, Central and peripheral anticholinergic potency of some drugs antagonistic to anticholinesterase poisoning, *Can. J. Physiol. Pharmacol.* **46**:559.

Mikikits, W., Mortara, A., and Spector, R. G., 1970, Effect of drugs on red cell fragility, *Nature* (*Lond.*) **225**:1150.

Mitchell, J. F., 1963, The spontaneous and evoked release of acetylcholine from the cerebral cortex, *J. Physiol.* (*Lond.*) **165**:98.

Molenaar, P. C., and Polak, R. L., 1970, Stimulation by atropine of acetylcholine release and synthesis in cortical slices from rat brain, *Brit. J. Pharmacol.* **40**:406.

Molinoff, P. B., and Potter, L. T., 1972, Isolation of the cholinergic receptor protein of *Torpedo* electric tissue, *Advan. Biochem. Psychopharmacol.* **6**:111.

Monti, J. H., Sala, M. A., Otegui, J. T., Benedetti, W. L., and Grino, E., 1970, Inhibition of ovarian compensatory hypertrophy by implants of atropine in the hypothalamus, *Experientia* **26**:1263.

Morisset, J., and Webster, P. D., 1970, Effects of atropine on pigeon pancreas, *Am. J. Physiol.* **219**:1286.

O'Brien, R. D., 1960, *Toxic Phosphorus Esters*, Academic Press, New York.

O'Brien, R. D., Gilmour, L. P., and Eldefrawi, M. E., 1970, A muscarone-binding material in electroplax and its relation to the acetylcholine receptor. II. Dialysis assay, *Proc. Natl. Acad. Sci.* **65**:438.

O'Brien, R. D., Eldefrawi, M. E., Eldefrawi, A. T., and Farrow, J. T., 1971, Binding of cholinergic ligands to electroplaxes and brain tissues, in: *Cholinergic Ligand Interactions* (D. J. Triggle, ed.) pp. 49–65, Academic Press, New York.

O'Brien, R. D., Eldefrawi, M. E., and Eldefrawi, A. T., 1972, Isolation of acetylcholine receptors, *Ann. Rev. Pharmacol.* **12**:19.

O'Brien, R. D., Eldefrawi, M. E., and Eldefrawi, A. T., 1973, Isolation of functional acetylcholine receptor, in: *Drug Receptors* (H. P. Rang, ed.), Macmillan, London.

O'Brien, R. D., Thompson, W. R., and Gibson, R. E., 1974, A comparison of acetylcholine and α-bungarotoxin binding to soluble *Torpedo* receptor, in: *Neurochemistry of Cholinergic Receptors* (E. De Robertis and J. Schacht, eds.) Raven Press, New York.

Orozlau, S. I., and Maengweyn-Davies, G. D., 1962*a*, The binding of atropine to bovine serum albumin, *Biochem. Pharmacol.* **11**:1203.

Orozlau, S. I., and Maengweyn-Davies, G. D., 1962*b*, The influence of acetylcholine on the binding of atropine to bovine serum albumin, *Biochem. Pharmacol.* **11**:1213.

Paton, W. D. M., and Rang, H. P., 1966, The uptake of atropine and related drugs by intestinal smooth muscle of the guinea-pig in relation to acetylcholine receptors, *Proc. Roy. Soc. Lond. Ser. B* **163**:2.

Phillis, J. W., 1970, *The Pharmacology of Synapses*, Pergamon Press, Oxford.

Pickering, J. W., 1896, Experiments on the hearts of mammalian and chick-embryos with special reference to action of electric currents, *J. Physiol.* (*Lond.*) **20**:165.

Polak, R. L., 1971, Stimulating action of atropine on the release of acetylcholine by rat cerebral cortex *in vitro, Brit. J. Pharmacol.* **41**:600.

Purcell, M., 1966, Atropine poisoning in infancy, *Brit. Med. J.* **5489**:738.

Quigley, J. P., 1937, Diminished effectiveness of second administration of atropine or novatropine: Mechanism of recovery, *Proc. Soc. Exptl. Biol. Med.* **36**:450.

Rinaldi, F., 1965, Direct action of atropine on the cerebral cortex of the rabbit, *Prog. Brain Res.* **16**:229.

Rinaldi, F., and Himwich, H. E., 1955, Alerting responses and actions of atropine and cholinergic drugs, *A.M.A. Arch. Neurol. Psychiat.* **73**:387.

Rosenblum, I., and Rosenblum, G., 1969, Effect of drugs and chemicals on subcellular organelles: Mitochondrial shrinking and autonomic agents, *Arch. Int. Pharmacodyn. Therap.* **181**:394.

Rudick, J., Werther, J. L., Chapman, M. L., and Janowitz, H. D., 1970, Ionic flux across the gastric mucosa: Effects of atropine on the permeability of fundus and antrum, *Proc. Soc. Exptl. Biol. Med.* **135**:605.

Schleifer, L. S., and Eldefrawi, M. E., 1974, Identification of the nicotinic and muscarinic acetylcholine receptors in subcellular fractions of mouse brain, *Neuropharmacol.*, **13**:53.

Schuberth, J. S., and Sundwall, A., 1967, Effects of some drugs on the uptake of acetylcholine in cortex slices of mouse brain, *J. Neurochem.* **14**:807.

Sheu, Y -S., George, R., and Jenden, D. J., 1969, Comparison of the effects of atropine sulfate and procaine hydrochloride on nerve conduction, *Experientia* **25**:1053.

Soldani, G., del Tacca, M., Gïacomelli, A., and Creme, C., 1970, Nerve mediated response of the guinea-pig colon *in situ*: Activity of some anticholinergic drugs, *Arch. Int. Pharmacodyn. Therap.* **187**:329.

Spector, W. S., ed., 1956, *Handbook of Toxicology*, Vol. I, W. B. Saunders, Philadelphia.

Spehlmann, R., 1969, Acetylcholine facilitation, atropine block of synaptic excitation of cortical neurons, *Science* **165**:404.

Szerb, J. C., 1964, The effect of tertiary and quaternary atropine on cortical acetylcholine output and on the electroencephalogram in cats, *Can. J. Physiol. Pharmacol.* **42**:303.

Takagi, K. T., and Takahashi, A. T., 1968, Studies of separation and characterization of acetylcholine receptor labeled with tritiated dibenamine, *Biochem. Pharmacol.* **17**:1609.

Triggle, D. J., 1965, *Chemical Aspects of the Nervous System*, Academic Press, New York.

Webster, P. D., and Morisset, J., 1971, Effect of atropine on pigeon pancreas, *Proc. Soc. Exptl. Biol. Med.* **136**:245.

Wood, D. J., 1972, Excitation of intestinal muscle by atropine, tetrodotoxin and xylocaine, *Am. J. Physiol.* **222**:118.

Chapter 5

Neurotoxic Amino Acids

Graham A. R. Johnston

Department of Pharmacology
Australian National University
Canberra, Australia

I. INTRODUCTION

Some 200 amino acids have been isolated from plants, but only about 10% of these are normal constituents of mammalian nervous tissue. Many of the other 90% structurally resemble certain of those present in nervous tissue, such that they may compete with the corresponding "normal" amino acid at one or more of its receptor sites, with consequent adverse effects on the nervous system. These receptor sites for amino acids may be on enzymes, transport carriers, or synaptic membranes. With the increasing acceptance of the concept of particular amino acids, especially γ-aminobutyric acid (GABA), glycine, and glutamic and aspartic acids, functioning as major synaptic transmitters in the mammalian central nervous system (Curtis and Johnston, 1974), it appears likely that the neurotoxicity of certain plant amino acids results from interference with amino acid-mediated synaptic transmission. The "antimetabolite" properties of toxic amino acids, particularly in microorganisms, have been extensively studied and have been reviewed by Fowden *et al.* (1967); this chapter is concerned with some amino acids of plant and fungal origin that adversely influence the mammalian central nervous system after systemic administration.

The central nervous system is protected from amino acids in the circulation by what is loosely called the blood–brain barrier. This "barrier" is less efficient in immature than in mature mammals, and in mammals in certain states, e.g., malnutrition, than in healthy mammals. Thus both age and health influence the susceptibility of mammals to potentially neurotoxic amino acids. Elevation of the normal concentrations of certain amino acids in the central nervous system by systemic administration of relatively large amounts may also produce neurotoxic effects. These amino acids occur, often in very large amounts, in plant foodstuffs, and although their ingestion by healthy adults usually presents no problems, there may be some cause for concern when neonates or ill adults are involved.

As isolation and identification techniques improve, new amino acids continue to be discovered in natural products. It is likely that many of these substances, in addition to the amino acids reviewed here, contribute to the neurotoxic properties of the natural products. The Specialist Reports of The Chemical Society on *Amino-Acids, Peptides and Proteins*, published annually since 1968, list the structures of new naturally occurring amino acids, but information regarding the pharmacological–toxicological properties of these substances is more difficult to obtain.

II. ACIDIC AMINO ACIDS

Many amino acids having one amino and two carboxylic groups, or their equivalents, may be described as "excitant" amino acids, as they excite most single neurons when administered locally by microelectrophoretic techniques (Curtis and Watkins, 1965; Curtis and Crawford, 1969). Furthermore, these amino acids cause convulsions when administered either intraventricularly to adult mammals (Crawford, 1963) or intraperitoneally to immature mammals (Johnston, 1973) and also produce degeneration of brain neurons when administered subcutaneously to immature mammals (Olney *et al*., 1971). Discussed in the following section are (A) β-*N*-oxalyl-L-α,β-diaminopropionic acid (Fig. 1), which is one of the most powerful neuronal excitants known and which may contribute to the clinical manifestations of neurolathyrism, and (B) L-glutamic acid, which is probably a major excitatory synaptic transmitter in the mammalian central nervous system.

$HOOCCONHCH_2CH(NH_2)COOH$	$HOOCCH_2CH_2CH(NH_2)COOH$
β-N-OXALYL-L-α, β-DIAMINOPROPIONIC ACID	L-GLUTAMIC ACID

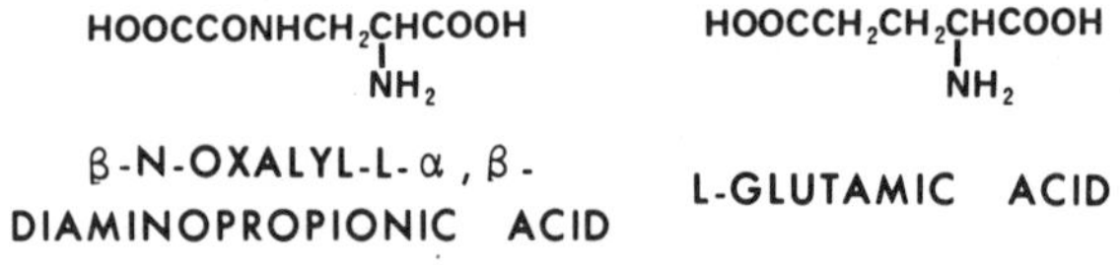

Fig. 1. Neurotoxic acidic amino acids.

A. β-*N*-Oxalyl-L-α,β-diaminopropionic Acid

Consumption of the seeds of the chick pea *Lathyrus sativus* can lead to the crippling disease known as lathyrism (Ganapathy and Dwivedi, 1961; Dastur, 1962; Sarma and Padmanaban, 1969, Rao *et al.*, 1969). This disease, referred to in the ancient Hindu treatise *Bravaprakasa*, and by Hippocrates, Pliny, and Galen, continues to be a public health problem in the central parts of India, especially during famine when *Lathyrus sativus* seeds form the main part of the diet. It is prevalent among horses and cattle as well as humans. *Lathyrus sativus* is a hardy winter crop, growing on almost all types of soil even under conditions of drought. This disease is not to be confused with *osteolathyrism* or *experimental lathyrism* terms, which refer to skeletal changes following ingestion of the sweet pea *Lathyrus odoratus*. Cyano derivatives (see Section IV), which are not found in *Lathyrus sativus*, appear to be responsible for osteolathyrism. Selye (1957) has used the term *neurolathyrism* to distinguish the classical disease produced by *Lathyrus sativus* from osteolathyrism.

Neurolathyrism is characterized by muscular rigidity, spastic paralysis of the legs, and in extreme cases death. In most cases on record, the onset of the disease is relatively sudden. It generally appears whenever a diet consisting of one-third to one-half of *Lathyrus sativus* seeds is consumed for a period of 3–6 months. Various claims have been made regarding the factor(s) responsible for the disease, but no adequate proof has been advanced to substantiate any one claim. It is possible that many factors are involved, perhaps with synergistic actions. These factors include (1) an acidic amino acid, β-*N*-oxalyl-L-α,β-diaminopropionic acid (Rao *et al.*, 1964, Murti *et al.*, 1964), (2) a phenol compound of unknown structure whose neurotoxic effects are potentiated by certain amino acids (Nagarajan *et al.*, 1966), and (3) a glycoside, which may be *N*-β-D-glycopyranosyl-*N*-α,L-arabinosyl-α,β-diaminopropionitrile (Rukmini, 1968). The following discussion is restricted to β-*N*-oxalyl-L-α,β-diaminopropionic acid (ODAP), which is present in the *Lathyrus sativus* seeds in concentrations ranging from 0.5 to 2% of the dry weight and is neurotoxic when administered to mammals.

1. *Chemistry*

The structure of ODAP (Fig. 1) isolated from *Lathyrus sativus* seeds has been determined unequivocally by degradation to, and synthesis from, L-α,β-diaminopropionic acid and oxalic acid moieties (Rao *et al.*, 1964; Murti *et al.*, 1964). The apparent pK values at 20°C for ODAP are 1.95, 2.95, and 9.25 (Rao *et al.*, 1964) and indicate that it is a stronger acid than glutamate. It can be converted into an approximately equimolar mixture of α- and β-*N*-oxalyl derivatives by heating at 80°C for 17 hr in aqueous solution (Bell and O'Donovan, 1966). Analytical procedures for the detection and estimation of ODAP have usually involved paper electrophoresis and development of a purple ninhydrin color (Sarma and Padmanaban, 1969), but the gas chromatographic analysis of trimethylsilyl or *N*-trifluoroacetyl derivatives of ODAP might provide a more precise procedure (Mehta *et al.*, 1972).

2. *Metabolism*

a. Plants. ODAP is synthesized in *Lathyrus sativus* seeds from oxalyl-coenyzme A and L-α,β-diaminopropionic acid (Malathi *et al.*, 1967, 1968, 1970; Johnston and Lloyd, 1967). The specificity of the oxalyl transferase reaction for L-α,β-diaminopropionic acid is questionable: amino groups other than the β-amino group of L-α,β-diaminopropionic acid, and also hydroxyl groups, can be oxalylated by extracts of *Lathyrus sativus* (Johnston and Lloyd, 1967; Malathi *et al.*, 1968, 1970). *O*-Oxalylhomoserine has been isolated from *Lathyrus sativus* (Przybylska and Pawelkiewicz, 1965), and there is some evidence for the occurrence of oxalyl derivatives of alanine, glycine, and serine (Rukmini, 1968) and the α-*N*-oxalyl isomer of ODAP (Bell and O'Donovan, 1966). Serine is not a precursor of ODAP in germinating seeds of *Lathyrus sativus* (Roy, 1969). Oxalyl-coenzyme A is synthesized from oxalic acid, ATP, and coenzyme A by the action of an oxalyl-coenzyme A synthetase, which appears to be very similar to an enzyme found in extracts of pea seeds, *Pisum sativum* (Giovanelli, 1966).

b. Mammals. Neither ODAP nor oxalyl-coenzyme A synthetase activity has been detected in extracts of cat and rat brain (Johnston and Lloyd, 1967). ODAP appears to be a substrate for rat kidney L-aspartate:2-oxoglutarate aminotransferase, and some 5–10% of ODAP administered to adult rats undergoes transamination to yield *N*-oxalyl-β-aminopyruvic acid, while 50–70% is extracted unchanged in the urine within 24 hr (Cheema *et al.*, 1971a). In adult rats, only traces of ODAP can be found in the brain after intraperitoneal injection, whereas appreciable amounts are found in the brain of immature rats so treated (Cheema *et al.*, 1969*a*, 1971*b*).

3. *Occurrence*

ODAP is generally confined to the genus *Lathyrus*, where it occurs in more than 20 species (Bell, 1964; Bell and O'Donovan, 1966), and appears to be absent from the related genus *Vicia*, though α,β-diaminopropionic acid has been found in *Vicia baicalensis* (Bell and Tirimanna, 1965). The occurrence of ODAP in two species of *Crotalaria* raises the possibility that the toxicity of these plants may not be due solely to the presence of pyrrolizidine alkaloids (Bell, 1968).

4. *Toxicity*

a. Adult Animals. Healthy adult animals appear to tolerate intraperitoneal injection of ODAP (Rao *et al.*, 1964) but succumb to ODAP if the blood–brain barrier is effectively bypassed by the route of administration. Thus approximately 0.006 mmol/kg (1mg/kg) of ODAP administered intraventricularly to adult mice produces convulsions (Watkins *et al.*, 1966; Rao *et al.*, 1969), as does approximately 0.01 mmol/kg administered intracranially to adult rats (Rao *et al.*, 1969). Approximately 0.024 mmol/kg administered intrathecally to adult monkeys results in a flaccid paralysis of the hind limbs (Mani *et al.*, 1971), in distinct contrast to the spastic paralysis which characterizes neurolathyrism. Acidotic adult rats convulse following intraperitoneal injection of approximately 2.2 mmol/kg of ODAP, presumably as a consequence of a lower blood–brain barrier compared to that of healthy adult rats (Cheema *et al.*, 1969*b*).

b. Immature Animals. ODAP produces convulsions in 1- to 2-day-old chicks and 10- to 12-day-old rats in doses of 1–3 mmol/kg administered intraperitoneally (Rao *et al.*, 1964; Murti *et al.*, 1964; Cheema *et al.*, 1969*a*; Lakshmanan *et al.*, 1971; Johnston, 1973). The convulsions induced by ODAP are of the clonic flexor type with extensor spasms; subconvulsive doses produce a gross hyperactivity with running and leaping movements (Rao *et al.*, 1969). ODAP also affects young pups and guinea pigs, producing an ataxic gait, dragging of the legs, and rigidity of the neck (Rao *et al.*, 1969).

5. *Mechanism of Action*

a. Excitation of Central Neurons. When administered extracellularly, ODAP excites Betz cells in the cerebral cortex and interneurons in the spinal cord of cats anesthetized with pentobarbitone sodium (Watkins *et al.*, 1966). The amino acid is more effective than L-glutamic acid and is in fact the most potent excitant amino acid yet tested that occurs naturally, only the synthetic *N*-methyl-D-aspartic acid being more potent. From structure–activity studies of a series of convulsant and excitant amino acids, it appears likely that the ability of ODAP to produce convulsions when administered intraperitoneally to immature rats and the excitant action of ODAP on feline neurons have the same basic mechanism, the direct depolarization of central neurons.

b. Effects on Levels of Various Brain Constituents. Immature rats during ODAP-induced convulsions have, compared to normal rats, elevated levels of glutamine, inorganic phosphate, and lactic acid, decreased levels of acetylcholine, glycogen, and phosphocreatine, and unchanged levels of aspartic acid, GABA, glutamic acid, and urea (Cheema *et al.*, 1969*a*; 1970). It has been suggested that these changes are typical of the convulsant state (Cheema *et al.*, 1970) and thus do not necessarily reflect the mechanism(s) whereby ODAP induces this state.

c. Effects on Brain Enzymes. ODAP administered to immature rats causes increased apparent activities of acid protease, adenylic acid deaminase, aspartate:2-oxoglutarate aminotransferase, aspartate:pyruvate aminotransferase, glutaminase, and transglutaminase and does not influence the apparent activities of adenosine deaminase, glutamic acid decarboxylase, glutamic acid dehydrogenase, glutamine synthetase, and guanosine deaminase (Cheema *et al.*, 1971*b*). Tracer studies indicate that these effects were observed when the overall concentration of ODAP in the brain was 7×10^{-5} M. In studies of these enzymatic activities *in vivo*, 10^{-4}M ODAP did not affect any of the measured activities (Cheema *et al.*, 1971*b*; Mehta *et al.*, 1972). Thus, as with the alterations in brain constituents, the changes in enzymatic activities in the brain induced *in vivo* by ODAP may be secondary rather than direct effects of this neurotoxin.

ODAP, at 5×10^{-4} M, has been reported to stimulate the glutaminase activity of rat brain mitochondria (Duque-Magalhaes and Packer, 1972) and, at 5×10^{-2} M, to inhibit the glutamate decarboxylase, GABA:2-oxoglutarate and alanine:2-oxoglutarate aminotransferases in homogenates of 1-day-old chick brain (Jacob *et al.*, 1967).

d. Effects on Transport Systems. ODAP appears to be a competitive inhibitor (K_i approximately 0.6×10^{-3} M) of glutamic acid uptake in rat brain mitochondria (Duque-Magalhaes and Packer, 1972) and of glutamic acid uptake (K_i 10^{-4} M) in resting yeast cells (Mehta *et al.*, 1972). ODAP, at 10^{-4} M, did not influence the high-affinity uptake of glutamic acid by rat brain slices (Balcar and Johnston, 1972).

e. Effect on Brain Lysosomes. ODAP, *in vivo* following intraperitoneal injection (2 mmol/kg) and also *in vitro* at 10^{-4} M, causes a significant liberation of degradative enzymes from 2-day-old chick brain lysosomes, perhaps as a result of damage to the lysosomal membrane (Lakshmanan *et al.*, 1971). Lysosomal damage has been reported in a variety of neurological diseases (Holtzman, 1969).

6. *Conclusion*

ODAP may mimic the postsynaptic action of natural excitatory transmitters in the CNS. The gross convulsant action of ODAP may result primarily from a direct excitant action on central neurons, and this may lead to a series of secondary changes in various brain constituents, enzymatic activities, transport systems, and cellular organelles. At present, it is not known whether ODAP actually enters cells in the CNS: ODAP could cause metabolic changes inside cells as a result of its extracellular action on neurons. The more subtle neurotoxic effects of ODAP, such as those which follow prolonged ingestion, have not been satisfactorily investigated. Nevertheless, it is highly probable that ODAP does contribute to the clinical manifestations of lathyrism.

B. L-Glutamic Acid

L-Glutamic acid in the form of its monosodium salt has been used in Far Eastern cookery since ancient times as the dried powder of an indigenous seaweed; it was characterized as the active principle and its flavor described as the "glutamic taste" by Ikeda (1912). Monosodium glutamate is also widely used in Western cooking as a taste enhancer, and thousands of tons are consumed yearly. This widespread use does not appear to present a problem to healthy adults when consumed in a balanced diet. There are reasons, however, to consider the consumption of excessive amounts of glutamic acid by infants as a possible cause of brain damage, the effects of which may not be apparent until later in life (Olney, 1969, 1971; but see also Prabhu and Oester, 1971). It must be remembered that glutamic acid is the most abundant amino acid in human milk, which contains 0.8–2 mM glutamic acid, and thus the breast-fed infant normally receives appreciable quantities (Stegink *et al.*, 1972). Furthermore, glutamic acid was at one time considered beneficial in the treatment of epilepsy (Waelsch and Price, 1944) and of mental retardation (Albert *et al.*, 1956).

1. *Chemistry and Biochemistry*

L-Glutamic acid (Fig. 1) has *p*K values of 2.16, 4.32, and 9.96 at 20°C (Neuberger, 1936). The metabolism of glutamic acid in the CNS is exceedingly complex. There are at least two major metabolic "pools" of glutamic acid (van den Berg, 1973; Balázs *et al.*, 1973), and at least two kinetically distinct transport systems take up extracellular glutamic acid in the CNS (Logan and Synder, 1972; Balcar and Johnston, 1972). Glutamic acid is also transported into brain mitochondria (Azzi *et al.*, 1967). *De novo* synthesis of glutamic acid occurs by transamination of the tricarboxylic acid intermediate 2-oxoglutaric acid with a variety of amino donors, and glutamic acid can be metabolized reversibly to glutamine, peptides such as glutathione, proteins, and intermediates of the tricarboxylic acid and urea cycles. Of particular interest in the CNS is the decarboxylation of glutamic acid to the inhibitory transmitter GABA.

2. *Toxicity*

a. Adult Animals. In common with other acidic amino acids which excite neurons, glutamic acid produces convulsions in adult animals when administered in such a way as to bypass or overcome the blood–brain barrier. Intraventricular glutamic acid (approximately 0.04 mmol/kg, 6 mg/kg) produces hyperactivity in mice (Crawford, 1963), and intracisternal glutamic acid (0.025–0.05 mmol/kg) results in seizures in rats (Hennecke and Wiechert, 1970). Intraperitoneal glutamic acid (20 mmol/kg) produces seizures in rats: EEG recordings show that while pyridoxine-deficient animals exhibit higher amplitudes of responses, no difference is apparent in the susceptibility to or the rate of onset of seizures between deficient and normal rats (Stewart, Coursin and Bhagavan, 1972).

Oral glutamic acid (7 mmol/kg) does not appear to influence the threshold for metrazole-induced convulsions in mice and rats, nor does intraperitoneal glutamic acid (20 mmol/kg) modify the seizure threshold in cats and monkeys (Goodman *et al.*, 1946); however, intraperitoneal glutamic acid (7 mmol/kg) has been reported to decrease this threshold in mice (Prabhu and Oester, 1971). Intraperitoneal glutamic acid (2 mmol/kg) in mice reduces the rate of uptake of glucose from the blood by the brain (Creasey and Malawista, 1971).

b. Immature Animals. Intraperitoneal glutamic acid (14–20 mmol/kg) produces convulsions in 7- to 15-day-old rats, the intragastric dose to produce similar effects being approximately double the intraperitoneal dose (Mushahwar and Koeppe, 1971; Johnston, 1973). Subcutaneous or oral glutamic acid (6–24 mmol/kg) results in acute degeneration of cells of the inner layer of the retina (Lucas and Newhouse, 1957; Potts *et al.*, 1960; Cohen, 1967; Olney, 1969) and of the arcuate nucleus of the hypothalamus (Olney, 1969; 1971; Arees and Mayer, 1970; Burde *et al.*, 1971). Immature monkeys are similarly affected by subcutaneous or oral glutamic acid (Olney and Sharpe, 1969; Oser *et al.*, 1971; Olney *et al.*, 1971).

The acute degeneration of neurons produced in these brain regions by glutamic acid, and by other excitant amino acids such as aspartic, cysteic, and homocysteic acids, is characterized by massive swelling and organelle degeneration in postsynaptic elements of the neuron cell body and dendrites. These changes become apparent within an hour of subcutaneous injection, and within 5 hr pyknosis of the neuronal cell nuclei occurs. No changes are detected in glial or vascular components of these brain regions, and the presynaptic components of the neurons also appear to remain intact histologically (Olney and Sharpe, 1969; Olney *et al.*, 1971; Burde *et al.*, 1971; but see also Arees and Mayer, 1970).

3. *Mechanism of Action*

a. Excitation of Central Neurons. L-Glutamic acid, administered microelectrophoretically, excites neurons in all regions of the central nervous system (Curtis and Crawford, 1969) and may be the major excitatory synaptic transmitter (Curtis and Johnston, 1974). This excitant action is the result of depolarization of the neurons caused by a change in membrane permeability, which includes a tetrodotoxin-insensitive influx of sodium ions. Structure–activity studies show that there is a close parallel between (1) ability to excite neurons, (2) ability to produce convulsions, and (3) ability to produce degeneration of neurons (Curtis and Watkins, 1965; Olney *et al.*, 1971; Johnston, 1973). The anatomical changes in the immature brain induced by the excitant amino acids appear to be consistent with a prime site of action being the postsynaptic elements of neurons.

b. Effects of Levels on Various Brain Constituents and Enzymatic Activities. Increased dietary glutamic acid for 16 weeks following weaning leads to elevated succinate, decreased GABA, and no change in glutamic acid, glutamine, aspartic acid, DNA, and protein levels of glutamic acid decarboxylase activity in rat brain (Prosky and O'Dell, 1971). On the other hand, systemic administration of glutamic acid to immature rats and mice produces elevated levels of glutamine and unchanged levels of glutamic acid, GABA, 2-oxoglutaric acid, ATP, glucose, glycogen inorganic phosphate, lactic acid, and phosphocreatinine (Mushahwar and Koeppe, 1971; Thurston and Warren, 1971). As equivalent doses of glycine also elevate brain glutamine, it is unlikely that the toxicity of glutamic acid is due to this change in glutamine level (Mushahwar and Koeppe, 1971).

In general, the gross brain levels of glutamic acid are *not* appreciably influenced by systematically administered glutamic acid. Himwich and Himwich (1955) showed that systemic glutamic acid (13 mmol/kg intraperitoneal) could raise the brain levels of glutamic acid in 1-day-old rats but not in 9- to 11-day-old rats, and Perez and Olney (1972) found that similar doses of glutamic acid administered subcutaneously to 4-day-old mice produced an approximately fourfold increase in the glutamic acid levels of the arcuate nucleus and only a small change in the glutamic acid levels of the ventromedial hypothalamus and lateral thalamus. The time course of the changes in glutamic acid levels in the plasma and the arcuate nucleus suggested that this nucleus was actively accumulating glutamic acid. It is in the arcuate nucleus that neuronal degeneration is first noted following glutamic acid administration (Olney *et al.*, 1971), and clearly future neurochemical studies of glutamic acid action should include detailed examination of this brain region.

c. In Vitro Studies. Glutamic acid (10^{-3} M) and related excitant amino acids inhibit protein synthesis in rat brain slices, but not in rat kidney slices (Orrego and Lipmann, 1967). In contrast, glutamic acid (5×10^{-3} M) stimulates protein synthesis in cell-free extracts of immature rat brain (Tewari and Baxter, 1969). Glutamic acid (10^{-3} to 10^{-2} M) depletes the ATP content of brain slices (Banay-Schwartz *et al.*, 1971; Gruener, 1972). Glutamic acid ($1–5 \times 10^{-3}$ M) and related excitant amino acids promote a rapid influx of sodium and calcium ions and an efflux of potassium ions from slices of neocortex (Harvey and McIlwain, 1968; Ramsey and McIlwain, 1970). Tetrodotoxin partially inhibits the effects of glutamic acid on ion movements in brain slices (McIlwain *et al.*, 1969; Ramsey and McIlwain, 1970), and there is evidence to indicate that the effect of glutamic acid on sodium ion movements in such slices is not restricted to neurons but may include glia (Okamoto and Quastel, 1970). L-Glutamic acid is taken up into brain slices and homogenates by at least two kinetically distinct transport systems (Logan and Snyder, 1972), and the processes of uptake, neuronal depolarization, and tetrodotoxin-sensitive sodium ion influx appear to be separate processses, as judged by apparent differences in substrate specificity and susceptibility to inhibitors (Balcar and Johnston, 1972).

It is clear from these *in vitro* studies that glutamic acid could directly and indirectly influence a variety of metabolic processes.

d. L-Glutamic Acid and Spreading Depression. Glutamic acid (10^{-2} M) applied topically to the cerebral cortex produces spreading depression (Van Harreveld, 1959; but see Do Carmo and Leão, 1972). The increase in transparency of the isolated retina produced by glutamic acid (0.2 to 5×10^{-3} M) may also be related to spreading depression (Van Harreveld and Fifkova, 1971). Spreading depression appears to be due to a reduction in cell excitability, perhaps due to excessive depolarization induced by L-glutamic acid, both the exogenous amino acid and that released synaptically. Inhibition is also likely to be involved, as many neurons are depressed without undergoing any initial apparent excitation (Phillis and Ochs, 1971).

e. Monosodium L*-Glutamate and the "Chinese Restaurant Syndrome."* Recent popular interest in monosodium L-glutamate as a neurotoxic amino acid stems from the report of Ho Man Kwok (1968) regarding what has become known as the "Chinese restaurant syndrome." This syndrome is characterized by a numbness or a burning sensation at the back of the neck, general weaknesses, and palpitations and results within 20 min from ingestion of monosodium glutamate in various food preparations (Schaumburg *et al.*, 1969). There is considerable variation (1.5–12 g) in the oral threshold doses among individuals. Due to the lack of experimental evidence, it is difficult to rationalize the mechanism(s) by which oral ingestion of monosodium glutamate produces the "Chinese restaurant syndrome" in susceptible individuals. The site of action is unknown and may be peripheral rather than central. Indeed, one study has suggested that the symptoms are due to parasympathomimetic effects of acetylcholine (Ghadimi and Kumar, 1972).

The taste-potentiating properties of monosodium glutamate may involve depolarization of peripheral taste receptors, analogous to the depolarization of central neurons by excitant amino acids, many of which can act as taste potentiators.

4. Conclusion

The neurotoxic properties of large doses of L-glutamic acid administered to experimental animals indicate that in human beings the ingestion of *excessively large amounts* of this amino acid by infants, or by ill adults may be unwise. This also probably applies to any of the excitant amino acids, e.g., ibotenic acid (see Section VA), which may be used as food additives, since both the taste-potentiating and neurotoxic properties are likely to have the same basis, i.e., membrane depolarization.

III. BASIC AMINO ACIDS

At least two basic amino acids that occur in toxic plants, L-α,γ-diaminobutyric and β-*N*-methyl-L-α,β-diaminopropionic acids (Fig. 2), produce neurological symptoms on administration to experimental animals.

A. L-α,γ-Diaminobutyric Acid

L-α,γ-Diaminobutyric acid (DAB) has been detected in 13 species of Lathyrus but is apparently absent in *Lathyrus sativus* and others implicated in neurolathyrism (Ressler *et al.*, 1961; Bell, 1964; Bell and O'Donovan,

$NH_2CH_2CH_2CHCOOH$ (with NH_2 on the α-carbon)

L-α,γ-DIAMINO BUTYRIC ACID

$CH_3NHCH_2CHCOOH$ (with NH_2 on the α-carbon)

β-N-METHYL-L-α,β-DIAMINOPROPIONIC ACID

Fig. 2. Neurotoxic basic amino acids.

1966). In ten of these species, DAB is accompanied by its α- and γ-N-oxalyl derivatives (Bell and O'Donovan, 1966). DAB is also found in a species of *Vicia* (Bell and Tirimanna, 1965) and in a large number of other species, especially those belonging to the Leguminosae and Cruciferae families (see Nigam and Ressler, 1966). In *Lathyrus sylvestris*, DAB appears to be synthesized from both aspartic acid and homoserine (Nigam and Ressler, 1966).

DAB has been found in very low amounts of bovine brain (Nakajima *et al.*, 1967). In rats, labeled DAB is oxidized to carbon dioxide, and β-alanine appears to be a major metabolite (Mushahwar and Koeppe, 1963).

Administration of DAB (0.5 mmol/kg, 50 mg/kg, subcutaneous) to rats produces characteristic neurological signs and death within 5 days (Vivanco *et al.*, 1966). L-Thyroxine administered simultaneously prevents development of these effects, which include hyperirritability, paralysis of the hind limbs, motor incoordination, and convulsions. Similar effects are also produced when DAB is administered to rats by stomach tube (Ressler *et al.*, 1961) or by intraperitoneal injection (O'Neal *et al.*, 1968) and are always delayed in onset at least 24 hr after DAB administration. Appreciable amounts of DAB and increased levels of GABA and glutamine can be detected in the brain at the time when neurological signs are observed (Vivanco *et al.*, 1966; O'Neal *et al.*, 1968; Chen *et al.*, 1972), although it has been suggested that the neurotoxicity of DAB is due primarily to effects on urea synthesis in the liver (O'Neal *et al.*, 1968).

DAB is an α-amino derivative of GABA, and thus it is not unexpected that DAB can interact with specific components of the GABA system in the CNS. Perhaps the increased GABA levels in the brain reflect this. DAB is a comparatively weak substrate for the GABA aminotransferase activity in extracts of beef brain (Baxter and Roberts, 1958) and a comparatively strong noncompetitive inhibitor of GABA uptake by rat brain slices (Iverson and Johnston, 1971). It is a weak depressant of the firing of feline spinal interneurons, which may indicate that it can activate the postsynaptic receptors for GABA on these neurons (Curtis and Watkins, 1960). Furthermore, the fact that DAB is found in the brain, albeit in very low concentration, may mean that it does have a function in the normal operation of the brain.

B. β-*N*-Methyl-L-α,β-diaminopropionic Acid

β-*N*-Methyl-L-α,β-diaminopropionic acid has been found in six species of *Cycas* (Polsky *et al.*, 1972), including *Cycas circinalis* from which it was isolated and characterized as the L-isomer (Vega *et al.*, 1968). The ingestion of cycad plant material by cattle causes ataxia with a characteristic "goose-stepping" gait; demyelination of isolated fibers in the spinal cord is found 2–4 weeks after development of these signs (Mason and Whiting, 1966). Furthermore, the incidence of amyotrophic lateral sclerosis among native people of Guam has been related to the use of the seeds of *C. circinalis* as a source of starch (Whiting, 1963). Administration of β-*N*-methyl-L-α,β-diaminopropionic acid (3–7 mmol/kg, 350–800 mg/kg, intraperitoneal) to young chicks produces convulsions within 6–8 hr, whereas the D-isomer is inactive at doses up to 14 mmol/kg (Vega *et al.*, 1968). The low concentration of the free and bound amino acid in *C. circinalis*, however, indicates, that it is unlikely to be the prime cause of the neurological disease (Polsky *et al.*, 1972).

IV. CYANOAMINO ACIDS

A. Effects

Amino acids containing a cyano substituent are usually toxic. β-(γ-L-Glutamyl)-aminopropionitrile appears to be the agent in the sweet pea *Lathyrus odoratus* responsible for osteolathyrism, which involves skeletal deformities rather than effects on the CNS (see Sarma and Padmanaban, 1969). While β-aminopropionitrile also exhibits osteolathyrogenic activity, the structurally related compound β-cyano-L-alanine (Fig. 3) has neurotoxic properties.

B. β-Cyano-L-alanine

β-Cyano-L-alanine occurs in the seeds of the common vetch *Vicia sativa* (Ressler, 1962) and in 15 other species of *Vicia* (Bell and Tirimanna,

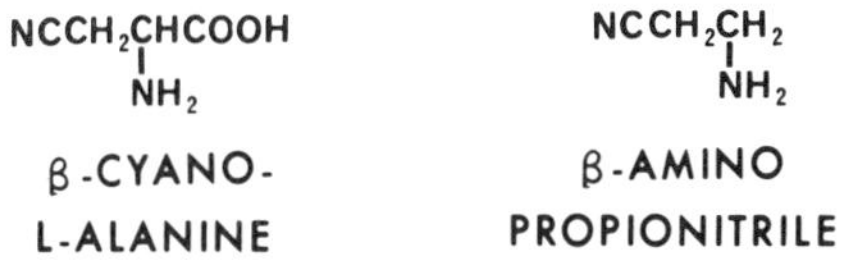

$NCCH_2CH(NH_2)COOH$	$NCCH_2CH_2NH_2$
β-CYANO-L-ALANINE	β-AMINO PROPIONITRILE

Fig. 3. Toxic cyanoamino acids.

1965). The γ-glutamyl derivative of β-cyano-L-alanine is also found in these *Vicia* species (Ressler *et al.*, 1963; Bell and Tirimanna, 1965). Neither compound occurs in any species of *Lathyrus* (Rao *et al.*, 1969). Experimental animals fed diets containing *Vicia sativa* develop abnormal neurological signs. β-Cyano-L-alanine (1.3 mmol/kg, 150 mg/kg, intragastric or 2 mmol/kg subcutaneous) administered to weanling rats causes hyperactivity, convulsions, and rigidity from which the rats recover after 4 hr; the γ-glutamyl derivative is equally active (Ressler, 1962; Ressler *et al.*, 1963). β-Cyano-L-alanine is a weak inhibitor of bacterial glutamic acid decarboxylase activity (Ressler and Koga, 1971).

V. HETEROCYCLIC AMINO ACIDS

Certain fungi contain neurotoxic substances which may be classified structurally as heterocyclic amino acids. In muscimol and related compounds (Fig. 4), the acidic part of the amino acid structure is associated with the 3-hydroxyisoxazole moiety, whereas in imidazole-4-acetic acid it is the amino function that is associated with the heterocyclic moiety.

A. Muscimol and Related Compounds

Mushrooms of the genus *Amanita* contain numerous biologically active substances (Wieland, 1968; Wieland and Wieland, 1972). Perhaps the most well known of these is muscarine, which is responsible for the excitatory effects on the parasympathetic nervous system after ingestion of *Amanita muscaria* mushrooms (fly agaric), but muscarine is not

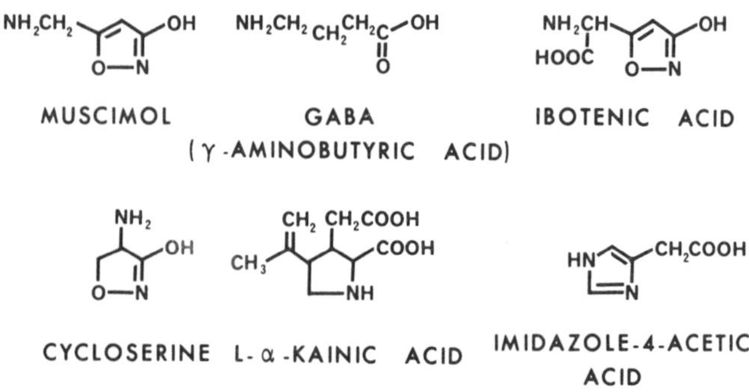

Fig. 4. GABA and some toxic heterocyclic amino acids.

responsible for the hallucinogenic effects of these mushrooms. The CNS effects of fly agaric appear to be due to the isoxazoles muscimol (also known as pantherin or agarin) and ibotenic acid and the oxazole muscazone (Waser, 1967; Benedict, 1972). The chemistry of these substances has been reviewed by Eugster (1969). Muscimol appears to be the most active of these heterocycles. In mice, CNS effects are evident after 0.01 mmol/kg (1mg/kg) of muscimol injected intraperitoneally or 0.02 mmol/kg administered orally. In man, 10–15 mg of muscimol orally results in considerable disturbance of psychic functions—toxic psychosis with confusions, illusions of color vision, sleep with dreams, etc. (Waser, 1967). Ibotenic acid in higher doses produces similar effects which may be due to conversion to muscimol by decarboxylation (Theobald *et al.*, 1968).

1. Muscimol

Muscimol is 5-aminomethyl-3-hydroxyisoxazole. It bears a remarkable structural similarity to GABA (Johnston *et al.*, 1968; Kier and Truitt, 1970; Brehm *et al.*, 1972), and like GABA is a powerful inhibitor of the firing of central neurons, an action that can be antagonized by the convulsant alkaloid bicuculline (see Chapter 6; Curtis *et al.*, 1971*a,b*). Unlike GABA, however, muscimol exerts pronounced central effects when administered to healthy adult mammals (see above). Studies on snail neurons also indicate that muscimol can activate GABA receptors (Walker *et al.*, 1971). The effects of muscimol on the EEG and the spontaneous conditioned behavior of cats, rabbits, and rats have been studied (Scotti de Carolis *et al.*, 1969). Like LSD, muscimol and ibotenic acid increase the levels of 5-hydroxytryptamine in certain parts of the brain (König-Bersin *et al.*, 1970). *In vitro* studies show that muscimol is unlikely to be a substrate for brain GABA aminotransferase activity (Beart and Johnston, 1973) or for the GABA uptake system in brain, and it has been suggested that inefficient removal of muscimol from the environment of GABA receptors may be an important factor contributing to the central effects of muscimol (Johnston, 1971).

2. Ibotenic Acid

Ibotenic acid is α-amino-α-(3-hydroxy-5-isoxazolyl)-acetic acid. It is structurally related to glutamate in the same way that muscimol is related to GABA. Like glutamate, ibotenic acid is a powerful excitant of cat and rat central neurons (Johnston *et al.*, 1968; Shinozaki and Konishi, 1970), is an inhibitor of the firing of snail ganglionic neurons (Walker *et al.*, 1971), and convulses immature rats when administered (1 mmol/kg, 160 mg/kg) by intraperitoneal injection (Johnston, 1973).

3. *Tricholomic Acid*

Tricholomic acid, erythro-α-amino-α-(3-oxo-5-isoxazolidinyl)-acetic acid, a compound with insecticidal properties obtained from the mushroom *Tricholoma muscarium* (Kamiya, 1969), is a dihydro derivative of ibotenic acid. It is also a powerful excitant of rat central neurons (Shinozaki and Konishi, 1970). Both ibotenic acid and tricholomic acid were discovered in Japan as a result of investigations on the fly-killing properties of certain mushrooms. The accidental finding (!) that these substances have taste-potentiating properties some 20 times more potent that those of monosodium glutamate has led to interest in their possible use as food additives (see Wieland, 1968). For the reasons outlined in Section IA care should be exercised in such use.

4. L-α-*Kainic Acid*

L-α-Kainic acid, a derivative of pyrrolidine-2-carboxylic acid isolated from the seaweed *Digenea simplex* (Murayama *et al.*, 1965) and an anthelmintic, is also a powerful excitant of rat and cat central neurons (Shinozaki and Konishi, 1970; D. R. Curtis, unpublished). It is an inhibitor of the uptake of L-glutamic acid by rat brain slices, whereas ibotenic acid is inactive (Balcar and Johnston, 1972, and unpublished). It convulses 10-day-old rats within 7 min of intraperitoneal injection of 0.05 mmol/kg (11 mg/kg) (A. Stephanson and G. A. R. Johnston, unpublished) and is thus the most potent of the convulsant amino acids yet tested (Johnston, 1973).

5. *Cycloserine*

Cycloserine, 4-amino-3-hydroxyisoxazoline, is an antibiotic whose clinical use in tuberculosis has been limited by its side-effects in the CNS, which include convulsions, hallucinations, and behavioral disorders (Leston *et al.*, 1970). It is structurally related to the spinal inhibitory transmitter glycine in a manner similar to that in which muscimol and GABA are related, and its CNS effects can be mediated by interaction with the glycine system, particularly if it is oxidized *in vivo* to 4-amino-3-hydroxyisoxazole. When administered electrophoretically, cycloserine inhibits the firing of cat spinal neurons (D. R. Curtis, unpublished). Cycloserine is known to inhibit various pyridoxal-dependent enzymes in brain extracts, including glutamic acid decarboxylase, GABA aminotransferase, and serine hydroxymethyltransferase (Sashchenko *et al.*, 1968; Severin *et al.*, 1968; Davies and Johnston, 1973).

B. Imidazole-4-acetic Acid

Imidazole-4-acetic acid (IAA) is found in the mushrooms *Polyporus sulfureus* and *Caprinus atramentarius* (List and Menssen, 1959; List and Reith, 1960). It is a metabolite of histamine in animal tissues (Kahlson and Rosengren, 1971) and structurally resembles GABA. It could be an inhibitory synaptic transmitter in the mammalian CNS.

Following parenteral administration (1–3 mmol/kg, 100–400 mg/kg, intraperitoneal) to mice and rats, it has mixed excitant and depressant effects which resemble those of γ-hydroxybutyric acid (Marcus *et al.*, 1971; Tunnicliff *et al.*, 1972; Clifford *et al.*, 1973). Such administration increases the levels of GABA and 5-hydroxytryptamine in the brain, the increased GABA levels probably resulting from the noncompetitive (K_i 3×10^{-4} M) inhibition of GABA aminotransferase (Clifford *et al.*, 1973). IAA is a relatively weak inhibitor of brain glutamate decarboxylase activity (Small *et al.*, 1970) and of the uptake of GABA into slices of spinal cord (Balcar and Johnston, 1973). It is an uncompetitive activator of brain cyclic 3′,5′-nucleotide phosphodiesterase activity (Roberts and Simonsen, 1970). When administered near single neurons in the cat cerebral cortex, medulla, and spinal cord, IAA is a bicuculline-sensitive inhibitor of firing, comparable in potency to GABA (Curtis *et al.*, 1971*a,b*; Haas *et al.*, 1972).

VI. SULFUR-CONTAINING AMINO ACIDS

A number of sulfur-containing amino acids might be classed as neurotoxic. Unlike most of the amino acids discussed in the earlier sections, these sulfur-containing amino acids (Fig. 5) do not have direct actions on neuronal firing, though they might be converted *in vivo* into compounds that do not have such an action. The abnormal metabolism of endogenous sulfur-containing amino acids is often associated with brain dysfunction (Gaull, 1972).

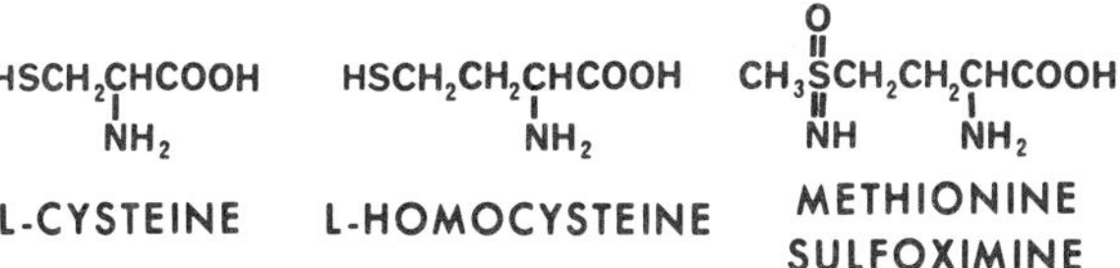

Fig. 5. Neurotoxic sulfur-containing amino acids.

A. Cysteine and Related Amino Acids

L-Cysteine (12 mmol/kg, 1.5 mg/kg, subcutaneous) administered to infant mice produces neuronal lesions in the brain similar to those produced by administration of MSG and related excitant amino acids (Olney *et al.*, 1971). L-Cysteine is the only compound to produce such lesions that does not have a direct excitant action on neuronal firing, and it is likely that it is oxidized to L-cysteic acid or L-cysteine sulfinic acid, both neuronal excitants (Curtis and Watkins, 1960), which may be responsible for the lesions (Olney *et al.*, 1971). Intraventricular injection of L-cysteine produces an EEG activatin in *encéphale isolé* cats and markedly increased spontaneous motor activity in chronic cats; these effects are inhibited by administration of cystathionine (Key and White, 1970). Cysteine, cysteic acid, cysteine sulfinic acid, and cystathionine all occur in the mammalian CNS and are metabolically interrelated (Gaitonde, 1970). Cysteic and cysteine sulfinic acids may act as excitatory transmitters in the CNS, and cystathionine may be an inhibitory transmitter.

DL-Homocysteine (5–7 mmol/kg, 675–950 mg/kg, intraperitoneal) convulses adult rats, whereas the related amino acids homocystine, homoserine, and cysteine are apparently inactive at these doses (Sprince *et al.*, 1969*a,b*). This effect could be due to conversion to DL-homocysteic acid, which is known to produce convulsions in immature animals after intraperitoneal injection of as little as 0.5 mmol/kg (Johnston, 1973) and is a potent neuronal excitant (Curtis and Watkins, 1965).

Cysteine and homocysteine are widely distributed in plants and appear to be metabolized by a variety of pathways (see, e.g., Giovanelli and Mudd, 1967).

B. Methionine Sulfoximine

Ingestion of flour made from wheat bleached with Agene (nitrogen chloride) may result in seizures. The toxic agent is methionine sulfoximine produced by the action of the gas on methionine (see Wolfe and Elliott, 1962, for a review of the early literature). Only one of the four possible stereoisomers of methionine sulfoximine, L-methionine *S*-sulfoximine, is a convulsant (Rowe and Meister, 1970).

DL-Methionine *SR*-sulfoximine (2 mmol/kg, 400 mg/kg, intraperitoneal) produces convulsions 4–6 hr after injection into mature and immature rats (Lamar and Sellinger, 1965; Johnston, 1973), causes considerable swelling of nerve endings and loss of synaptic vesicles, and strongly inhibits brain alanine aminotransferase and glutamine synthetase activities (De Robertis *et al.*, 1967). L-Methionine *SR*-sulfoximine antagonizes the excitant action of L-glutamic acid and L-aspartic acid, but not that of acetylcholine, on the firing of neurons in the cat CNS (Curtis *et al.*, 1972), but it is difficult to relate this action to its action as a convulsant. Methionine sulfoximine is structurally related to glutamic acid. L-Methionine *SR*-sulfoximine does not influence the transport of L-glutamic acid by either the high- or the low-affinity system in rat brain slices (Balcar and Johnston, 1972) or the activity of any of the following brain enzymes: choline acetylase, acetylcholinesterase, monoamine oxidase, glutamic acid dehydrogenase, aspartate aminotransferase, and GABA aminotransferase (De Robertis *et al.*, 1967).

The inhibition of brain glutamine synthetase activity by methionine sulfoximine has been extensively studied. Of the four isomers, only the convulsant isomer, L-methionine *S*-sulfoximine, inhibits the activity of this enzyme (Manning *et al.*, 1966). The inhibition in the presence of ATP and Mg^{2+} (or Mn^{2+}) is irreversible and involves tight binding of L-methionine *S*-sulfoximine phosphate and ADP to the enzyme (Rowe *et al.*, 1969). Several authors have noted that there is little correlation *in vivo* between the onset of or recovery from the seizures and the gross changes in glutamine synthetase activity or glutamine levels in the brain (Sellinger *et al.*, 1968; Lamar, 1968), but as with monosodium glutamate it may be discrete regions of the brain, e.g., the arcuate nucleus, that are affected by methionine sulfoximine, and there is a clear need for more detailed neurochemical studies.

The "small pool" of glutamic acid metabolism in the brain is characterized by high glutamine synthetase activity (van den Berg, 1973; Balázs *et al.*, 1973). This pool may be associated with glial cells and may represent "inactivated" glutamic acid taken up from the synaptic cleft after synaptic release (Curtis and Johnston, 1974). It is possible that inhibition by methionine sulfoximine of glutamine synthetase activity might reduce the turnover of glutamic acid in the "small pool" and thus reduce the rate of removal of glutamic acid from the synaptic cleft, resulting in more prolonged activation of the postsynaptic receptors for this excitatory transmitter.

VII. CONCLUSIONS

Most of the neurotoxic amino acids of plant and fungal origin are structurally related to the amino acids that are likely to function as important synaptic transmitters in the mammalian CNS. Thus β-*N*-oxalyl-L-α,β-diaminopropionic acid, ibotenic acid, homocysteine, and methionine sulfoximine are related to glutamic acid; α,γ-diaminobutyric acid, muscimol, and imidazole-4-acetic acid are related to GABA; and β-cyano-L-alanine and cysteine are related to aspartic acid. Though the thesis that these neurotoxic amino acids do in fact act as "antimetabolites" to the transmitter amino acids is far from substantiated, it does serve as a valuable stimulus for further investigations.

ACKNOWLEDGMENTS

The author is grateful to Mrs. A. Stephanson and Mrs. H. Walsh for invaluable assistance, and to Professor D. R. Curtis for helpful advice.

VIII. REFERENCES

Albert, K., Hoch, P., and Waelsch, H., 1946, Preliminary report on the effect of glutamic acid administration in mentally retarded subjects, *J. Nerv. Ment. Dis.* **104**:263.

Arees, E., and Mayer, J., 1970, Monosodium glutamate-induced brain lesions, electron microscopic examination, *Science* **1970**:549.

Azzi, A., Chappell, J. B., and Robinson, B. H., 1967, Penetration of the mitochondrial membrane by glutamate and aspartate, *Biochem. Biophys. Res. Commun.* **29**:148.

Balázs, R., Patel, A. J., and Richter, D., 1973, Metabolic compartments in the brain: Their properties and relation to morphological structures, in: *Metabolic Compartmentation in the Brain* (R. Balázs and J. E. Cremer, eds.) pp. 167–184, Macmillan, London.

Balcar, V. J., and Johnston, G. A. R., 1972, Glutamate uptake by brain slices and its relation to the depolarization of neurones by acidic amino acids, *J. Neurobiol.* **3**:295.

Balcar, V. J., and Johnston, G. A. R., 1973, High affinity uptake of transmitters: Studies on the uptake of L-asparate, GABA, L-glutamate and glycine in cat spinal cord, *J. Neurochem.* **20**:529.

Banay-Schwartz, M., Piro, L., and Lajtha, A., 1971, Relationship of ATP levels to amino acid transport in slices of mouse brain, *Arch. Biochem. Biophys.* **145**:199.

Baxter, C. F., and Roberts, E., 1958, The γ-aminobutyric acid-α-ketoglutaric acid transaminase of beef brain, *J. Biol. Chem.* **233**:1135.

Beart, P. M., and Johnston, G. A. R., 1973, Transamination of analogues of γ-aminobutyric acid by extracts of rat brain mitochondria, *Brain Res.* **49**:459.

Bell, E. A., 1964, Relevance of biochemical taxonomy to the problem of lathyrism, *Nature* (*Lond.*) **203**:378.

Bell, E. A., 1968, Occurrence of the neurolathyrogen α-amino-β-oxalylaminopropionic acid in two species of *Crotalaria, Nature* (*Lond.*) **218**:197.

Bell, E. A., and O'Donovan, J. P., 1966, The isolation of α- and γ-oxalyl derivatives of α,γ-diaminobutyric acid from seeds of *Lathyrus latifolius*, and the detection of the α-oxalyl-isomer of the neurotoxin α-amino-β-oxalylaminopropionic acid in this and other species, *Phytochemistry* **5**:1211.

Bell, E. A., and Tirimanna, A. S. L., 1965, Association of amino acids and related compounds in the seeds of forty-seven species of *Vicia*: Their taxonomic and nutritional significance, *Biochem. J.* **97**:104.

Benedict, R. G., 1972, Mushroom toxins other than *Amanita*, in: *Microbial Toxins*, Vol. 8 (S. Kadis, A. Ciegler, and S. J. Ajl, eds.) pp. 281–320, Academic Press, New York.

Brehm, L., Hjeds, H., and Krogsgaard-Larsen, P., 1972, The structure of muscimol, a GABA analogue of restricted conformation, *Acta Chem. Scand.* **26**:1298.

Burde, R. M., Schainker, B., and Kayes, J., 1971, Acute effect of oral and subcutaneous administration of monosodium glutamate on the arcuate nucleus of the hypothalamus in mice and rats, *Nature* (*Lond.*) **233:58.**

Cheema, P. S., Malathi, K., Padmanaban, G., and Sarma, P. S., 1969*a*, The neurotoxicity of β-*N*-oxalyl-L-α,β-diaminopropionic acid, the neurotoxin from the pulse *Lathyrus sativus, Biochem. J.* **112**:29.

Cheema, P. S., Padmanaban, G., and Sarma, P. S., 1969*b*, Neurotoxic action of β-*N*-oxalyl-L-α,β-diaminopropionic acid in acidotic adult rats, *Indian J. Biochem. Biophys.* **6**:146.

Cheema, P. S., Padmanaban, G., and Sarma, P. S., 1970, Biochemical characterization of β-*N*-oxalyl-L-α,β-diaminopropionic acid, the *Lathyrus sativus* neurotoxin as an excitant amino acid, *J. Neurochem.* **17**:1295.

Cheema, P. S., Padmanaban, G., and Sarma, P. S., 1971*a*, Transamination of β-*N*-oxalyl-L-α,β-diaminopropionic acid, the *Lathyrus sativus* neurotoxin, in tissues of the rat, *Indian J. Biochem. Biophys.* **8**:16.

Cheema, P. S., Padmanaban, G., and Sarma, P. S., 1971*b*, Mechanism of action of β-*N*-oxalyl-L-α,β-diaminopropionic acid, the *Lathyrus sativus* neurotoxin, *J. Neurochem.* **18**:2137.

Chen, C. H., Flory, W., and Koeppe, R. E, 1972, Variation of neurotoxicity of L- and D-2,4-diaminobutyric acid with route of administration, *Toxicol. Appl. Pharmacol.* **23**:334.

Clifford, J. M., Taberner, P. V., Tunnicliff, G., Rick, J. T., and Kerkut, G. A., 1973, Biochemical and pharmacological actions of imidazoleacetic acid, *Biochem. Pharmacol.* **22**:535.

Cohen, A. I., 1967, An electron microscopic study of the modification by monosodium glutamate of the retinas of normal and "rodless" mice, *Am. J. Anat.* **120**:319.

Crawford, J. M., 1963, The effect upon mice of intraventricular injection of excitant and depressant amino acids, *Biochem. Pharmacol.* **12**:1443.

Creasey, W. A., and Malawista, S. E., 1971, Monosodium L-glutamate–inhibition of glucose uptake in brain as a basis for toxicity, *Biochem. Pharmacol.* **20**:2917.

Curtis, D. R., and Crawford, J. M., 1969, Central synaptic transmission—Microelectrophoretic studies, *Ann. Rev. Pharmacol.* **9**:209.

Curtis, D. R., and Johnston, G. A. R., 1974, Amino acid transmitters in the mammalian central nervous system, *Ergeb. Physiol. Biol. Chem. Exptl. Pharmakol.* **69**:97.

Curtis, D. R., and Watkins, J. C., 1960, The excitation and depression of spinal neurones by structurally related amino acids, *J. Neurochem.* **6**:117.

Curtis, D. R., and Watkins, J. C., 1965, The pharmacology of amino acids related to γ-aminobutyric acid, *Pharmacol. Rev.* **17**:347.

Curtis, D. R., Duggan, A. W., Felix, D., and Johnston, G. A. R., 1971*a*, Bicuculline, an antagonist of GABA and synaptic inhibition in the spinal cord, *Brain Res.* **32**:69.

Curtis, D. R., Duggan, A. W., Felix, D., Johnston, G. A. R., and McLennan, H., 1971*b*, Antagonism between bicuculline and GABA in the cat brain, *Brain Res.* **33**:57.

Curtis, D. R., Duggan, A. W., Felix, D., Johnston, G. A. R., Tebēcis, A. K., and Watkins, J. C., 1972, Excitation of mammalian central neurones by acidic amino acids, *Brain. Res.* **41**:283.

Dastur, D. K., 1962, Lathyrism, *World Neurol.* **3**:721.

Davies, L. P., and Johnston, G. A. R., 1973, Serine hydroxymethyltransferase in the central nervous system: Regional and subcellular distribution studies, *Brain Res.* **54**:149.

De Robertis, E., Sellinger, O. Z., Rodriguez de Lores Arnaiz, G., Alberici, M., and Zieher, L. M., 1967, Nerve endings in methionine sulphoximine convulsant rats, a neurochemical and ultrastructural study, *J. Neurochem.* **14**:81.

Do Carmo, R. J., and Leão, A. A. P., 1972, On the relation of glutamic acids and some allied compounds to cortical spreading depression, *Brain Res.* **39**:515.

Duque-Magalhaes, M. C., and Packer, L., 1972, Action of the neurotoxin β-*N*-oxalyl-L-α,β-diaminopropionic acid on glutamate metabolism of brain mitochondria, *FEBS Letters* **23**:188.

Eugster, C. H., 1969, Chemie der Wirkstoffe aus dem Fliegenpilz (*Amanita muscaria*), *Fortschr. Chem. Org. Naturst.* **27**:261.

Fowden, L., Lewis, D., and Tristram, H., 1967, Toxic amino acids: Their actions as antimetabolites, *Advan. Enzymol. Relat. Areas Mol. Biol.* **29**:89.

Gaitonde, M. K., 1970, Sulfur amino acids, in: *Handbook of Neurochemistry*, Vol. 3 (A. Lajtha, ed.) pp. 225–287, Plenum Press, New York.

Ganapathy, K. T., and Dwivedi, M. P., 1961, *Studies on Clinical Epidemiology of Lathyrism*, Lathyrism Enquiry Field Unit, Indian Council of Medical Research, Gandhi Memorial Hospital, Rewa.

Gaull, G. E, 1972, Abnormal metabolism of sulfur-containing amino acids associated with brain dysfunction, in: *Handbook of Neurochemistry,* Vol. 7 (A. Lajtha, ed.) pp. 169–190, Plenum Press, New York.

Ghadimi, H., and Kumar, S., 1972, Current status of monosodium glutamate, *Am. J. Clin. Nutr.* **25**:643.

Giovanelli, J., 1966, Oxalyl-coenzyme A synthetase from pea seeds, *Biochim. Biophys. Acta.* **118**:124.

Giovanelli, J., and Mudd, S. H., 1967, Synthesis of homocysteine and cysteine by enzyme extracts of spinach, *Biochem. Biophys. Res. Commun.* **27**:150.

Goodman, L. S., Swinyard, E. A., and Toman, J. E. P., 1946, Effects of *l*(+)glutamic acid and other agents on experimental seizures, *Arch. Neurol. Psychiat.* **56**:20.

Gruener, N., 1972, Effect of glutamic acid on ATP levels in the neuron, *Israel J. Med. Sci.* **8**:101.

Haas, H. L., Anderson, E. G. and Hösli, L., 1972, Histamine and metabolites: Their effects and interactions with convulsants on brain stem neurones, *Brain. Res.* **51**:269.

Harvey, J. A., and McIlwain, H., 1968, Excitatory acidic amino acids and the cation content and sodium ion flux of isolated tissues from the brain, *Biochem. J.* **108**:269.

Hennecke, H., and Wiechert, P., 1970, Seizures and the dose of L-glutamic acid in rats, *Epilepsia* **11**:327.

Himwich, H. E., and Himwich, W. A,. 1955, The permeability of the blood–brain barrier to glutamic acid in the developing brain, in: *Biochemistry of the Developing Nervous System* (H. Waelsch, ed.) pp. 202–207, Academic Press, New York.

Holtzman, E., 1969, Lysosomes in the physiology and pathology of neurons, in: *Lysosomes in Biology and Pathology* (J. T. Dingle and H. B. Fell, eds.) pp. 192–216, North-Holland, Amsterdam.

Ho Man Kwok, R., 1968, Letter to the editor, *New Engl. J. Med.* **278**:796.

Ikeda, K., 1912, The taste of the salt of glutamic acid, *Orig. Com. 8th Internat. Congr. Appl. Chem.* **18**:147; *Chem. Abst.* **6**:3134.

Iversen, L. L., and Johnston, G. A. R., 1971, GABA uptake in rat central nervous system: Comparison of uptake in slices and homogenates and the effects of some inhibitors, *J. Neurochem.* **18**:1939.

Jacob, E., Patel, A. J., and Ramakrishnan, C. V., 1967, Effect of neurotoxin from the seeds of *Lathyrus sativus* on glutamate metabolism in chick brain, *J. Neurochem.* **14**:1091.

Johnston, G. A. R., 1971, Muscimol and the uptake of γ-aminobutyric acid by rat brain slices, *Psychopharmacologia* **22**:230.

Johnston, G. A. R., 1973, Convulsions induced in 10-day-old rats by intraperitoneal injection of monosodium glutamate and related amino acids, *Biochem. Pharmacol.* **22**:137.

Johnston, G. A. R., and Lloyd, H. J., 1967, Oxalyl-coenzyme A synthetase and the neurotoxin β-N-oxalyl-L-α,β-diaminopropionate, *Aust. J. Biol. Sci.* **20**:1241.

Johnston, G. A. R., Curtis, D. R., de Groat, W. C., and Duggan, A. W., 1968, Central actions of ibotenic acid and muscimol, *Biochem. Pharmacol.* **17**:2488.

Kahlson, G., and Rosengren, E,. 1971, *Biogenesis and Physiology of Histamine*, Edward Arnold, London.

Kamiya, T. 1969, Synthesis of tricholomic acid. VII. Synthesis of four optically active isomers of tricholomic acid, *Chem. Pharm. Bull.* **17**:890.

Key, B. J., and White, P. R., 1970, Neuropharmacological comparison of cystathionine, cysteine, homoserine and alpha-ketobutyric acid in cats, *Neuropharmacology* **9**:349.

Kier, L. B., and Truitt, E. B., 1970, Molecular orbital studies on the conformation of γ-aminobutyric acid and muscimol, *Experientia* **29**:988.

König-Bersin, P., Waser, P. G., Langmann, H., and Lichtensteiger, W., 1970, Monoamines in the brain under the influence of muscimol and ibotenic acid, two psychoactive principles of *Amanita muscaria, Psychopharmacologia* **18**:1.

Lakshmanan, J., Cheema, P. S., and Padmanaban, G., 1971, Effects of β-N-oxalyl-L-α,β-diaminopropionic acid on chick brain lysosomes, *Nature New Biol.* **234**:156.

Lamar, C., 1968, The duration of the inhibition of glutamine synthetase by methionine sulphoximine, *Biochem. Pharmacol.* **17**:636.

Lamar, C., and Sellinger, O. Z., 1965, The inhibition *in vivo* of cerebral glutamine synthetase and glutamine transferase by the convulsant methionine sulphoximine, *Biochem. Pharmacol.* **14**:489.

Leston, J. M., Rey, J. C., Gonzales Montaner, L. J., Grondona, A., and Zavalla, P. N., 1970, Psychosomatic reactions to cycloserine in the treatment of tuberculosis, *Scand. J. Resp. Dis.* (*Suppl.*) **71**:231.

List, P. H., and Menssen, H. G., 1959, Basic constituents of mushrooms, IV. Biogenic amines of *Polyporus sulfureus, Arch. Pharm.* **292**:260.

List, P. H., and Reith, H., 1960, Basic constituents of fungi. X. Imidazole derivatives in ink cap, *Coprinus atroamentarius Bull. Hoppe–Seyler's Physiol. Chem.* **319**:17.

Logan, W. J., and Synder, S. H., 1972, High affinity uptake systems for glucine, glutamic and aspartic acids in synaptosomes of rat central nervous tissue, *Brain. Res.* **42**:413.

Lucas, D. R., and Newhouse, J. P., 1957, The toxic effect of sodium -glutamate on the inner layers of the retina, *Arch. Ophthalmol.* **58**:193.

Malathi, K., Padmanaban, G., Rao, S. L. N., and Sarma, P. S., 1967, Studies on the biosynthesis of β-N-oxalyl-L-α,β-diaminopropionic acid, the *Lathyrus sativus* neurotoxin, *Biochem. Biophys. Acta* **141**:71.

Malathi, K., Padmanaban, G., and Sarma, P. S., 1968, Oxalylation of some amino acids by an enzyme preparation from *Lathyrus sativus, Indian J. Biochem. Biophys.* **5**:184.

Malathi, K., Padmanaban, G., and Sarma, P. S., 1970, Biosynthesis of β-N-oxalyl-L-α,β-diaminopropionic acid, the *Lathyrus sativus* neurotoxin, *Phytochemistry* **9**:1603.

Mani, K. S., Sriramachari, S., Rao, S. L. N., and Sarma, P. S., 1971, Experimental neurolathyrism in monkeys, *Indian J. Med. Res.* **59**:880.

Manning, J. M., Moore, S., Rowe, W. B., and Meister, A., 1969, Identification of L-methionine-S-sulfoximine as the diastereoisomer of L-methionine-SR-sulfoximine that inhibits glutamine synthetase, *Biochemistry,* **8**:2681.

Marcus, R. J., Winters, W. D., Roberts, E., and Simonsen, D. G., 1971, Neuropharmacological studies of imidazole-4-acetic acid actions in the mouse and rat, *Neuropharmacology* **10**:203.

Mason, M. M., and Whiting, M. G., 1966, Demyelination in the bovine spinal cord caused by zamia neurotoxicity, *Fed Proc.* **25**:533.

McIlwain, H., Harvey, J. A., and Rodriguez, G., 1969, Tetrodotoxin on the sodium and other ions of cerebral tissues, excited electrically and with glutamate, *J. Neurochem.* **16**:363.

Mehta, T., Hsu, A.-F., and Haskell, B. E., 1972, Specificity of the neurotoxin from *Lathyrus sativus* as an amino acid antagonist, *Biochemistry* **11**:4053.

Murayama, K., Morimura, S., Nakamura, Y., and Sunagawa, G., 1965, Synthesis of pyrrolidine derivatives. II. Synthesis of kainic acid and its derivatives by Wittig reaction, *Yakugaku Zasshi* **85**:757.

Murti, V. V. S., Seshadri, T. R., and Venkitasubramanian, T. A., 1964, Neurotoxic compounds of the seeds of *Lathyrus sativus, Phytochemistry* **3**:73.

Mushahwar, I. K., and Koeppe, R. E., 1963, Concerning the metabolism of D- and L-α,γ-diaminobutyric acid-2-C^{14} in rats, *J. Biol. Chem.* **238**:2460.

Mushahwar, I. K., and Koeppe, R. E., 1971, The toxicity of monosodium glutamate in young rats, *Biochem. Biophys. Acta* **244**:318.

Nagarajan, V., Mohan, V. S., and Gopalan, C., 1966, Further studies on the toxic factor in *Lathyrus sativus*—Potentiation of a toxic fraction from the seed by some amino acids, *Indian J. Biochem. Biophys.* **3**:130.

Nakajima, T., Wolfram, F., and Clark, W. G., 1967, Identification of 1,4-methylhistamine, 1, 3-diaminopropane and 2,4-diaminobutyric acid in bovine brain, *J. Neurochem.* **14**:1113.

Neuberger, A., 1936, Dissociation constants and structures of glutamic acid and its esters, *Biochem. J.* **30**:2085.

Nigam, S. N., and Ressler, C., 1966, Biosynthesis of 2,4-diaminobutyric acid from L-[^{3}H]homoserine and DL-[1-^{14}C]aspartic acid in *Lathyrus sylvestris* W., *Biochemistry* **5**:3426.

Okamoto, K., and Quastel, J. H., 1970, Tetrodotoxin-sensitive uptake of ions and water by slices of rat brain *in vitro, Biochem. J.* **120**:37.

Olney, J. W., 1969, Brain lesions, obesity, and other disturbances in mice treated with monosodium glutamate, *Science* **164**:719.

Olney, J. W., 1971, Glutamate-induced neuronal necrosis in the infant mouse hypothalamus, *J. Neuropathol. Exptl. Neurol.* **30**:75.

Olney, J. W., and Sharpe, L. G., 1969, Brain lesions in an infant rhesus monkey treated with monosodium glutamate, *Science* **166**:386.

Olney, J. W., Ho, O. L., and Rhee, V., 1971, Cytotoxic effects of acidic and sulphur containing amino acids on the infant mouse central nervous system, *Exptl. Brain Res.* **14**:61.

O'Neal, R. M., Chen, C.-H., Reynolds, C. S., Meghal, S. K., and Koeppe, R. E., 1968, The "neurotoxicity" of L-2,4-diaminobutyric acid, *Biochem. J.* **106**:699.

Orrego, F., and Lipmann, F., 1967, Protein synthesis in brain slices, *J. Biol. Chem.* **242**:665.

Oser, B. L., Carson, S., Vogin, E. E., and Cox, G. E., 1971, Oral and subcutaneous administration of monosodium glutamate to infant rodents and dogs, *Nature* (*Lond.*) **229**:411.

Perez, V. J., and Olney, J. W., 1972, Accumulation of glutamic acid in the arcuate nucleus of the hypothalamus of the infant mouse following subcutaneous administration of monosodium glutamate, *J. Neurochem.* **19**:1777.

Phillis, J. W., and Ochs, S., 1971, Excitation and depression of cortical neurones during spreading depression, *Exptl. Brain Res.* **12**:132.

Polsky, F. I., Nunn, P. B., and Bell, E. A., 1972, Distribution and toxicity of α-amino-β-aminopropionic acid, *Fed. Proc.* **31**:1473.

Potts, A. M., Modrell, K. W., and Kingsbury, C., 1960, Permanent fractionation of the electroretinogram by sodium glutamate, *Am. J. Ophthalmol.* **50**:900.

Prabhu, V. G., and Oester, Y. T., 1971, Neuromuscular functions of mature mice following neonatal monosodium glutamate, *Arch. Int. Pharmacodyn. Therap.* **189**:59.

Prosky, L., and O'Dell, R. G., 1971, Effect of dietary monosodium L-glutamate on some brain and liver metabolites in rats, *Proc. Soc. Exptl. Biol. Med.* **138**:517.

Przybylskā, J., and Pawelkiewicz, J., 1965, *O*-Oxalylhomoserine, a new homoserine derivative in young pods of *Lathyrus sativus, Bull. Acad. Pol. Sci.* **13**:327.

Ramsey, R. L., and McIlwain, H., 1970, Calcium content and exchange in neocortical tissues during the cation movements induced by glutamates, *J. Neurochem.* **17**:781.

Rao, S. L. N., Adiga, P. R., and Sarma, P. S., 1964, The isolation and characterization of β-*N*-oxalyl-L-α,β-diaminopropionic acid: A neurotoxin from the seeds of *Lathyrus sativus, Biochemistry* **3**:432.

Rao, S. L. N., Malathi, K., and Sarma, P. S., 1969, Lathyrism, *World Rev. Nutr. Diet.* **10**:214.

Ressler, C., 1962, Isolation and identification from common vetch of the neurotoxin β-cyano-L-alanine, a possible factor in neurolathyrism, *J. Biol. Chem.* **237**:733.

Ressler, C., and Koga, T., 1971, α-Cyanoamino acids and related nitriles as inhibitors of glutamate decarboxylase, *Biochim. Biophys. Acta* **242**:473.

Ressler, C., Redstone, P. A., and Erenberg, R. H., 1961, Isolation and identification of a neuroactive factor from *Lathyrus latifolius, Science* **134**:188.

Ressler, C., Nigam, S. N., Giza, Y.-H., and Nelson, J., 1963, Isolation and identification from common vetch of γ-L-glutamyl-β-cyano-L-alanine, a bound form of the neurotoxin β-cyano-L-alanine, *J. Am. Chem. Soc.* **85**:3311.

Roberts, E., and Simonsen, D. G., 1970, Some properties of cyclic 3′,5′-nucleotide phosphodiesterase of mouse brain: Effects of imidazole-4-acetic acid, chlorpromazine, cyclic 3′,5′-GMP and other substances, *Brain Res.* **24**:91.

Rowe, B. W., and Meister, A., 1970, Identification of L-methionine-*S*-sulphoximine as the convulsant isomer of methionine sulphoximine, *Proc. Natl. Acad. Sci.* **66**:500.

Rowe, W. B., Ronzio, R. A., and Meister, A., 1969, Inhibition of glutamine synthetase by methionine sulfoximine: Studies on methionine sulfoximine phosphate, *Biochemistry* **8**:2674.

Roy, D. N., 1969, Biosynthesis of β-oxalylaminoalanine: Evidence that serine is not the precursor, *Indian J. Biochem. Biophys.* **6**:147.

Rukmini, C., 1968, Isolation and purification of a new toxic factor from *Lathyrus sativus, Indian J. Biochem. Biophys.* **5**:182.

Sarma, P. S., and Padmanaban, G., 1969, Lathyrogens, in: *Toxic Constituents of Plant Foodstuffs* (I. E., Liener, ed.) pp. 267–291, Academic Press, New York.

Sashchenko, L. P., Severin, E. S., and Khomutov, R. M., 1968, Inhibition of L-glutamic acid decarboxylase by hydroxylamine derivatives, *Biokhimiya* **33**:142.

Schaumburg, H. H., Byck, R., Gerstl, B. R., and Mashman, J. H., 1969, Monosodium L-glutamate: Its pharmacology and role in the Chinese restaurant syndrome, *Science* **163**:826.

Scotti de Carolis, A., Lipparini, F., and Longo, V. G., 1969, Neuropharmacological investigations on muscimol, a psychotropic drug extracted from *Amanita muscaria Psychopharmacologia* **15**:186.

Sellinger, O. Z., Azcurra, J. M., and Ohlsson, W. G., 1968, Methionine sulfoximine seizures. VIII. Dissociation of the convulsant and glutamine synthetase inhibitory effects, *J. Pharmacol. Exptl. Therap.* **164**:212.

Selye, H., 1957, Lathyrism, *Rev. Can. Biol.* **16**:1.

Severin, E. A., Sashchenko, L. P., Kovaleva, G. K., and Khomutov, R. M., 1968, An effective inhibitor of γ-aminobutyrate transaminase, *Biokhimiya* **33**:1210.

Shinozaki, H., and Konishi, S., 1970, Actions of several anthelmintics and insecticides on rat cortical neurones, *Brain Res.* **24**:368.

Small, N. A., Holton, J. B., and Ancill, R. J., 1970, *In vitro* inhibiton of serotonin and γ-aminobutyric acid synthesis in rat brain by histidine metabolites, *Brain. Res.* **21**:55.

Sprince, H., Parker, C. M., and Josephs, J. A., 1969*a*, Homocysteine-induced convulsions in the rat: Protection by homoserine, serine, betaine, glycine and glucose, *Agents Actions* **1**:9.

Sprince, H., Parker, C. M., Josephs, J. A., and Magazino, J., 1969*b*, Convulsant activity of homoserine and other short-chain mercaptoacids: Protection therefrom, *Ann. N.Y. Acad. Sci.* **166**:323.

Stegink, L. D., Filer, L. J., and Baker, G. L., 1972, Monosodium glutamate: Effect on plasma and breast milk amino acid levels in lactating women, *Proc. Soc. Exptl. Biol. Med.* **140**:836.

Stewart, C. N., Coursin, D. B., and Bhagavan, H. N., 1972, Electroencephalographic study of L-glutamate induced seizures in rats, *Toxicol. Appl. Pharmacol.* **23**:635.

Tewari, S., and Baxter, C. F., 1969, Stimulatory effect of γ-aminobutyric acid upon amino acid incorporation into protein by a ribosomal system from immature rat brain, *J. Neurochem.* **16**:171.

Theobald, W., Büch, O., Kuntz, H. A., Krupp, P., Stenger, E. G., and Heimann, H., 1968, Pharmakologische und experimentalpsychologische Untersuchungen mit 2 Inhaltsstoffen des Fliegenpilzes (*Amanita muscaria*), *Arzneim.-Forsch.* **18**:311.

Thurston, J. H., and Warren, S. K., 1971, Permeability of the blood–brain barrier to monosodium glutamate and effects on the components of the energy reserve in newborn mouse brain, *J. Neurochem.* **18**:2241.

Tunnicliff, G., Wein, J., and Roberts, E., 1972, Effects of imidazole-acetic acid on brain amino acids and body temperature in mice, *J. Neurochem.* **19**:2017.

van den Berg, C. J., 1973, A model of compartmentation in mouse brain based on glucose and acetate metabolism, in: *Metabolic Compartmentation in the Brain* (R. Balázs and J. E. Cremer, eds.) pp. 129–136, Macmillan, London.

Van Harreveld, A., 1959, Compounds in brain extracts causing spreading depression of cerebral cortical activity and contraction of crustacean muscle, *J. Neurochem.* **3**:300.

Van Harreveld, A., and Fifkova, E., 1971, Effects of glutamate and other amino acids on the retina, *J. Neurochem.* **18**:2145.

Vega, A., Bell, E. A., and Nunn, P. B., 1968, The preparation of L- and D-α-amino-β-methylaminopropionic acids and the identification of the compound isolated from *Cycas circinalis* as the L-isomer, *Phytochemistry* **7**:1885.

Vivanco, F., Ramos F., and Jimenez-Diaz, C., 1966, Determination of γ-aminobutyric acid and other free amino acids in whole brains of rats poisoned with β,β'-iminodipropionitrile and α,γ-diaminobutyric acid with, or without, administration of thyroxine, *J. Neurochem.* **13**:1461.

Waelsch, H., and Price, J.C., 1944, Biochemical aspects of glutamic acid therapy for epilepsy, *Arch. Neurol. Psychol.* **51**:393.

Walker, R. J., Woodruff, G. N., and Kerkut, G. A., 1971, The effect of ibotenic acid and muscimol on single neurons of the snail *Helix aspera, Comp. Gen. Pharmacol.* **2**:168.

Waser, P. G., 1967, The pharmacology of *Amanita muscaria,* in: *Ethnopharmacological Search for Psychoactive Drugs* (D. H. Efron, B. Holmstedt, and N. S. Kline, eds. pp. 419–438. U.S. Public Health Service Publication No. 1645, Washington, D.C.

Watkins, J. C., Curtis, D. R., and Biscoe, T. J., 1966, Central effects of β-*N*-oxalyl-α,β-diaminopropionic acid and other *Lathyrus* factors, *Nature* (*Lond.*) **211**:637.

Whiting, M. G., 1963, Toxicity of cycads, *Econ. Bot.* **17**:271.

Wieland, T., 1968, Poisonous principle of mushrooms of the genus *Amanita, Science* **159**:946.

Wieland, T., and Wieland, O,. 1972, The toxic peptides of *Amanita* species, in: *Microbial Toxins,* Vol. 8, (S. Kadis, A. Ciegler, and S. J. Ajl, eds.) pp. 249–280, Academic Press, New York.

Wolfe, L. S., and Elliott, K. A. C., 1962, Chemical studies in relation to convulsive disorders, in: *Neurochemistry* (K. A. C. Elliott, I. H. Page, and J. H. Quastel, eds.) pp. 694–727,

Chapter 6

Convulsant Alkaloids

D. R. Curtis and G. A. R. Johnston

Deparment of Pharmacology
Australian National University
Canberra, Australia

I. INTRODUCTION

This chapter is concerned with convulsants of biological origin which are used experimentally in neurobiology. It is not intended to provide detailed descriptions of the general actions of these agents when administered to different animals, and the presentation is restricted to effects which have been investigated at the cellular level, particularly in relation to studies of the nature of inhibitory synaptic transmitters and the membrane receptors for them.

It is noteworthy that the majority of convulsants investigated in this fashion interfere with transmitter action at inhibitory synapses. As yet, no clear evidence has been provided for convulsants which enhance transmitter action at excitatory synapses, although the convulsions which follow the systemic administration of certain acidic amino acids when the blood–brain barrier is defective may be associated with the activation of receptors normally concerned with excitatory transmission by aspartate and glutamate (Johnston, Chapter 5).

The natural products chosen for discussion are grouped together on the basis of their pharmacological action in mammals. The majority are alkaloids, a group of compounds which have been of considerable and predominantly chemical interest for many years. A substantial amount of historical, chemical, and pharmacological information is provided by Henry (1949). The series edited by Manske (*The Alkaloids*, Academic Press, 14 volumes to 1973) and the Specialist Reports of The Chemical Society on *The Alkaloids* (annually since 1971) are concerned primarily with chemistry. Plant sources of the alkaloids are detailed by Raffauf (1970).

A number of convulsants have not been considered, including nicotine (Ryall, Chapter 2), anticholinesterases (Tower, 1969), and agents producing convulsions either as a consequence of metabolic derangements (Stone, 1972) or as a manifestation of an abstinence or withdrawal syndrome (Essig, 1972).

II. STRYCHNINE AND RELATED SUBSTANCES

A. Chemistry

Strychnine, an indole alkaloid (Fig. 1), was first isolated in crystalline form from the beans of *Strychnos ignatii* and *Strychnos nux-vomica*. It occurs in other species of *Strychnos* and is commercially available as a variety of salts. In view of the following discussion (Section IIB1) of the antagonism which has been demonstrated between strychnine and glycine, it is of interest that this amino acid is a precursor of strychine in *S. nux-vomica* (Maier and Gröger, 1971).

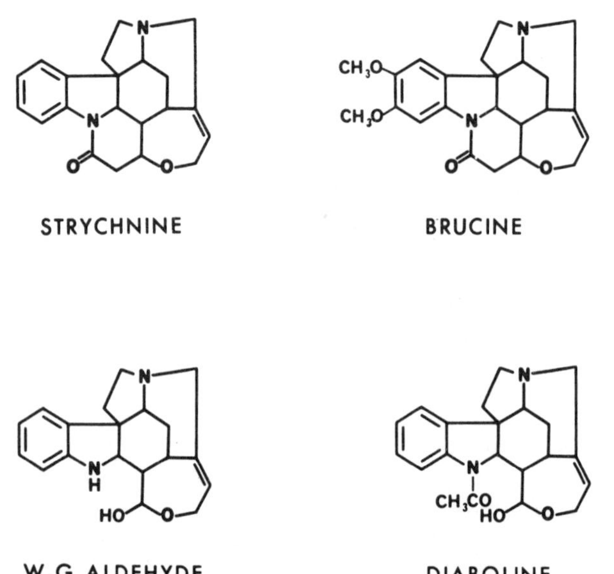

Fig. 1. Structures of strychnine, brucine, the Wieland-Gümlich aldehyde, and diaboline.

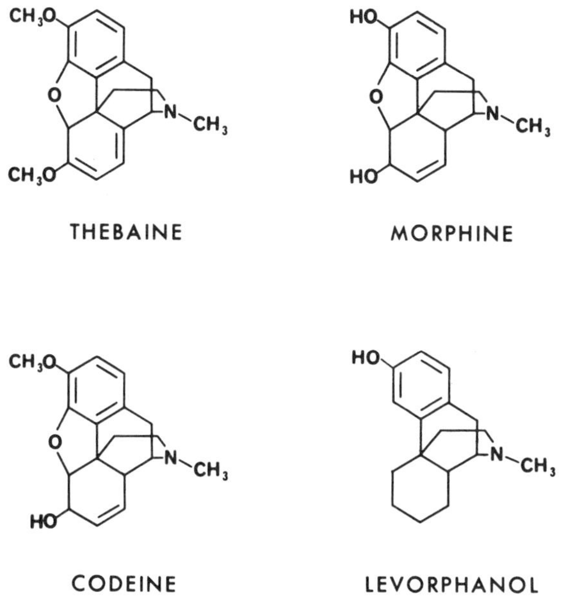

THEBAINE MORPHINE

CODEINE LEVORPHANOL

Fig. 2. Structures of thebaine, morphine, codeine, and levorphanol.

Strychnine hydrochloride is a dihydrate (MW 406.9) readily soluble in water up to a concentration of 10^{-1} M. The elucidation of the chemical structure of strychnine, reviewed by Robinson (1952), represents one of the great classics of organic chemistry and resulted in the publication of more than 250 papers, mainly from the laboratories of Leuchs and of Robinson. The absolute configuration of strychnine, which contains six asymmetrical centers, was determined by X-ray crystallography (Peerdeman, 1956). The total synthesis of strychnine was achieved by Woodward et al. (1963), who described this alkaloid as "for its molecular size . . . the most complex substance known."

Brucine, a dimethoxy derivative of strychnine (Fig. 1), is found together with strychnine in *S. nux-vomica* and *S. ignatii*. It is commercially available as free base (MW 394.5), which is only sparingly soluble in water and is used extensively in synthetic chemistry for the resolution of opticallly active acids, and as the sulfate (MW 1013.1), which is readily soluble in water.

The chemistry of strychnine, brucine, and related substances such as diaboline and the Wieland-Gümlich aldehyde (Fig. 1), has been extensively reviewed by Smith (1965).

Thebaine, morphine, and codeine (Fig. 2) are morphine alkaloids, a class of alkaloids biosynthetically derived from the benzylisoquinoline alkaloids (Robinson, 1968). The chemistry of the morphine alkaloids has been extensively reviewed by Bentley (1954, 1971). The X-ray crystal structure of morphine has been determined by Mackay and Crowfoot Hodgkin (1955). The synthetic substance levorphanol (Fig. 2, (−)-3-hydroxyl-*N*-methylmorphinan, MW 257.4) possesses the same absolute steric configuration as the natural alkaloids (Corrodi *et al*., 1959).

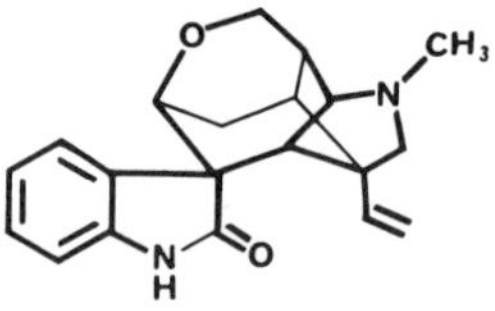

GELSEMINE

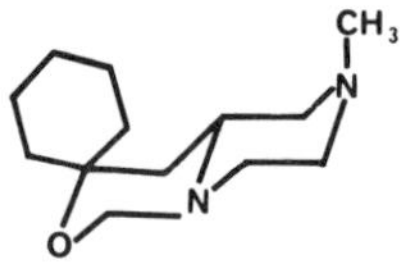

C.O.P.

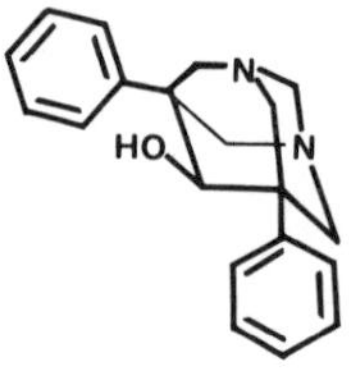

1757 I.S.

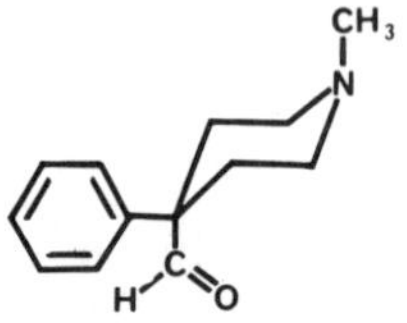

1762 I.S.

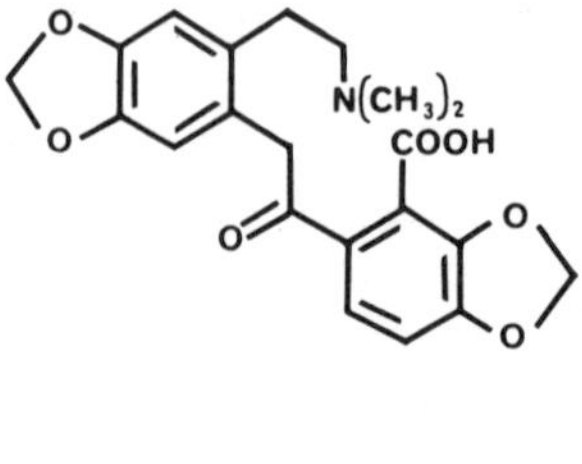

N-METHYL-BICUCULLEINE

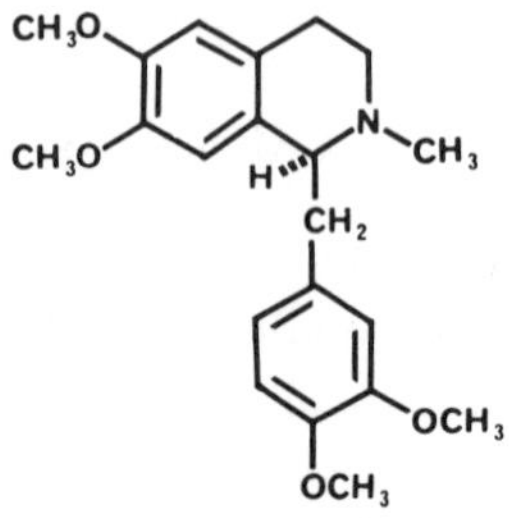

LAUDANOSINE

Fig. 3. Structures of gelsemine, COP, 1757 I.S., 1762 I.S., *N*-methylbicuculleine, and laudanosine.

The free bases of these alkaloids are sparingly soluble in water, but the salts, e.g., thebaine hydrochloride (MW 365.8), morphine hydrochloride (MW 375.8), and codeine hydrochloride (MW 371.9), are freely soluble.

Gelsemine (Fig. 3) is an indole alkaloid (MW 322.4) isolated from the roots of *Gelsemium sempervirens* (Chou, 1931). Its structure was determined by chemical and spectroscopic studies (Conroy and Chakrabarti, 1959) and by X-ray crystallography (Lovell *et al.*, 1959). The chemistry of gelsemine and related *Gelsemium* alkaloids has been reviewed by Saxton (1965).

Laudanosine (Fig. 3) in a benzylisoquinoline alkaloid (MW 357.4) found in opium, *Papaver somniferum*. The chemistry of laudanosine and related alkaloids has been reviewed by Burger (1954), Bentley (1965), and Kametani (1969).

B. Neuropharmacology

1. Strychnine

Although long known as a central, and especially spinal, convulsant (see Dusser de Barenne, 1933; Curtis, 1963), it is only relatively recently that a specific central effect of strychnine (Fig. 1) has been demonstrated in the vertebrate nervous system. Observations of the selective antagonism of certain types of spinal inhibition by low concentrations of strychnine (Bradley *et al.*, 1953) were a direct outcome of earlier proposals by Sherrington concerning the modification of spinal reflexes by the alkaloid (Sherrington, 1905, 1907; Owen and Sherrington, 1911; Liddell and Sherrington, 1925; see also Bremer, 1944). The experimental methods available up to the late 1940s were, however, inadequate to differentiate between effects on excitatory and inhibitory synaptic mechanisms. Furthermore, the investigation of spinal reflexes is complicated by the presence in the cord of two inhibitory processes, one reduced by strychnine (Curtis, 1963), the other apparently enhanced (Schmidt, 1971).

The finding of Eccles and his associates that the short-latency "direct" inhibition of biceps-semitendinosus motoneurons by afferent volleys in low-threshold afferent in the cat's quadriceps muscle nerve was reduced by subconvulsive doses of strychnine was the first demonstration of a selective effect of low concentrations of the alkaloid. This was subsequently confirmed with intracellular studies of the effects of strychnine on direct and recurrent inhibitory postsynaptic potentials: these potentials could be reduced in magnitude in the absence of changes of excitatory postsynaptic potentials, resting membrane potential, and conductance (Eccles *et al.*,

Koketsu, 1954; Coombs *et al.*, 1955; Curtis, 1962; Fuortes and Nelson, 1963; Araki, 1965; Curtis *et al.*, 1968*a,b*; Larson, 1969). Such an effect can now be interpreted in terms of antagonism between strychnine and the probable inhibitory transmitter, glycine.

Major problems in analzying the central effects of strychnine have been the concentrations used and the methods of administration. Systemic or topical administration is generally not suitable for determining the effect of strychnine on synaptic processes influencing particular neurons which belong to a complex interneuronal network, although much has been learned from the effects of strychnine on the operation of simple systems such as those of direct or recurrent inhibition of spinal motoneurons. Furthermore, strychnine has a variety of effects on neuronal membrane which are dose dependent, have been determined on a number of different tissues (see Curtis *et al.*, 1971*c*), and may not all be relevant to the effects produced in mammals by doses of the order of 0.01–0.2 mg/kg, which, if uniformly distributed throughout body water, would produce concentrations of the order of $2.5\text{–}50 \times 10^{-7}$ M. Use has been made of relatively high concentrations of strychnine to trace cortical pathways, but direct excitation of neurons is presumably the basis of strychnine neuronography (Dusser de Barenne and McCulloch, 1939; Chang, 1951; Frankenhaeuser, 1951; Wall and Horwitz, 1951; Ajmone-Marsan, 1969), particularly as strychnine-sensitive inhibiton has not been rigorously demonstrated to be present in the cerebral cortex.

There is now a considerable body of neurochemical and neurophysiological evidence that glycine is an inhibitory transmitter in the spinal cord and medulla at synapses sensitive to strychnine (reviewed by Aprison and Werman, 1968; Curtis and Johnston, 1974). Electrophoretic glycine hyperpolarizes spinal neurons, and the ionic conductance increase producing this hyperpolarization appears to be identical to that of short-latency synaptically evoked inhibition. The intraspinal distribution of glycine is compatible with its transmitter role, and at a number of sites within the nervous system strychnine is a reversible and selective antagonist of the inhibitory action of glycine, the similar action of γ-aminobutyric acid (GABA) being relatively resistant to strychnine.

The site of action of strychnine is most likely to be in the vicinity of inhibitory synapses releasing glycine. The alkaloid, after systemic administration, does not influence the firing of inhibitory interneurons of either the direct or the recurrent inhibitory pathways to motoneurons, inhibitory processes sensitive to strychnine (Eccles *et al.*, 1954; Curtis, 1962, 1967; Larson, 1969), and when administered electrophoretically near motoneurons strychnine reduces a number of spinal inhibitions influencing these cells. Suppression of transmitter synthesis seems unlikely since the latency of strychnine action is extremely short after intravenous or electrophoretic administration, and although evidence has been presented that strychnine can alter the excitability of primary afferent terminals within the spinal cord (Wall *et al.*, 1955; see also Curtis and Ryall, 1966), a difference between the properties of preterminal excitatory and inhibitory fibers has not been demonstrated which would account for the selective effect of strychnine on inhibitory transmission. No direct evidence has been obtained to support the proposal that strychnine interferes with the cholinergic excitation of inhibitory nerve terminals, a process suggested as necessary for transmitter release (McKinstry and Koelle, 1967); in fact, concentrations of strychnine adequate to suppress the inhibition of spinal Renshaw cells facilitate transmission at the cholinergic axon collateral terminals which excite these neurons (Curtis, 1967).

Since both glycine and the inhibitory transmitter at synapses affected by strychnine appear to produce an identical change in postsynaptic membrane permeability, it seems reasonable to conclude that glycine receptors on spinal neurons could be identical with those activated by the transmitter, and that strychnine interferes with the action of glycine and the transmitter by a common mechanism. This proposal gained support by the finding that a number of alkaloids and synthetic substances which all suppress spinal inhibitions of the strychnine-sensitive type are also glycine antagonists when administered electrophoretically, and the relative potencies for these two actions are similar. These substances are less effective glycine antagonists than strychnine; the majority alter inhibition after systemic administration, and in addition to alkaloids listed in subsequent sections include the following synthetic compounds (Fig. 3): 4-phenyl-4-formyl-*N*-methylpiperidine (1762 I.S.); 5,7-diphenyl-1,3-diazadamantan-6-ol (1757 I.S.); hexahydro-2′-methylspiro[cyclohexane-1,8′(6*H*)-oxazino(3,4-*A*) pyrazine] (COP) (see Longo and Chiavarelli, 1962; Curtis *et al.*, 1968*a*); and *N*-methylbicuculleine (Johnston *et al.*, 1972).

Antagonism between glycine and strychnine has been demonstrated when both were administered electrophoretically, and also when strychnine was administered systemically, both in the spinal cord (Curtis *et al.*, 1971*c*) and in the cuneate nucleus (Kelly and Renaud, 1973*b*). Results obtained in both kinds of experiments are of limited value in determining the nature of the strychnine–glycine interaction (see Curtis *et al.*, 1971*c*), but a number of possibilities can be excluded. Mere physicochemical interaction which reduces the subsynaptic concentration of glycine is unlikely since *in vitro* studies have not demonstrated the formation of stable strychnine–glycine complexes other than simple salts, and effective concentrations of strychnine are probably of the order of 1% of those of glycine (see Curtis *et al.*, 1971*c*).

Modification by strychnine of the ionic conductance change induced by glycine in the postsynaptic membrane of spinal neurons also seems improbable. Both hyperpolarizing and depolarizing inhibitory potentials (depolarizing after manipulation of intracellular ion concentrations) are blocked by strychnine (Coombs *et al.*, 1955; Curtis *et al.*, 1968*b*; Larson, 1969); the "reversal" potential for the inhibitory potential is not altered by strychnine (Larson, 1969); and although both glycine and GABA induce the same change in ionic permeability, the action of glycine is much more sensitive to strychnine than that of GABA (Curtis *et al.*, 1968*a,b*; Larson, 1969). Higher concentrations of strychnine may affect the nature of the change in ionic permeability induced by amino acids and other substances (Araki, 1965; Pollen and Lux, 1966), providing in part an explanation for the modification of the inhibitory effects of GABA, dopamine, and norepinephrine on a variety of central neurons (Phillis and York, 1967; Phillis and Tebēcis, 1967; Davidoff *et al.*, 1969; Johnson *et al.*, 1970). Even higher concentrations may involve changes in sodium permeability, accounting for excitation and depression of nerve cell activity. Changes in the properties of cortical neurons induced by topically administered strychnine, which have been interpreted in terms of alterations in sodium ion permeability (Pollen and Ajmone-Marsan, 1965; Stefanis and Jasper, 1965), may not necessarily have arisen from a direct action of strychnine at inhibitory synapses on pyramidal tract neurons. The inhibitions studied were polysynaptic in nature, the postsynaptic potentials recorded probably consisted of a mixture of excitatory and inhibitory potentials, and strychnine may have modified the operation of inhibitory and excitatory interneurons synapsing with pyramidal cells. The conclusion of Araki (1965) concerning the abolition of a potassium conductance change by strychnine is not supported by the observation that low concentrations do not affect the hyperpolarization of motoneurons by GABA.

From the foregoing, it is probable that strychnine interacts with membrane structures at or in the vicinity of glycine receptors on neurons, so preventing effective access of the amino acid. The antagonism is possibly competitive in type (Johnson *et al.*, 1970; Curtis *et al.*, 1971*c*), and investigations are currently in progress of those structural features of strychnine and strychnine-like molecules which permit interaction wtih glycine receptors yet are relatively inactive at GABA receptors. When tests are carried out on spinal neurons in the cat (Curtis *et al.*, 1968*a,b*, 1971*a*) and rat (Biscoe *et al.*, 1972), there is a clear-cut distinction between glycine-like amino acids (glycine, α-alanine, β-alanine, serine, cystathionine, β-aminoisobutyric acid, taurine, and proline), the effects of which are reduced by strychnine, and the GABA-like amino acids (GABA, γ-amino-β-hydroxybutryic acid, 3-aminopropane sulfonic acid, δ-aminovaleric acid, ϵ-

aminocaproic acid, imidazoleacetic acid, muscimol). An identical classification emerged from a study of the effects of bicuculline, which blocks only the effects of GABA-like amino acids on spinal neurons without modifying strychnine-sensitive inhibitions. The distribution between the two classes of depressant amino acids based on the effects of strychnine and bicuculline (see also cuneate nucleus; Kelly and Renaud, 1973*a,b*) is, however, not so sharp in supraspinal areas (Curtis *et al.*, 1971*b*; Biscoe *et al.*, 1972).

Thus the pharmacological importance of strychnine is its use in determining the nature of mammalian central inhibitory transmitters. Taken in conjunction with neurochemical evidence, an inhibitory process sensitive to low concentrations of strychnine probably involves glycine (or a glycine-like amino acid) as the transmitter, particularly if the effects of strychnine on the inhibitory process can be demonstrated at the cellular level. This last point is of importance since the effects of systemically administered strychnine on one neuron in a multineuronal network may be complex and unrelated to inhibitory synapses on that neuron.

The action of strychnine at spinal inhibitory synapses of amphibia is probably similar to that occuring in mammals (Kuno, 1967; Tebēcis and Phillis, 1969). A strychnine-sensitive inhibition of the goldfish Mauthner cell has been described (Furukawa *et al.*, 1964), but the relevance of this to the possible involvement of glycine as the transmitter has been questioned (Diamond *et al.*, 1973). Strychnine is generally considered not to have a specific postsynaptic action at peripheral inhibitory junctions in crayfish stretch receptors (Washizu *et al.*, 1961), crayfish muscle (Parnas and Atwood, 1966; Kano and Ishikawa, 1972) and hermit crab muscle (Earl and Large, 1972), and has complex effects on ganglion cells of *Aplysia* (Klee *et al.*, 1973) and on Retzius cells of the leech (Pritchard, 1971) which are probably related more to the excitatory effects demonstrated on mammalian neurons than to the specific effects at inhibitory synapses.

2. *Analogues*

The convulsant and lethal doses of brucine (Fig. 1) for mice are higher than those of strychnine (factor of 40, intravenous, Warnat, 1931; 120, subcutaneous, Sandberg and Kristianson, 1970). Brucine, administered intravenously (D. R. Curtis, unpublished observations) or electrophoretically (Curtis, 1962), reduces spinal inhibitions which are sensitive to strychnine. Furthermore, brucine is a glycine antagonist (Curtis *et al.*, 1968*a*).

Several studies have been made of congeners of strychnine and brucine. Of a number of reduction products (Rees and Smith, 1967), some are relatively weak convulsants (H. Smith, personal communication), and these and others of the series are weak glycine antagonists (D. R. Curtis and G. A. R. Johnston, unpublished). The convulsant dose (mice, subcutaneous) of 4-hydroxystrychnine is only slightly lower than that of strychnine (Sandberg and Kristianson, 1970), and the LD_{50} values for a variety of *Strychnos* alkaloids are listed for rats by Amann *et al.* (1943) and for mice by Warnat (1931) and Sandberg and Kristianson (1970). Although the latter authors indicate that diaboline, a tertiary base (Fig. 1) from *Strychnos diaboli* (see West, 1937), did not convulse mice within 1 hr of the subcutaneous administration of 250 mg/kg, West (1937) reported convulsive activity in both rabbits and cats of slow onset after intravenous doses of 100 mg/kg and 20–200 mg/kg, respectively. Furthermore, in cats anesthetized with pentobarbitone, both diaboline (intravenous, 9 mg/kg) and the closely related Wieland-Gümlich aldehyde (Fig. 1) (3.2 mg/kg) reduced the direct inhibition of hind limb flexor monosynaptic reflexes by aproximately 50% within 5 min (D. R. Curtis and D. Felix, unpublished observations), and both compounds when administered electrophoretically reduced the inhibitory effects of glycine on spinal neurons and the synaptic inhibition of Renshaw cells (D. R. Curtis and G. A. R. Johnston, unpublished).

3. Thebaine, Morphine, and Codeine

When administered intravenously, thebaine (Fig. 2) is a convulsant (Tatum *et al.*, 1929) and is approximately one-fifth to one-tenth as effective as strychnine as an antagonist of the direct inhibition of feline spinal motorneurons (Fatt, 1954; Pinto Corrado and Longo, 1961). Antagonism of the inhibitory action of glycine has been demonstrated, and again thebaine was less potent than strychnine (Curtis *et al.*, 1968*a*).

Although the action is probably unrelated to the analgesic effects of morphine and structurally related alkaloids, morphine (Fig. 2) is a convulsant when administered in relatively large doses (McGuigan and Ross, 1915; Jöel and Arndts, 1925; Tatum *et al.*, 1929; Wikler, 1944; Chernov and Woods, 1965). Probably largely because of the influence of morphine on the cardiopulmonary system, differing results have been reported regarding the effect of this alkaloid on spinal inhibition (Kruglov, 1964; Curtis and Duggan, 1969; Felpel *et al.*, 1970). However, both direct and recurrent inhibition of extensor monosynaptic reflexes can be reduced by morphine given intravenously in large doses (20–60 mg/kg; Curtis and Duggan, 1969), and the apparently greater susceptibility of recurrent inhibition (Kruglov, 1964; Felpel *et al.*, 1970) does not appear to result from antagonism at cholinergic excitatory synapses on Renshaw cells (Felpel *et al.*, 1970; Curtis and Duggan, 1969; Duggan and Curtis, 1972), although when administered electrophoretically some depression of acetylcholine release from axon collateral terminals has been demonstrated (Duggan and Curtis, 1972). Electrophoretic morphine also reduced the inhibitory action of glycine but not that of GABA on spinal interneurons (Curtis and Duggan, 1969). Morphine was less effective in this respect than thebaine, and codeine (Fig. 2), having a similar action, was in turn less effective than morphine. This relatively weak action of codeine as a glycine antagonist probably accounts for its central effects after systemic administration (Pinto Corrado and Longo, 1961), including reduction of spinal recurrent inhibition (Kruglov, 1964). Levorphanol (Fig. 2) also selectively reduced the inhibitory action of glycine on spinal neurons and was less potent than morphine (D. R. Curtis, A. W. Duggan, and G. A. R. Johnston, unpublished observations). Little selectivity could be demonstrated for 7-keto-*d*-dehydrothebaine methyl enolate (sinomenine; Kreuger, 1955) as an antagonist of the effects of glycine and GABA on spinal interneurons and Renshaw cells in the rat (T. J. Biscoe, A. W. Duggan, and D. Lodge, unpublished observations).

4. Gelsemine

Earlier findings regarding the pharmacology of gelsemine (Fig. 3) are summarized in Henry (1949). Although used therapeutically as a component of sedative mixtures, particularly in treating migraine and trigeminal neuralgia, a weak strychnine-like effect has been demonstrated in the cat spinal cord. Electrophoretic gelsemine reduced the inhibitory effect of glycine but not that of GABA on spinal interneurons and Renshaw cells (Curtis *et al.*, 1971*a*). The intravenous administration of 6.6 mg gelsemine hydrochloride per kilogram did not, however, affect spinal direct inhibition. The toxicity of gelsemine appears not to be as high as that of other constitutents of *Gelsemium* (see Moore, 1910; Henry, 1949: Saxton, 1965).

5. Laudanosine

The convulsant dose of laudanosine (Fig. 3) in dogs (dose not stated) was ascribed to effects in the spinal cord (Mercier and Delphaut, 1935). In contrast to bicuculline, to which it is structurally related, laudanosine (5 mg/kg) reduced the direct inhibition of hind limb flexor reflexes in cats anesthetized with pentobartitone, and when administered electrophoretically reduced the inhibitory action of glycine, but not that of GABA, on spinal interneurons (Curtis *et al.*, 1971*a*). The central action of laudanosine thus resembles that of strychnine.

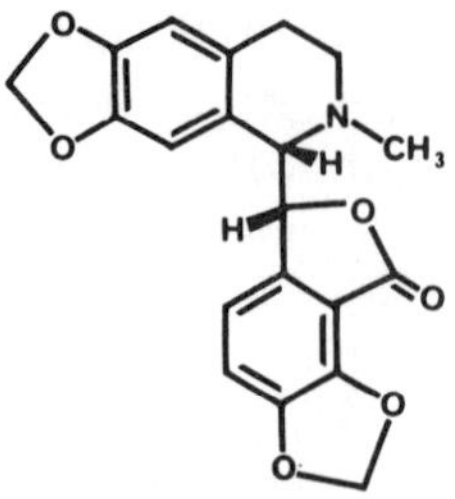

BICUCULLINE

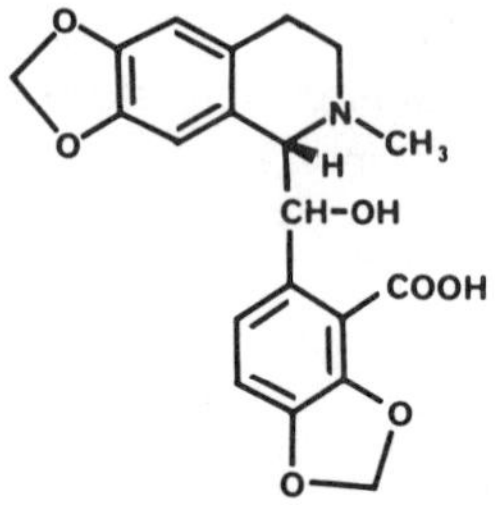

BICUCINE

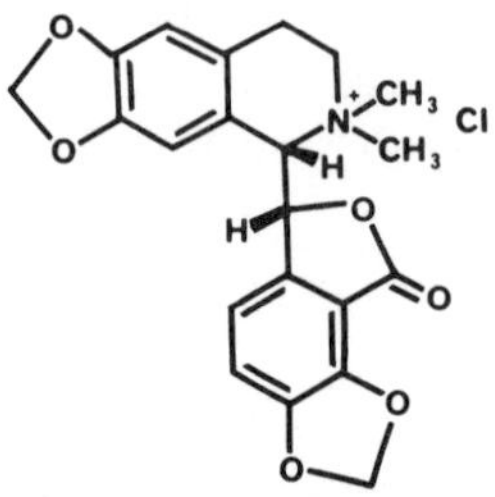

BICUCULLINE METHOCHLORIDE

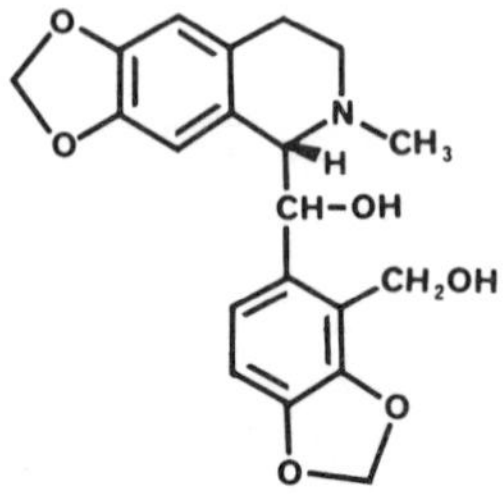

BICUCULLINE DIOL

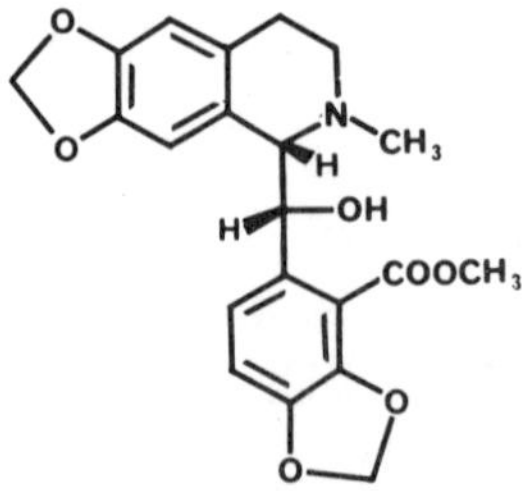

BICUCINE METHYL ESTER

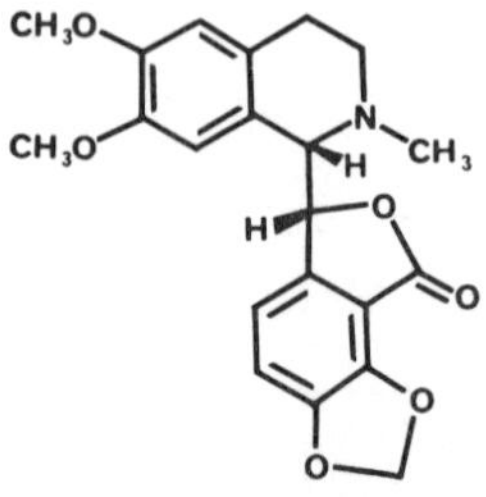

CORLUMINE

Fig. 4. Structures of bicuculline, bicucine, bicuculline methochloride, bicuculline diol, bicucine methyl ester, and corlumine.

III. BICUCULLINE AND RELATED SUBSTANCES

A. Chemistry

Bicuculline (Fig. 4) is a phthalide isoquinoline alkaloid first isolated from *Dicentra cucullaria* (Manske, 1932) and subsequently from a variety of species of *Corydalis, Dicentra*, and *Adlumia* (Kametani, 1969). The basic structure of bicuculline was established by Manske (1933*a*) and its synthesis achieved by Groenewoud and Robinson (1936). Its relative configuration was determined by degradative (Bláha *et al.*, 1964) and proton magnetic resonance procedure (Safe and Moir, 1964). The absolute configuration (1*S*,9R) was deduced from optical rotatory dispersion and circular dichroism measurements (Snatzke *et al.*, Swan, 1969). Incorrect absolute configurations of bicuculline have been illustrated in Chemical Abstracts Subject Indices (*68*:5575; *69*:5055; corrected in *72*:6085), Kametani (1969), Curtis *et al.*, (1972), and Kier and George (1973). Molecular orbital calculations indicate that preferred conformations of bicuculline exist (Andrews and Johnston, 1973; Kier and George, 1973). Bicuculline is dextrorotary; its optical antipode (–)-bicuculline has been isolated from *Corydalis sewerzowi* (Yunousov and Yunousov, 1968) and synthesized and its X-ray crystal structure has been determined (Teitel *et al.*, 1972).

Bicuculline free base (MW 367.3) is sparingly soluble in water, with a pK_a of 6.48 determined by potentiometric titration of a 10^{-4} M solution of the hydrochloride (Andrews and Johnston, 1973); i.e., at physiological *p*H, bicuculline exists predominantly (approximately 89%) as its free base. For microelectrophoretic studies, bicuculline is usually prepared as a 5×10^{-3} M solution of the hydrochloride at *p*H 3 in 165×10^{-3} M sodium chloride (Curtis *et al.*, 1971*a*); no heating is necessary to prepare this solution. Indeed, heating should be avoided to ensure that there is no acid-catalyzed opening of the phthalide ring system which yields the hydroxy acid bicucine (Fig. 4; Manske, 1933*b*), a much less potent convulsant than bicuculline (Welch and Henderson, 1934*b*).

Quaternary salts of bicuculline are more water soluble than bicuculline hydrochloride. Bicuculline methiodide (MW 509.3) is easily prepared from bicuculline, and neutral aqueous solutions up to 4×10^{-2} M are obtained (Pong and Graham, 1973). Bicuculline methochloride (Fig. 4) (MW 417.8) is easily prepared from the methiodide and is more soluble (up to 2.5×10^{-1} M) than the latter (Johnston *et al.*, 1972).

Other synthetic materials derived from bicuculline and examined for pharmacological activity include (1) *N*-methylbicuculleine (Fig. 3), prepared by Hofmann degradation of bicuculline (Manske, 1933*a*); (2) bicuculline diol (Fig. 4), prepared by lithium aluminum hydride reduction of bicuculline (Snatzke *et al.*, 1969); and (3) bicucine methyl ester (Fig. 4), prepared by methylation of bicucine with diazomethane (Johnston *et al.*, 1972).

Corlumine (Fig. 4) isolated by Manske (1936) from *Dicentra cucullaria* and subsequently found in several species of *Corydalis* (Kametani, 1969), has the same absolute configuration (1*S*,9R) as bicuculline. Phthalide isoquinoline alkaloids with different absolute configurations include (−)-β-hydrastine (1R,9*S*), (−)-adlumine (1R,9R), and (+)-adlumine (1*S*,9*S*).

The chemistry of the phthalide isoquinoline alkaloids is reviewed by Stanek and Manske (1954), Stanek (1967), Kametani (1969), and Śantavý (1970).

B. Neuropharmacology

1. Bicuculline

Although the convulsant action of bicuculline (Fig. 4) and some related phthalide isoquinoline alkaloids was first described by Welch and Henderson some 40 years ago (1934*a,b*), the central effects of these substances have only recently been investigated in detail (Curtis *et al.*, 1970*b,c*) and use made of bicuculline as an experimental convulsant (Meldrum and Horton, 1971, 1973; Uhlemann and Neims, 1972). The effects of a number of simple isoquinoline derivatives had been described earlier by Laidlaw (1911).

The convulsant dose of bicuculline (intravenous) for laboratory mammals is of the order of 0.1–0.4 mg/kg, approximately $3–10 \times 10^{-7}$ M if uniformly distributed in body water: baboon and rhesus monkey, 0.1–0.4 mg/kg (Meldrum and Horton, 1971); rabbits, 0.2 mg/kg (Welch and Henderson, 1934*a*); anesthetized cats, 0.2–0.5 mg/kg (Curtis *et al.*, 1971*a*); mice, 0.1–0.2 mg/kg (Curtis *et al.*, 1971*a*; Johnston *et al.*, 1972); rats, 0.07 mg/kg (Johnston and Mitchell, 1971; 4.4 mg/kg, intraperitoneal).

Bicuculline is thus approximately as effective a convulsant as strychnine, and the major importance of recent investigations in cats and amphibia is that, unlike strychnine (Section II), bicuculline is a readily reversible antagonist of the central inhibitory effects of γ-aminobutyric acid (GABA). The use of this alkaloid has in fact been of considerable value in distinguishing those central inhibitory synapses which operate by releasing this particular amino acid from those which use glycine as a transmitter (see Curtis and Johnston, 1974).

A considerable number of publications from different laboratories now support this proposal, although there has been some controversy regarding bicuculline–GABA antagonism in the mammalian central nervous system. This has arisen in microelectrophoretic experiments largely because of the use of solutions of low convulsant potency (Godfraind *et al.*, 1970), perhaps resulting from hydrolysis to bicucine during preparation, or from difficulties associated with the interpretation of nonequilibrium "dose–response" measurements (Straughan *et al.*, 1971; Hill and Simmonds, 1973). The recent availability of quaternary salts or bicuculline which are more soluble than the hydrochloride may overcome some of these investigational difficulties. Bicuculline methiodide ("*N*-methylbicuculline;" Pong and Graham, 1972) is a more potent convulsant than bicuculline when administered intracisternally to rats, and both this salt (frog; Davidoff *et al.*, 1973) and the methochloride (Fig. 4) (cat; Johnston *et al.*, 1972) are GABA antagonists.

Bicuculline hydrochloride (10^{-4} M) does not alter the activity of bacterial or brain glutamic acid decarboxylase and GABA transaminase (Beart and Johnston, 1972; see also Davies and Comis, 1971; Straughan *et al.*, 1971), and both this and higher concentrations do not modify the transport of GABA into rat brain slices (Curtis *et al.*, 1970*b*; Straughan *et al.*, 1971; Peck *et al.*, 1973) or slices of cat spinal cord (Balcar and Johnston, 1973). The binding of bicuculline to synaptic membranes of rat cerebellar cortical tissue (Peck *et al.*, 1973) may underlie the reduction by bicuculline of the inhibitory action of GABA on mammalian central neurons, although further study of the specificity of such binding is warranted.

In a number of regions of the feline central nervous system, bicuculline has been demonstrated to be a more effective antagonist of the inhibitory action of electrophoretically administered GABA (and GABA-like amino acids; see Curtis *et al.*, 1968*a*, 1971*a,b*) than of glycine (and glycine-like amino acids): spinal cord (Curtis *et al.*, 1971*a*), cuneate nucleus (Kelly and Renaud, 1973*a*), medullary reticular formation (Tebēcis *et al.*, 1971; Tebēcis, 1973), hypoglossal nucleus (Duggan *et al.*, 1973), Deiters' nucleus (Curtis *et al.*, 1971*b*), hypothalamus (Nicoll and Barker, 1971; Dreifuss and Matthews, 1972), thalamic ventrobasal complex (Curtis *et al.*, 1971*b*), lateral geniculate nucleus (Curtis and Tebēcis, 1972), cerebellar interpositus nucleus (Kawaguchi and Ono, 1973), cerebellar, cerebral, and hippocampal cortices (Curtis *et al.*, 1971*b*), and the olfactory bulb (Felix and McLennan, 1971; Nicoll, 1971). Similar observations have been made in the spinal cord and cerebral cortex of the rat, although bicuculline displayed little specificity as an amino acid antagonist in the cerebral cortex (Biscoe *et al.*, 1972). A similar apparent reduction in specificity toward different amino acids was also observed in the cat thalamus and cerebral and cerebellar cortices (Curtis *et al.*, 1971*b*), and possibly indicates differences in both amino acid receptors and the importance of different amino acid transmitters in these regions in comparison with the cord.

Observations of this bicuculline–GABA antagonism together with the effects of electrophoretic or systemically administered bicuculline on synaptic inhibitory processes have been used to support other evidence (see Curtis and Johnston, 1974) which favors a role of GABA as the inhibitory transmitter of a number of central pathways in the spinal cord (Curtis *et al.*, 1971*a*; Huffman and McFadden, 1972; Levy and Anderson, 1972; Benoist *et al.*, 1972), cuneate nucleus (Kelly and Renaud, 1973*c*; Davidson and Reisine, 1971; Banna *et al.*, 1972), brain stem nuclei (Precht *et al.*, 1973), Deiters' nucleus (Curtis *et al.*, 1970*a*), thalamus (Duggan and McLennan, 1971; Curtis and Tebēcis, 1972), cerebellar nuclei (Kawaguchi and Ono, 1973), cerebellar (Curtis and Felix, 1971; Bisti *et al.*, 1971), hippocampal (Curtis *et al.*, 1970*d*), and cerebral (Curtis and Felix, 1971) cortices, and the olfactory bulb (Felix and McLennan, 1971; McLennan, 1971; Nicoll, 1971).

The depolarization by GABA of the superior cervical ganglion of the rat (Bowery and Brown, 1972) and cat (de Groat *et al.*, 1971), and of sensory ganglia of the cat (de Groat, 1972; de Groat *et al.*, 1972), is also suppressed by bicuculline. Bicuculline is also a GABA antagonist and blocks synaptic inhibitions in the frog cerebellum (Woodward *et al.*, 1971) and spinal cord (Davidoff, 1972*a*; Davidoff *et al.*, 1973; but see Pixner, 1973).

One important feature of the action of bicuculline in the mammal is the relatively short duration of action after systemic administration (Curtis *et al.*, 1971*a*; Bisti *et al.*, 1971; Levy and Anderson, 1972). That the molecule was rapidly detoxified was first suggested by Welch and Henderson (1934*a*), who noted the minimal effects in the rabbit resulting from the intravenous administration of fractions of the convulsive dose at intervals of 10–30 min.

The effects of bicuculline at GABA receptors in crustacea are somewhat controversial: although the alkaloid (1–3×10^{-4} M) suppressed the inhibitory action of both GABA and impulses in inhibitory nerve fibers on the stretch receptor of the crayfish *Eustacus armatus*, and was more potent in these effects than picrotoxinin (McLennan, 1970), bicuculline was less potent than picrotoxinin as a GABA antagonist at the neuromuscular junction of the crayfish *Cambarus clarkii* (Takeuchi and Onodera, 1972), and was reported as inactive (5×10^{-5} M) at the neuromuscular junction of the hermit crab *Eupagarus bernhardus* (Earl and Large, 1972). Picrotoxinin was ten times more potent than bicuculline as a GABA antagonist in the snail *Helix aspersa*, but five times less potent in the cockroach *Periplaneta americana* (Walker *et al.*, 1971). Such differences suggest that the GABA receptors of these various creatures have different properties, and that pharmacological findings in any one species regarding GABA antagonists need not necessarily be applicable to another species.

2. *Analogues*

The number of convulsant phthalide isoquinoline alkaloids which have been tested as antagonists of the central effects of amino acids is relatively small, largely because of low aqueous solubility. Potent members of this series of compounds such as bicuculline are convulsants when administered intravenously at doses less than 1 mg/kg; doses of relatively inactive compounds exceed 10–20 mg/kg. Factors to be considered in such differences include effectiveness at central receptors and also the access to these sites. Thus, for example, although bicuculline methochloride is more effective as a GABA antagonist than bicuculline when both are administered electrophoretically (Johnston *et al.*, 1972), the convulsant doses of the methochloride when administered systemically (mouse, intravenous, 12 mg/kg; 10-day-old rat, intraperitoneal, 10 mg/kg) exceed those of the parent alkaloid (0.2 mg/kg and 1 mg/kg), presumably because a diffusional barrier hinders the access of the quaternary compound to neurons. Thus a true assessment of the structure–activity relationship of bicuculline analogues can only be obtained when all are administered in the vicinity of neurons, although there may also be considerable interpretational difficulties in such analyses.

The convulsant dose of bicucine (Fig. 4) in rabbits is of the order of 15–20 mg/kg (intravenous; Welch and Henderson, 1934*b*), and modification of the inhibitory effects of either glycine or GABA could not be demonstrated in microelectrophoretic studies (Johnston *et al.*, 1972). Bicuculline diol (Fig. 4) and (−)-bicuculline were also without effect microelectrophoretically (Johnston *et al.*, 1972, and unpublished). On the other hand, bicucine methyl ester (Fig. 4) reduced the inhibitory effect of GABA, but not that of glycine, on spinal interneurons and was of similar potency to bicuculline (Johnston *et al.*, 1972). In contrast, *N*-methylbiculleine (Fig. 3) was a glycine antagonist (Johnston *et al.*, 1972).

Corlumine (Fig. 4) was a less potent convulsant than bicuculline (rabbits, intravenous, 3 mg/kg; cats, subcutaneous, 5 mg/kg; Rice, 1938). When administered electrophoretically, corlumine blocked the inhibition of spinal interneuron firing by GABA without affecting that produced by glycine (Johnston *et al.*, 1972).

IV. PICROTOXININ AND RELATED SUBSTANCES

A. Chemistry

Picrotoxin is an equimolar mixture of picrotoxinin (MW 292.3) and picrotin (MW 310.3) (Fig. 5) and was first isolated by Boullay in 1812 from *Anamirta cocculus* and related poisonous plants of the moonseed family.

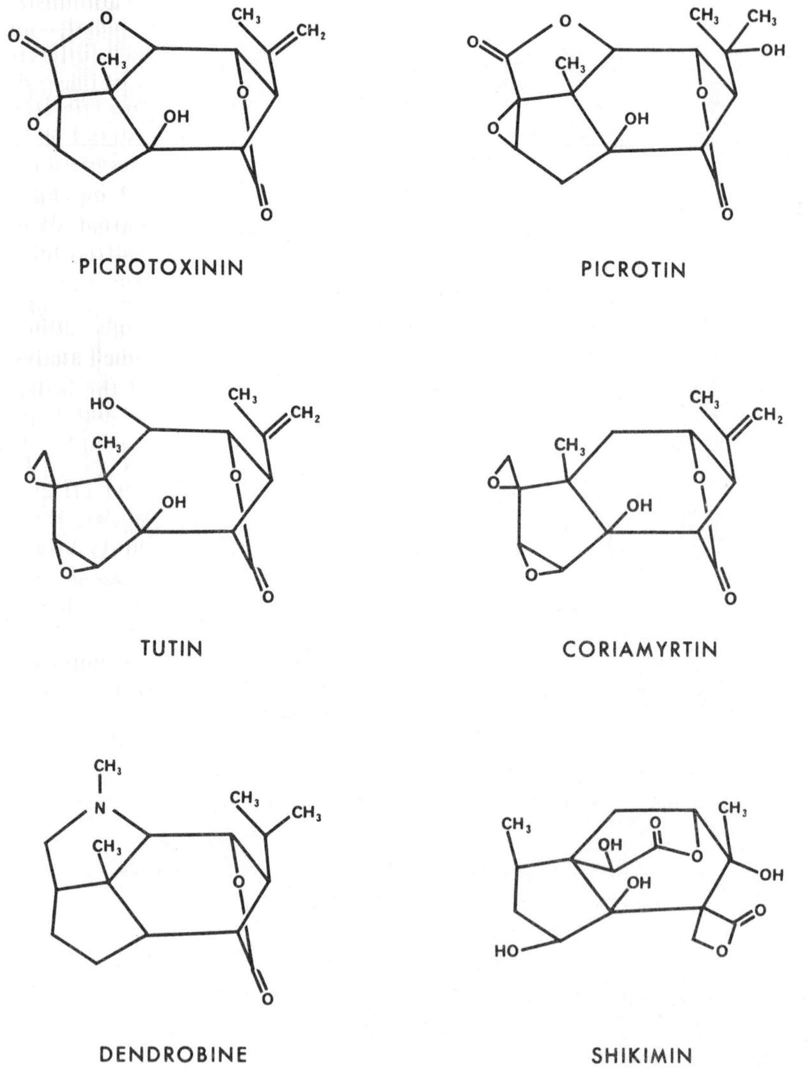

PICROTOXININ

PICROTIN

TUTIN

CORIAMYRTIN

DENDROBINE

SHIKIMIN

Fig. 5. Structures of picrotoxinin, picrotin, tutin, coriamyrtin, dendrobine, and shikimin.

The commercially available picrotoxin can be separated readily into its components by column chromatography on silica gel (Jarboe and Porter, 1965). A saturated aqueous solution of picrotoxin is approximately 10^{-2} M (based on a mean MW of 301.3). The *p*H of freshly prepared solutions slowly decreases with little apparent change in potency, whereas elevation of the *p*H beyond about 9.5 markedly reduces the convulsant potency (Ramwell and Shaw, 1963).

Tutin (Fig. 5) (MW 294.3) is structurally related to picrotoxinin. It is the poisonous constituent of the New Zealand species of *Coriaria*, known collectively as "tutu," and was first isolated by Easterfield and Aston (1901). It is some five times more soluble in water than is picrotoxin (Curtis *et al.*, 1974).

Coriamyrtin (Fig. 5) (MW 278.3), which lacks the secondary hydroxyl group of tutin, was first isolated from the European *Coriaria myrtifolia* (Riban, 1864, 1867) and subsequently found in the Japanese *Coriaria japonica.*

The determination of the absolute structures of picrotoxinin, picrotin, tutin, and coriamyrtin has been reviewed in detail by Porter (1967).

Dendrobine (Fig. 5) (MW 264.4) was first isolated from the Szechuan variety of the Chinese herbal preparation Chin-Shih-Hu (Chen and Chen, 1935*a*). The plant responsible for the presence of dendrobine in this preparation is probably the ornamental orchid *Dendrobium nobile.* The alkaloid is structurally related to picrotoxinin and tutin. Aspects of its chemistry are discussed by Porter (1967). Recently, the absolute configuration has been determined (Behr and Leander, 1972) and a total synthesis achieved (Inubushi *et al.*, 1972).

B. Neuropharmacology

1. Picrotoxinin

Until 1963, descriptions of the pharmacology of picrotoxinin (Fig. 5) were largely devoted to the convulsive phenomena, which in mammals appear to involve predominantly supraspinal regions (see Hahn, 1960). Some attempts had been made, however, to correlate these effects with a transmitter function of GABA. This proposal was based on the antagonism between picrotoxin and GABA which had been demonstrated in crustacea, and which presumably underlies the excitatory effects of picrotoxin on these creatures (Florey, 1951; Gerschenfeld, 1973).

In relatively low concentrations (10^{-6} to 10^{-5} M), picrotoxin blocks synaptic inhibition and the effects of GABA in a number of different crustacean preparations: crayfish heart (Florey, 1957); crayfish stretch receptor (Elliott and Florey, 1956; Kuffler, 1960; Iwasaki and Florey, 1969; McLennan, 1970); and the inhibitory neuromuscular junctions of the crayfish (Robbins and Van der Kloot, 1958; Robbins, 1959; Van der Kloot, 1960; Takeuchi and Takeuchi, 1969), lobster (Grundfest *et al.*, 1958), and crab (Epstein and Grundfest, 1970; Earl and Large, 1972). Antagonism of synaptic inhibition and the inhibitory effects of GABA has been demonstrated in insects (Usherwood and Grundfest, 1965), and picrotoxin also reduced the depolarization by GABA of amphibian spinal afferent fibers *in vitro* (Tebēcis and Phillis, 1969; Barker and Nicoll, 1973) and of mammalian autonomic (de Groat, 1970; Bowery and Brown, 1972) and sensory (de Groat, 1972; de Groat *et al.*, 1972) ganglia *in vivo*. Since most of these tissues are relatively insensitive to inhibitory amino acids other than GABA, the specificity of picrotoxin as a GABA antagonist could not be determined, but in the isolated amphibian spinal cord picrotoxin blocked the depolarization of afferent fibers by both GABA and L-glutamate (Tebēcis and Phillis, 1969).

A detailed analysis of the reversible effects of picrotoxin at the crayfish neuromuscular junction led to the suggestion that the antagonism was noncompetitive in type, one molecule of picrotoxin decreasing the conductance increase induced by two molecules of GABA, either by preventing the access of the amino acid to receptor sites or by interfering with the movement of ions through the synaptic membrane (Takeuchi and Takeuchi, 1969). The latter mechanism was also proposed to explain the effect of relatively high concentrations of picrotoxin on the chloride permeability of the nonsynaptic membrane of crayfish muscle (Ozeki *et al.*, 1966). No explanation has been provided in terms of receptor or membrane mechanisms of the reported antagonism of the depolarization by 5-hydroxytryptamine of autonomic ganglia by picrotoxin, an effect not observed using bicuculline (de Groat and Lalley, 1973).

In 1963, Eccles *et al.* provided the first definitive evidence of the reduction by picrotoxin (intravenous, topical) of an inhibitory process in the mammalian spinal cord. A number of previous investigations (and numerous subsequent ones) had been concerned with this "presynaptic" inhibitory process (see Schmidt, 1971), in which reduction of excitatory synaptic transmission is accompanied by depolarization of the terminal portions of primary afferent fibers. GABA is now generally accepted as the transmitter involved in this process, the reduction by picrotoxin of both the inhibition of reflex activity and the terminal depolarization being explained in terms of antagonism between picrotoxin and GABA at inhibitory axodendritic synapses on motoneurons and/or depolarizing axoaxonic synapses on afferent terminals (see Curtis and Johnston, 1974). A number of other synaptic inhibitions in the vertebrate CNS are also reduced by picrotoxin and are not affected by strychnine. At many of these sites, bicuculline also interferes with the inhibitory mechanism, and there is reasonably convincing neurochemical and other evidence that GABA is the transmitter. In the majority of cases, the amino acid operates as a hyperpolarizing inhibitory transmitter, and the important inhibitions in the mammal which are sensitive to systemically administered picrotoxin include basket cell inhibition of Purkinje cells and Golgi cell inhibition of cerebellar granule cells (Bisti *et al.*, 1971); granule cell inhibition of olfactory mitral cells (Nicoll, 1971); caudonigral inhibition (Precht and Yoshida, 1971); Purkinje cell inhibition of vestibular (Obata *et al.*, 1970; Fukuda *et al.*, 1972) and cerebellar nuclei (Kawaguchi and Ono, 1973); vestibular inhibition of ocular motoneurons (Highstein *et al.*, 1971; Precht *et al.*, 1973; Highstein, 1973); and the long-latency and -duration inhibitions of cuneate (Banna and Jabbur, 1969; Davidson and Reisine, 1971; Kelly and Renaud, 1973*c*), medullary (Sauerland and Mizuno, 1969; Nakamura and Wu, 1970; Morimoto and Kawamura, 1972), and spinal (Eccles *et al.*, 1963; Kellerth and Szumski, 1966; Kellerth, 1968; Levy and Anderson, 1972; Besson *et al.*, 1971) neurons which are associated with afferent terminal depolarization. Such antagonism of inhibition throughout the nervous system, and presumably also at GABA-mediated inhibitory synapses in the cerebral (and hippocampal) cortices which have yet to be thoroughly investigated with picrotoxin, accounts for its effects when directly injected into brain tissue (Baker *et al.*, 1965; Banerjee *et al.*, 1970) or into the ventricles (Feldberg and Georgiev, 1970) and when administered systemically.

Despite this quite substantial evidence that picrotoxin interferes with the action of synaptically released GABA in the vertebrate central nervous system, the results of experiments in which microelectrophoretically administered picrotoxin has been tested as a GABA antagonist have been somewhat inconsistent. The major problem is probably technical, picrotoxin having a low solubility and being poorly ionized in aqueous solution. Most investigations have thus depended on the electroosmotic ejection of picrotoxin from saturated solutions in 165×10^{-3} M NaCl (see Curtis, 1964). In the cat cerebral cortex, picrotoxin has been reported to be inactive as a GABA antagonist (Krnjević *et al.*, 1966; Krnjević, 1971) and to be a reversible antagonist of the action of GABA in a high proportion of cells (Hill *et al.*, 1972*a*; Hill and Simmonds, 1973). In the rat cerebral cortex, no selectivity could be demonstrated for picrotoxin, which reduced the effects of GABA, glycine, and β-alanine on all cells tested (Biscoe *et al.*, 1972). In the cerebellar cortex of the cat, picrotoxin did not interfere markedly with the depression of Purkinje cell firing by GABA (Kawamura and Provini, 1970), although in the frog picrotoxin blocked the synaptic inhibition of Purkinje cells and the effects of GABA but not those of glycine (Woodward *et al.*, 1971).

Electrophoretic picrotoxin readily antagonized the inhibitory action of GABA, but not that of glycine, on 80% of mitral cells tested in the olfactory bulb of the rabbit, and reduced the inhibitory effects of granule cell excitation on mitral cells (Nicoll, 1971). Picrotoxin also suppressed both vestibular inhibition and the inhibitory action of GABA on oculomotor neurons in the rabbit (Obata and Highstein, 1970). Antagonism of the depressant effects of GABA has also been demonstrated in the supraoptic nucleus (Nicoll and Barker, 1971) and the hypoglossal nucleus (Bruggencate and Sonnhoff, 1972); in the latter region, the effects of glycine were unaltered. In Deiters' nucleus, selective antagonism of the inhibitory action of GABA was found for less than 20% of the cells tested (Bruggencate and Engberg, 1971), although in another investigation, in which picrotoxin was also shown to reduce the cerebellar inhibition of Deiters' cells, antagonism of the inhibitory effect of GABA without modification of that of glycine could be demonstrated with all cells tested with some micropipettes, and with none tested with others (Obata *et al.*, 1970). In the medullary reticular formation, picrotoxin slightly reduced the effects of GABA and glycine on less than 50% of cells tested (Hösli and Tebēcis, 1970), and although two reports suggest specific antagonism of the inhibition of cuneate neurons by GABA (Galindo, 1969; Kelly and Renaud, 1973*b*), another indicates significant antagonism of the effects of both GABA and glycine (Hill *et al.*, 1973).

The results of investigations made on spinal neurons are even more confusing, ranging from reduction of the effects of both glycine and GABA in 25% of cells (Curtis *et al.*, 1969; see also rat, Biscoe *et al.*, 1972), to selective antagonism of GABA in approximately 15% of cells (Engberg and Thaller, 1970), to antagonism of the effect of *glycine* on 95% of neurons tested (Davidoff and Aprison, 1969). It is reasonably clear from all of these observations that a more soluble picrotoxin-like molecule is required in order to fully assess the actions of this compound at central amino acid receptors.

Although a relatively long latency is said to be a characteristic feature of the enhanced excitability resulting from intravenous picrotoxin, a time reduced by increasing doses and by topical or intraarterial administration (Hahn, 1960; Ramwell and Shaw, 1963), the effects of microelectrophoretically administered picrotoxin are not unusually slower than those of strychnine or bicuculline. Many of the recent reports of the action of picrotoxin on specific inhibitory mechanisms do not include precise details of the time course, but doses of the order of 3 mg/kg significantly modify spinal dorsal root potentials and associated excitability changes in afferent fibers within minutes (Bell and Anderson, 1972; Levy and Anderson, 1972). Hence slow penetration of a blood–brain diffusional barrier, or even chemical modification of the picrotoxin molecule prior to its involvement with GABA receptors, seems an unlikely explanation for the latency of action, and this time probably reflects the complex interrelationships of inhibitory systems and neuronal pathways modified by this substance.

2. *Picrotin*

Picrotin (Fig. 5) is considerably less active as a convulsant than picrotoxinin. In mice, after intraperitoneal injections, the convulsant and lethal doses of picrotin are approximately 50 times those of picrotoxinin (Jarboe *et al*., 1968). The relative inactivity of picrotin has also been discussed by Ramwell and Shaw (1963), and picrotoxinin is generally assumed to be responsible for effects observed in investigations in which picrotoxin was used.

3. *Dendrobine*

The general pharmacology of dendrobine, a nitrogen-containing compound (Fig. 5), has been discussed by Chen and Chen (1935*b*). The convulsant dose for laboratory mammals (intravenous) is of the order of 20 mg/kg. When administered electrophoretically near spinal neurons, dendrobine was found to block the inhibitory action of *glycine* and not that of GABA. Furthermore, intravenous doses of 3 mg/kg reduced the direct inhibition of spinal flexor monosynaptic reflexes in the cat, but were much less effective than strychnine, 0.1 mg/kg (Curtis *et al*., 1971*a*).

4. *Tutin*

The convulsant action of tutin (Fig. 5) was first investigated by Marshall (1906, 1909), and an exhaustive study was made of its effects on a variety of animals by Fitchett and Malcolm (1909; see also Fitchett, 1908; Ford, 1910; Porter, 1967; Fastier, 1971) largely because of the detrimental effects on the New Zealand economy of stock losses resulting from the ingestion of the tutu plant.

Marshall considered that the effects were predominantly supraspinal in origin, whereas Fitchett and Malcolm indicated that there was convulsive activity below a spinal transection in the cat, as occurs with picrotoxinin. Subcutaneous doses of 1–2 mg/kg produce convulsions in laboratory mammals (Marshall, 1906; Fitchett and Malcolm, 1909; see also Jarboe *et al*., 1968), and in the spinal cat anesthetized with pentobarbitone sodium amounts exceeding 1.5 mg/kg (intravenous) reduce the prolonged (presynaptic) inhibition of gastrocnemius monosynaptic reflexes by repetitive stimulation of flexor muscle afferents and the dorsal root potentials generated by such an inhibiting volley. Doses exceeding 6 mg/kg also reduce spinal direct inhibition (Curtis *et al*., 1973).

It thus seems probable that tutin is a GABA antagonist, and would reduce GABA-mediated inhibition elsewhere in the nervous system. Direct evidence of this antagonism was obtained in microelectrophoretic studies on spinal neurons, although concentrations of tutin adequate to suppress the inhibitory action of GABA considerably reduced that of glycine (Curtis *et al.*, 1973). Thus despite the considerable advantage of tutin over both bicuculline and picrotoxinin in terms of aqueous solubility, this nonselectivity as an amino acid antagonist rather limits its usefulness in neuropharmacological investigations of amino acid inhibitory transmitters, although inhibitions modified by GABA would be expected to be affected to a greater extent than those which involve glycine as the transmitter.

5. *Coriamyrtin*

Coriamyrtin is a close structural analogue of tutin (Fig. 5) and appears to have very similar central effects (Marshall, 1912), although no reports have been published concerning its action on central inhibitory processes. Coriamyrtin is three to ten times more potent on a weight basis than picrotoxin as a convulsant of laboratory mammals, the convulsant dose (intravenous) in rabbits being 0.14 mg/kg (Maloney, 1936; Swanson and Chen, 1936). The effects are more rapid in onset and of shorter duration than those of picrotoxinin, and a study of repeated subconvulsive doses suggests that coriamyrtin is rapidly detoxified in the body. The toxicity of coriamyrtin in mice (subcutaneous) is similar to that of picrotoxinin and tutin (Jarboe *et al.*, 1968). Antagonism of the inhibitory effect of GABA, but not that of glycine, on spinal neurons has been observed in the cat (D. R. Curtis, J. Davies, G. A. R. Johnston, and R. M. McCulloch, unpublished), but the low solubility of coriamyrtin has hindered a thorough investigation of its effects at a cellular level.

6. *Shikimin*

The general pharmacology of shikimin (Fig. 5) has been reported by Kajimoto *et al.* (1955*b*). The convulsive dose (subcutaneous) in mice is between 290 and 300 mg/kg, convulsions being preceded by general paralysis. In the pentobarbitone-anesthetized cat, intravenous administration of 1–1.3 mg/kg results in salivation, dilation of the pupils, and oscillating increases in blood pressure, all changes similar to those produced by picrotoxinin, and reduction in the prolonged (presynaptic) inhibition of spinal reflexes, direct inhibition remaining unaffected (Curtis *et al.*, 1973).

V. MISCELLANEOUS SUBSTANCES

A. Benzylpenicillin

Benzylpenicillin (Fig. 6) (penicillin G, MW 334.4) is produced commercially from mutant strains of *Penicillium chrysogenum*. The chemistry

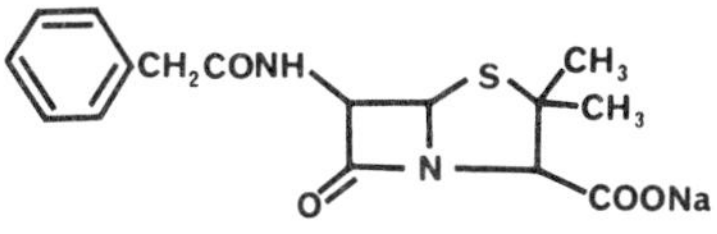

BENZYL PENICILLIN

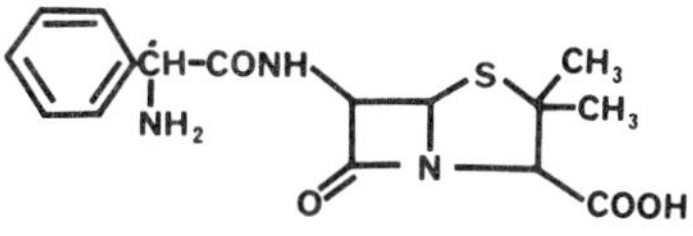

AMPICILLIN

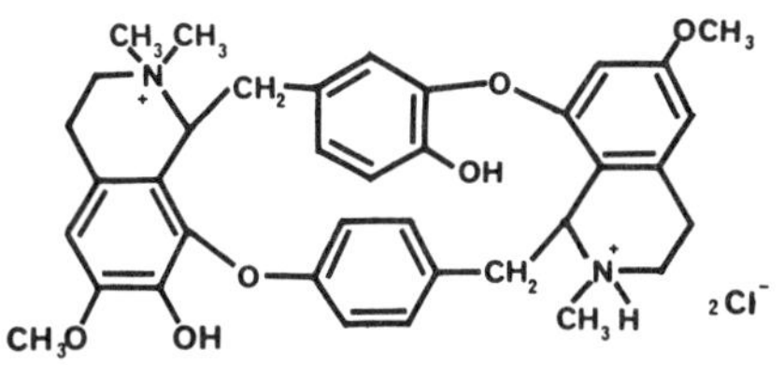

(+) -TUBOCURARINE

DIHYDROCHLORIDE

Fig. 6. Structures of benzylpenicillin, ampicillin, and (+)-tubocurarine dihydrochloride.

of this and related penicillins has been reviewed extensively in a book edited by Clarke *et al.*, (1949) and more recently by Doyle and Nayler (1964). The X-ray crystal structure of benzylpenicillin reported by Crowfoot *et al.* (1949) is the mirror image of the absolute structure (Crowfoot Hodgkin and Maslen, 1961).

Although benzylpenicillin is strictly neither of plant origin nor an alkaloid, its convulsant action is of considerable interest, both as a complication of penicillin therapy and as a means of establishing an experimental epileptiform focus (Gloor, 1969; Prince, 1972). Numerous publications have been concerned with the effects of penicillin on nervous tissue, both invertebrate (Ayala *et al.*, 1970, 1971; Earl and Large, 1973*b*; Meyer and Prince, 1973) and vertebrate (Prince, 1969; Walsh, 1971; Kao and Crill, 1972*a,b*; Spira and Bennett, 1972; Clarke and Hill, 1972; Ayala *et al.*, 1973). Most of these investigations were concerned with the possible enhancement of excitation by penicillin or with induced alteration of neuronal metabolism (Swanson, 1972; O'Connor *et al.*, 1972).

Recently, however, penicillin has been shown to reduce "presynaptic" inhibition and the depolarizing action of GABA on afferent terminals in the amphibian spinal cord, being approximately one-hundredth as effective as bicuculline (Davidoff, 1972*b*). Subsequent studies in the cat demonstrated reduction by intravenous sodium benzylpenicillin (0.9–1.8

g/kg) of prolonged (presynaptic) but not direct spinal inhibition, and diminution of dorsal root reflexes and potentials (Davidoff, 1972*c*; D. R. Curtis, C. J. A. Game, and R. M. McCulloch, unpublished observations). Furthermore, electrophoretic penicillin reversibly antagonized the inhibitory effect of GABA but not that of glycine on spinal neurons (Davidoff, 1972*b*; Curtis *et al.*, 1972) and of GABA on pericruciate neurons (Curtis *et al.*, 1972). Preliminary studies suggest that ampicillin (Fig. 6) is either very weak or inactive as a GABA antagonist, an observation consistent with this derivative being one-fifth as toxic as benzylpenicillin when injected intracerebrally into mice (Gerald *et al.*, 1973).

Although a blood–brain barrier may in part account for the relatively high doses of penicillin required to modify synaptic inhibition in the cord, the action of electrophoretic penicillin as a GABA antagonist is relatively weak when compared with that of bicuculline (Curtis *et al.*, 1972). Hence attempts at modifying synaptic inhibition in the cerebral and cerebellar cortices have not been successful largely because of difficulties in achieving adequate concentration of penicillin by electrophoretic administration. Topically administered penicillin has been observed to reduce cortical surface potentials generated by the recurrent inhibition of pyramidal tract neurons (van Duijn *et al.*, 1973), but the similar action of strychnine suggests that this effect may not necessarily indicate antagonism of synaptic inhibition. Nevertheless, antagonism of GABA seems undoubtedly an important factor in the epileptogenic action of penicillin.

B. Tubocurarine

(+)-Tubocurarine chloride (Fig. 6) is a bis-benzylisoquinoline alkaloid salt (MW 681.64) isolated from *Chondodendron tomentosum*. Originally thought to be a bis-quaternary derivative, recent chemical and spectroscopic studied have shown it to contain one tertiary and one quaternary nitrogen atom (Everett *et al.*, 1970). Reviews of the chemistry of bis-benzylisoquinoline alkaloids include those of Kulka (1954, 1960), Bentley (1965), and Kametani (1969).

Tubocurarine is included in this section because of the strychnine-like action of topically administered curare on the cerebral cortex (Chang, 1953; Feldberg *et al.*, 1957) and the curare-like action of strychnine at cholinergic junctions (Lanari and Luco, 1939; Alving, 1961; Landau, 1967). The use of curare or strychnine has not contributed, however, to the elucidation of the nature of the transmitters involved either in the cortex or at cholinergic junctions, respectively, and in general the concentrations used have been in excess of those for which relatively specific effects of these two alkaloids have been demonstrated.

In the cerebral (Bhargava and Meldrum, 1969; Banerjee *et al.*, 1970) and hippocampal (Feldberg and Lotti, 1970) cortices, no direct evidence has been provided that either strychnine or curare (and related alkaloids, toxiferine and alloferin; Bhargava and Meldrum, 1969) suppresses inhibitory mechanisms. Although a recent report suggests that the convulsant action of (+)-tubocurarine is due in part to antagonism of the inhibitory action of GABA on cortical neurons (Hill *et al.*, 1972*b*), the effects of glycine were apparently also antagonized in both the cortex (Hill *et al.*, 1972*b*) and the cuneate nucleus (Hill *et al.*, 1973). Furthermore, no antagonism has been found between (+)-tubocurarine and either of these amino acids in the feline spinal cord (D. R. Curtis, unpublished observations) and curare has not been found to block the inhibitory action of GABA at the crab neuromuscular junction (Earl and Large, 1973*a*).

Although depression of cholinergic transmission by strychnine has been demonstrated at the neuromuscular junction (Bouman, 1937, Alving, 1961; Landau, 1967), and in autonomic ganglia (Lanari and Luco, 1939), an effect which may in part be presynaptic (Takagi and Takayanagi, 1966; McKinstry and Koelle, 1967; Neal, 1967; Landau, 1967), no evidence has been obtained in the central nervous system that concentrations of strychnine sufficient to suppress synaptic inhibition interfere with either the release or the postsynaptic action of acetylcholine at nicotinic synapses on Renshaw cells (Curtis, 1967).

C. Pilocarpine, Arecoline, and Coniine

Correlations have been demonstrated between the effects of strychnine, thebaine, coniine, pilocarpine, and arecoline (Fig. 7) at central inhibitory synapses and at peripheral cholinergic synapses, of both the neuromuscular junction and the superior cervical ganglion (Ferguson *et al.*, 1970). These observations have been claimed to support a cholinergic link in postsynaptic central inhibition, a proposal which, however, has not gained support from more direct investigations of the inhibitory process. Such a cholinergic link is difficult to reconcile with the failure of either atropine sulfate (1–2 mg/kg) or dihydro-β-erythroidine hydrochloride (2–4 mg/kg) to diminish spinal direct inhibition (D. R. Curtis, unpublished observations; see also Fatt, 1954). Furthermore, neither coniine nor pilocarpine has been found to be a glycine antagonist (D. R. Curtis, A. W. Duggan, and G. A. R. Johnston, unpublished observations).

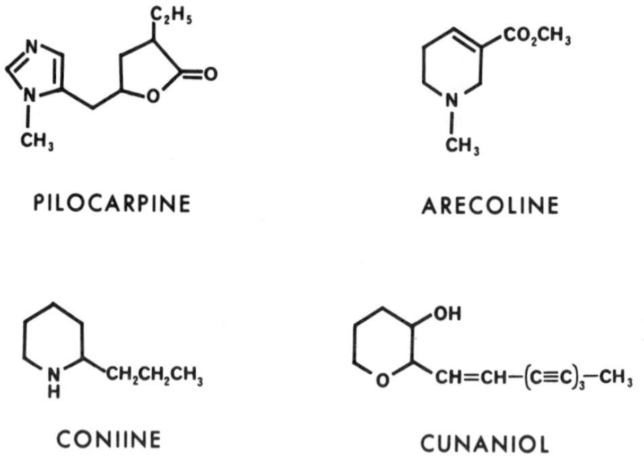

Fig. 7. Structures of pilocarpine, arecoline, coniine, and cunaniol.

1. Pilocarpine

Pilocarpine, a pyrrole derivative (Fig. 7) (MW 208.3) from the leaves of *Pilocarpus microphyllus* and related species, has both central excitatory and depressant effects when administered to rats and mice (Zablocka and Esplin, 1963), and after systemic administration reduced (80–160 mg/kg) direct inhibition and abolished (40–80 mg/kg) recurrent inhibition (Esplin and Zablocka, 1964) of spinal motoneurons in the cat. Subsequently, on the basis of the effects of pilocarpine on the threshold in mice for strychnine convulsions, at explanation has been provided for the action of pilocarpine at inhibitory synapses in terms of a presynaptic action releasing and depleting the store of inhibitory transmitter (Turkanis and Esplin, 1968).

2. Arecoline

Arecoline, a tetrahydropyridine derivative (Fig. 7) (MW 155.2) isolated from the seeds of the betel nut palm *Areca cathecu*, has behavioral effects in cats similar to those of pilocarpine, and the decrease of spinal postsynaptic inhibition by doses of 10–60 mg/kg has been ascribed to actions on the release mechanism of the inhibitory transmitter (Zablocka and Esplin, 1964).

3. Coniine

The complex central and peripheral effects of the various alkaloids from hemlock, including coniine (2-*n*-proplypiperidine, Fig. 7) (MW

127.2), have been described by Bowman and Sanghvi (1963). An increase in membrane permeability to potassium ions has been proposed (Sampson, 1966) as an explanation of the reduction by systemically administered coniine (25–30 mg/kg) of spinal direct and recurrent inhibition and the effects of the alkaloid on spinal reflexes (Sampson *et al.*, 1966). Differences between the actions of coniine and strychnine have also been suggested from observations of the effects of both compounds on olivocochlear inhibition (La Grutta and Desmedt, 1964), an inhibitory process reduced by strychnine (Desmedt and Monaco, 1962), which may however involve cholinergic transmission rather than an amino acid transmitter (Brown *et al.*, 1969; Guth and Bobbin, 1971).

D. Cunaniol

Cunaniol, a polyacetylenic alcohol from *Clibadium sylvestre*, is included because the actions on fish are similar to those of picrotoxin, cunaniol (Fig. 7) being ten times more potent in producing hyperactivity, loss of coordination, and eventually paralysis and death (Quilliam and Stables, 1968). Cunaniol is a convulsant in frogs and mice; the convulsant dose for mice (intraperitoneal), 4 mg/kg, is similar to that of picrotoxinin, but the effects of cunaniol are more rapid in onset (Quilliam and Stables, 1969). In the cat, microelectrophoretically administered cunaniol (saturated solution in 165 mM NaCl) reduces the effectiveness of GABA, relative to that of glycine, as a depressant of the firing of spinal neurons (D. R. Curtis and R. M. McCulloch unpublished).

VI. CONCLUSIONS

Certain substances which produce increased and abnormal activity of the mammalian central nervous system interfere with inhibitory synaptic processes.

Strychnine and a number of other compounds (Figs. 1–3) antagonize the action of glycine, an important inhibitory transmitter in the spinal cord. Bicuculline, picrotoxinin, and some related substances (Figs. 4 and 5) including benzylpenicillin (Fig. 6) reduce the action of GABA, a major inhibitory transmitter in both the brain and the spinal cord. In addition, picrotoxinin is a GABA antagonist at a number of invertebrate inhibitory synapses.

The use of these convulsants has aided analyses of inhibitory mechanisms, and further investigations of structurally related compounds are warranted, as a means of strengthening proposals regarding the molecular nature of the inhibitory transmitters and the receptors with which they interact.

It is unlikely that GABA and glycine are the only inhibitory transmitters in the central nervous system, and thus it seems very probable that further "classes" of convulsants that act as antagonists of central inhibition await investigation.

VII. REFERENCES

Ajmone-Marsan, C., 1969, Acute effects of topical epileptogenic agents, in: *Basic Mechanisms of the Epilepsies* (H. H. Jasper, A. A. Ward, Jr., and A. Pope, eds.) pp. 299–319, Little, Brown, Boston.

Alving, B. O., 1961, The action of strychnine at cholinergic functions, *Arch. Int. Pharmacodyn.* **131**:123.

Amann, A., Jaeger, K. H., and Jarisch, A., 1943, Vergleichende Untersuchungen über Strychnin und Strychninderivate, *Arch. Exptl. Pathol. Pharmakol.* **201**:161.

Andrews, P., and Johnston, G. A. R., 1973, Molecular orbital and proton magnetic resonance studies of bicuculline, *Nature New Biol.* **243**:29.

Aprison, M. H., and Werman, R., 1968, A combined neurochemical and neurophysiological approach to identification of central nervous system transmitters, in: *Neurosciences Research,* Vol. 1, (S. Ehrenpreis and P. C. Solnitzky, eds.) pp. 143–174, Academic Press, New York.

Araki, T., 1965, The effects of strychnine on the postsynaptic inhibitory action. *Excerpta Medica Foundation,* Amsterdam. In: *Lectures and Symposia, XXIII International Congress of Physiological Sciences,* pp. 96–97.

Ayala, G. F., Lin, S., and Vasconetto, C., 1970, Penicillin as epileptogenic agent: Its effect on an isolated neuron, *Science* **167**:1257.

Ayala, G. F., Spencer, W. A., and Gumnit, R. J., 1971, Penicillin as an epileptogenic agent: Effect on an isolated synapse, *Science* **171**:915.

Ayala, G. F., Dichter, M., Gumnit, R. J., Matsumoto, H., and Spencer, W. A., 1973, Genesis of epileptic interictal spikes: New knowledge of cortical feedback systems suggests a neurophysiological explanation of brief paroxysms, *Brain Res.* **52**:1.

Baker, W. W., Kratky, M., and Benedict, F., 1965, Electrographic responses to intrahippocampal injections of convulsant drugs, *Exptl. Neurol.* **12**:136.

Balcar, V. J., and Johnston, G. A. R., 1973, High affinity uptake of transmitters: Studies on the uptake of L-aspartate, GABA, L-glutamate and glycine in cat spinal cord, *J. Neurochem.* **20**:529.

Banerjee, U., Feldberg, W., and Georgiev, V. P., 1970, Microinjections of tubocurarine, leptazol, strychnine and picrotoxin into the cerebral cortex of anaesthetized cats, *Brit. J. Pharmacol.* **40**:6.

Banna, N. R., and Jabbur, S. J., 1969, Pharmacological studies on inhibition in the cuneate nucleus of the cat, *Internat. J. Neuropharmacol.* **8**:299.

Banna, N. R., Naccache, A., and Jabbur, S. J., 1972, Picrotoxin-like action of bicuculline, *Europ. J. Pharmacol.* **17**:301.

Barker, J. L., and Nicoll, R. A., 1973, The pharmacology and ionic dependency of amino acid responses in the frog spinal cord, *J. Physiol.* (*Lond.*) **288**:259.

Beart, P. M., and Johnston, G. A. R., 1972, Bicuculline and GABA-metabolising enzymes, *Brain Res.* **38**:226.

Behr, D., and Leander, K., 1972, Studies on Orchidaceae alkaloids. XXVIII. The absolute configuration of the dendrobine alkaloids, *Acta Chem. Scand.* **26**:3196.

Bell, J. A., and Anderson, E. G., 1972, The influence of semicarbazide-induced depletion of γ-aminobutyric acid on presynaptic inhibition, *Brain. Res.* **43**:161.

Benoist, J. M., Besson, J. M., Conseiller, C., and Le Bars, D., 1972, Action of bicuculline on presynaptic inhibition of various origins of the cat's spinal cord, *Brain Res.* **43**:672.

Bentley, K. W., 1954, *The Chemistry of the Morphine Alkaloids*, Oxford University Press, Oxford.

Bentley, K. W., 1965, *The Isoquinoline Alkaloids*, Pergamon Press, Oxford.

Bentley, K. W., 1971, The morphine alkaloids, in: *The Alkaloids*, Vol. XIII, pp. 1–163, Academic Press, New York.

Besson, J. M., Rivot, J. P., and Aleonard, P., 1971, Action of picrotoxin on presynaptic inhibition of various origins in the cat's spinal cord, *Brain Res.* **26**:212.

Bhargava, V. K., and Meldrum, B. S., 1969, The strychnine-like action of curare and related compounds on the somatosensory evoked response of the rat cortex, *Brit. J. Pharmacol.* **37**:112.

Biscoe, T. J., Duggan, A. W., and Lodge, D., 1972, Antagonism between bicuculline, strychnine and picrotoxin and depressant amino acids in the rat central nervous system, *Comp. Gen. Pharmacol.* **3**:423.

Bisti, S., Iosif, G., Marchesi, G. F., and Strata, P., 1971, Pharmacological properties of inhibitions in the cerebellar cortex, *Exptl. Brain Res.* **14**:24.

Bláha, K., Hrbek, J., Kovář, J., Pijewska, L., and Šantavý, F., 1964, Configuration of nitrogen-containing compounds. XVIII. Determination of relative and absolute configuration of phthalide isoquinoline alkaloids, *Coll. Czech. Chem. Commun.* **29**:2328.

Bouman, H. D., 1937, Experiments on the mechanism of strychnine "curarization," *J. Physiol. (Lond.)* **88**:328.

Bowery, N. G., and Brown, D. A., 1972, Depolarization of isolated rat ganglia by γ-aminobutyric acid and related compounds, *Brit. J. Pharmacol.* **45**:160P.

Bowman, W. C., and Sanghvi, I. S., 1963, Pharmacological actions of hemlock (*Conium maculatum*) alkaloids, *J. Pharm. Pharmacol.* **15**:1.

Bradley, K., Easton, D. M., and Eccles, J. C., 1953, An investigation of primary or direct inhibition, *J. Physiol. (Lond.)* **122**:474.

Bremer, F., 1944, Le mode d'action de la strychnine à la lumière de travaux récents, *Arch. Int. Pharmacodyn. Therap.* **69**:249.

Brown, R. D., Daigneault, E. A., and Pruett, J. R., 1969, The effects of selected cholinergic drugs and strychnine on cochlear responses and olivo-cochlear inhibition, *J. Pharmacol. Exptl. Therap.* **165**:300.

Bruggencate, G. Ten, and Engberg, I., 1971, Iontophoretic studies in Deiters' nucleus of the inhibitory actions of GABA and related amino acids and the interactions of strychnine and picrotoxin, *Brain Res.* **25**:431.

Bruggencate, G. Ten, and Sonnhof, U., 1972, Effects of glycine and GABA, and blocking actions of strychnine and picrotoxin in the hypoglossus nucleus, *Pflüger's Arch.* **334**:240.

Burger, A., 1954, The benzylisoquinoline alkaloids, in: *The Alkaloids*, Vol. IV (R. H. F. Manske, ed.) pp. 29–75, Academic Press, New York.

Chang, H., 1951, An observation on the effect of strychnine on local cortical potentials, *J. Neurophysiol.* **14**:23.

Chang, H., 1953, Similarity in action between curare and strychnine on cortical neurons, *J. Neurophysiol.* **16**:221.

Chen, K. K., and Chen, A. L., 1935*a*, The alkaloid of Chin-Shih-Hu, *J. Biol. Chem.* **111**:653.

Chen, K. K., and Chen, A. L., 1935*b*, The pharmacological action of dendrobine, the alkaloid of Chin-Shih-Hu, *J. Pharmacol. Exptl. Therap.* **55**:319.

Chernov, H. I., and Woods, L. A., 1965, Central nervous system distribution and metabolism of C^{14}-morphine during morphine-induced feline mania, *J. Pharmacol. Exptl. Therap.* **149**:146.

Chou, T. Q., 1931, The alkaloids of gelsemium. I. Gelsemine and gelsemicine, *Chin. J. Physiol.* **5**:131.

Clarke, G., and Hill, R. G., 1972, Effects of a focal penicillin lesion on responses of rabbit cortical neurones to putative neurotransmitters, *Brit. J. Pharmacol.* **44**:435.

Clarke, H. T., Johnson, J. R., and Robinson, R., 1949, *The Chemistry of Penicillin*, Princeton University Press, Princeton, N.J.

Conroy, H., and Chakrabarti, J. K., 1959, NMR spectra of gelsemine derivatives: The structure and biogenesis of the alkaloid gelsemine, *Tetrahedron Letters* **4**:6.

Coombs, J. S., Eccles, J. C., and Fatt, P., 1955, The inhibitory suppression of reflex discharges from motoneurons, *J. Physiol.* (*Lond.*) **130**:396.

Corrodi, H., Hellerbach, J., Züst, A., Hardegger, E., and Schnider, O., 1959, Die Konfiguration der Morphinane, *Helv. Chim. Acta* **42**:212.

Crowfoot, D., Bunn, C. W., Rogers-Low, B. W., and Turner-Jones, A., 1949, The X-ray crystallographic investigation of the structure of penicillin, in: *The Chemistry of Penicillin* (H. T. Clarke, J. R. Johnson, and R. Robinson, eds.) pp. 310–381, Princeton University Press, Princeton, N.J.

Crowfoot, Hodgkin, D., and Maslen, E. N., 1961, The X-ray analysis of the structure of cephalosporin C, *Biochem. J.* **79**:393.

Curtis, D. R., 1962, The depression of spinal inhibition by electrophoretically administered strychnine, *Internat. J. Neuropharmacol.* **1**:239.

Curtis, D. R., 1963, The pharmacology of central and peripheral inhibition, *Pharmacol. Rev.* **15**:333.

Curtis, D. R., 1964, Microelectrophoresis, in: *Physical Techiques in Biological Research*, Vol. 5 (W. L. Nastuk, ed.) pp. 144–190, Academic Press, New York.

Curtis, D. R., 1967, Acetylcholine, strychnine and spinal inhibition, *Nature* (*Lond.*) **215**:1503.

Curtis, D. R., and Duggan, A. W., 1969, The depression of spinal inhibition by morphine, *Agents Actions* **1**:14.

Curtis, D. R., and Felix, D., 1971, The effect of bicuculline upon synaptic inhibition in the cerebral and cerebellar cortices of the cat, *Brain Res.* **34**:301.

Curtis, D. R., and Johnston, G. A. R., 1974, Amino acid transmitters in the mammalian central nervous system, *Ergeb. Physiol. Biol. Chem. Exptl. Pharmacol.* **69**:97.

Curtis, D. R., and Ryall, R. W., 1966, Pharmacological studies upon spinal presynaptic fibres, *Exptl. Brain Res.* **1**:195.

Curtis, D. R., and Tebēcis, A. K., 1972, Bicuculline and thalamic inhibition, *Exptl. Brain Res.* **16**:210.

Curtis, D. R., Hösli, L., and Johnston, G. A. R., 1968*a*, A pharmacological study of the depression of spinal neurones by glycine and related amino acids, *Exptl. Brain Res.* **6**:1.

Curtis, D. R., Hösli, L., Johnston, G. A. R., and Johnston, I. H., 1968*b*, The hyperpolarization of spinal motoneurones by glycine and related amino acids, *Exptl. Brain Res.* **5**:235.

Curtis, D. R., Duggan, A. W., and Johnston, G. A. R., 1969, Glycine, strychnine, picrotoxin and spinal inhibition, *Brain Res.* **14**:759.

Curtis, D. R., Duggan, A. W., and Felix, D., 1970*a*, GABA and inhibition of Deiters' neurones, *Brain Res.* **23**:117.

Curtis, D. R., Duggan, A. W., Felix, D., and Johnston, G. A. R., 1970*b*, GABA, bicuculline and central inhibition, *Nature* (*Lond.*) **226**:1222.

Curtis, D. R., Duggan, A. W., Felix, D., and Johnston, G. A. R., 1970*c*, Bicucilline and central GABA receptors, *Nature* (*Lond.*) **228**:676.

Curtis, D. R., Felix, D., and McLennan, H., 1970*d*, GABA and hippocampal inhibition, *Brit. J. Pharmacol.* **40**:881.

Curtis, D. R., Duggan, A. W., Felix, D., and Johnston, G. A. R., 1971*a*, Bicuculline, an antagonist of GABA and synaptic inhibition in the spinal cord, *Brain Res.* **32**:69.

Curtis, D. R., Duggan, A. W., Felix, D., Johnston, G. A. R., and McLennan, H., 1971*b*, Antagonism between bicuculline and GABA in the cat brain, *Brain Res.* **33**:57.

Curtis, D. R., Duggan, A. W., and Johnston, G. A. R., 1971*c*, The specificity of strychnine as a glycine antagonist in the mammalian spinal cord, *Exptl. Brain Res.* **12**:547.

Curtis, D. R., Game, C. J. A., Johnston, G. A. R., McCulloch, R. M., and Maclachlan, R. M., 1972, Convulsive action of penicillin, *Brain Res.* **43**:242.

Curtis, D. R., Davies, J., Game, C. J. A., Johnston, G. A. R., and McCulloch, R. M., 1973, Central actions of shikimin and tutin, *Brain Res.* **63**:419.

Davidoff, R. A., 1972*a*, The effects of bicuculline on the isolated spinal cord of the frog, *Exptl. Neurol.* **35**:179.

Davidoff, R. A., 1972*b*, Penicillin and presynaptic inhibition in the amphibian spinal cord, *Brain Res.* **36**:218.

Davidoff, R. A., 1972*c*, Penicillin and inhibition in the cat spinal cord, *Brain Res.* **45**:638.

Davidoff, R. A., and Aprison, M. H., 1969, Picrotoxin antagonism of the inhibition of interneurones by glycine, *Life Sci.* **8**:107.

Davidoff, R. A., Aprison, M. H., and Werman, R., 1969, The effects of strychnine on the inhibition of interneurons by glycine and γ-aminobutyric acid, *Internat. J. Neuropharmacol.* **8**:191.

Davidoff, R. A., Silvey, G. E., Kobetz, S. A., and Spira, H. M., 1973, *N*-Methyl bicuculline and primary afferent depolarization, *Exptl. Neurol.* **38**:525.

Davidson, N., and Reisine, H., 1971, Presynaptic inhibition in cuneate blocked by GABA antagonists, *Nature New Biol.* **234**:223.

Davies, W. E., and Comis, S. D., 1971, Bicuculline and its effect on γ-aminobutyric acid transaminase in the guinea-pig brain stem, *Nature New Biol.* **231**:156.

De Groat, W. C., 1970, The actions of γ-aminobutyric acid and related amino acids on mammalian autonomic ganglia, *J. Pharmacol. Exptl. Therap.* **172**:384.

De Groat, W. C., 1972, GABA-depolarization of a sensory ganglion: Antagonism by picrotoxin and bicuculline, *Brain Res.* **38**:429.

De Groat, W. C., and Lalley, P. M., 1973, Interaction between picrotoxin and 5-hydroxytryptamine in the superior cervical ganglion of the cat, *Brit. J. Pharmacol.* **48**: 233.

De Groat, W. C., Lalley, P. M., and Block, M., 1971, The effects of bicuculline and GABA on the superior cervical ganglion of the cat, *Brain. Res.* **25**:665.

De Groat, W. C., Lalley, P. M., and Saum, W. R., 1972, Depolarization of dorsal root ganglia in the cat by GABA and related amino acids: Antagonism by picrotoxin and bicuculline, *Brain Res.* **44**:273.

Desmedt, J. E., and Monaco, P., 1962, in: *The Pharmacology of a Centrifugal Inhibitory Pathway in the Cat's Acoustic System* (W. D. M. Paton, ed.) pp. 183–188, Pergamon Press, Oxford.

Diamond, J., Roper, S., and Yasargil, G. M., 1973, The membrane effects, and sensitivity to strychnine, of neural inhibition of the Mauthner cell, and its inhibition by glycine and GABA, *J. Physiol.* (*Lond.*) **232**:87.

Doyle, F. P., and Nayler, J. H. C., 1964, Penicillins and related structures, *Advan. Drug. Res.* **1**:2.

Dreifuss, J. J., and Matthews, E. K., 1972, Antagonism between strychnine and glycine and bicuculline and GABA, in the ventromedial hypothalamus, *Brain Res.* **45**:599.

Duggan, A. W., and Curtis, D. R., 1972, Morphine and the synaptic activation of Renshaw cells, *Neuropharmacology* **11**:189.

Duggan, A. W., and McLennan, H., 1971, Bicuculline and inhibition in the thalamus, *Brain Res.* **25**:188.

Duggan, A. W., Lodge, D., and Biscoe, T. J., 1973, The inhibition of hypoglossal motoneurones by impulses in the glossopharyngeal nerve of the rat, *Exptl. Brain Res.* **17**:261.

Dusser de Barenne, J. G., 1933, The mode and site of action of strychnine in the nervous system, *Physiol. Rev.* **13**:325.

Dusser de Barenne, J. G., and McCulloch, W. S,. 1973, Physiological delimination of neurones in the central nervous system, *Am. J. Physiol.* **127**:620.

Earl, J., and Large, W. A., 1972, The effect of bicuculline, picrotoxin and strychnine on neuromuscular inhibition in hermit crabs (*Eupagurus bernhardus*), *J. Physiol.* (*Lond.*) **224**:45P.

Earl, J., and Large, W. A., 1973*a*, *d*-Tubocurarine does not antagonize the inhibitory effects of GABA at the crustacean neuromuscular junction, *Brain Res.* **49**:456.

Earl, J., and Large, W. A., 1973*b*, Effect of penicillin on the increase in membrane conductance induced by γ-aminobutyric acid at the crab neuromuscular junction, *Brit. J. Pharmacol.* **48**:318.

Easterfield, T. H., and Aston, B. C., 1901, XI. Tutu. Part I. Tutin and Coriamyrtin, *J. Chem. Soc.* **79**:120.

Eccles, J. C., Fatt, P,. and Koketsu, K., 1954, Cholinergic and inhibitory synapses in a pathway from motor-axon collaterals to motoneurones, *J. Physiol.* (*Lond.*) **126**:524.

Eccles, J. C., Schmidt, R. F., and Willis, W. D., 1963, Pharmacological studies on presynaptic inhibition, *J. Physiol.* (*Lond.*) **168**:500.

Elliott, K. A. C., and Florey, E., 1956, Factor I—An inhibitory factor from brain, *J. Neurochem.* **1**:181.

Engberg, I., and Thaller, A., 1970, On the interaction of picrotoxin with GABA and glycine in the spinal cord, *Brain Res.* **19**:151.

Epstein, R., and Grundfest, H., 1970, Desensitization of gamma aminobutyric acid (GABA) receptors in muscle fibres of the crab *Cancer borealis*, *J. Gen. Physiol.* **56**:33.

Esplin, D. W., and Zablocka, B., 1964, Pilocarpine blockade of spinal inhibition in cats, *J. Pharmacol. Exptl. Therap.* **143**:174.

Essig, C. F., 1972, Drug withdrawal convulsions in animals, in: *Experimental Models of Epilepsy* (D. P. Purpura, J. K. Penry, D. B. Tower, D. M. Woodbury, and R. D. Walter, eds.) pp. 495–508, Raven Press, New York.

Everett, A. J., Lowe, L. A., and Wilkinson, S., 1970, Revision of the structures of (+)-tubocurarine chloride and (+)-chondrocurine, *J. Chem. Soc. Sect. D* **16**:1020.

Fastier, F. N., 1971, Tutu poisoning, in: *Research in Physiology* (F. F. Kao, K. Koizumi, and M. Vassalle, eds.) pp. 653–659, Aulo Gaggi Publ., Bologna.

Fatt, P., 1954, Biophysics of junctional transmission, *Physiol. Rev.* **34**:674.

Feldberg, W., and Georgiev, V. P., 1970, Central effects of picrotoxin when acting from the liquor spaces in anaesthetized cats, *Brit. J. Pharmacol.* **40**:23.

Feldberg, W., and Lotti, V. J., 1970, Direct and indirect activation of the hippocampus by tubocurarine, *J. Physiol.* (*Lond.*) **210**:697.

Feldberg, W., Malcolm, J. L., and Darian Smith, I., 1957, Effect of tubocurarine on the electrical activity of the cat's brain under chloralose, *J. Physiol.* (*Lond.*.) **138**:178.

Felix, D., and McLennan, H., 1971, The effect of bicuculline on the inhibition of mitral cells of the olfactory bulb, *Brain Res.* **25**:661.

Felpel, L. P., Sinclair, J. G., and Yim, G. K. W., 1970, Effects of morphine on Renshaw cell activity, *Neuropharmacology* **9**:203.

Ferguson, R. K., Zablocka-Esplin, B., and Esplin, D. W., 1970, Peripheral cholinergic blockade by drugs that block postsynaptic central inhibition, *Arch. Int. Pharmacodyn. Therap.* **185**:298.

Fitchett, F., 1908, Physiological action of tutin, *Trans. New Zealand Inst.* **41**:286.

Fitchett, F., and Malcolm, J., 1909, Tutin, *Quart. J. Exptl. Physiol.* **2**:335.

Florey, E., 1951, Vorkommen und Funktion sensibler Erregungssubstanzen und die abbauender Fermente in Tierreich, *Z. Vergl. Physiol.* **33**:327.

Florey, E., 1957, Further evidence for the transmitter function of Factor I, *Naturwissenschaften* **44**:424.

Ford, W. W., 1910, On the toxicology of the tutin plant, *J. Pharmacol. Exptl. Therap.* **2**:73.

Frankenhaeuser, B., 1951, Limitations of method of strychnine neuronography, *J. Neurophysiol.* **14**:73.

Fukuda, J., Highstein, S. M., and Ito, M,. 1972, Cerebellar inhibitory control of the vestibulo-ocular reflex investigated in the rabbit IIIrd nucleus, *Exptl. Brain Res.* **14**:511.

Fuortes, M. G. F., and Nelson, P. G., 1963, Strychnine: Its action on spinal motoneurones of cats, *Science* **140**:806.

Furukawa, T., Fukami, Y., and Asada, Y., 1964, Effects of strychnine and procaine on collateral inhibition of the Mauthner cell of goldfish, *Jap. J. Physiol.* **14**:386.

Galindo, A., 1969, GABA–picrotoxin interaction in the mammalian central nervous system, *Brain Res.* **14**:763.

Gerald, M. C., Massey, J., and Spadaro, D. C., 1973, Comparative convulsant activity of various penicillins after intracerebral injections in mice, *J. Pharm. Pharmacol.* **25**:104.

Gerschenfeld, H. M., 1973, Chemical transmission in invertebrate central nervous systems and neuromuscular junctions, *Physiol. Rev.* **53**:1.

Gloor, P., 1969, Epileptogenic action of penicillin, *Ann N.Y. Acad. Sci.* **166**:350.

Godfraind, J. M., Krnjević, K., and Pumain, R., 1970, Doubtful value of bicuculline as a specific antagonist of GABA, *Nature* (*Lond.*) **228**:675.

Groenewoud, P. W. G,. and Robinson, R., 1936, Synthesis of bicuculline. Part I, *J. Chem. Soc.* **1936**:199.

Grundfest, A., Reuben, J. P., and Rickles, W. H., 1958, Electrophysiology and pharmacology of lobster muscle fibres, *Biol. Bull.* **115**:332.

Guth, P. S., and Bobbin, R. P., 1971, The pharmacology of peripheral auditory processes: Cochlear pharmacology, *Advan. Pharmacol. Chemotherap.* **9**:93.

Hahn, F., 1960, Analeptics, *Pharmacol. Rev.* **12**:447.

Henry, T. A., 1949, *The Plant Alkaloids*, Churchill, London.

Highstein, S. M., 1973, The organization of the vestibo-oculomotor and trochlear reflex pathways in the rabbit, *Exptl. Brain Res.* **17**:285.

Highstein, S. M., Ito, M., and Tsuchiya, T., 1971, Synaptic linkage in the vesibulo-ocular reflex pathway of rabbit, *Exptl. Brain Res.* **13**:306.

Hill, R. G., and Simmonds, M. A., 1973, A method for comparing the potencies of γ-aminobutyric acid antagonists on single cortical neurones using micro-iontophoretic techniques, *Brit. J. Pharmacol.* **48**:1.

Hill, R. G., Simmonds, M. A., and Straughan, D. W., 1972*a*, Antagonism of GABA by picrotoxin in the feline cerebral cortex, *Brit. J. Pharmacol.* **44**:807.

Hill, R. G., Simmonds, M. A., and Straughan, D. W., 1972*b*, Convulsive properties of *d*-tubocurarine and cortical inhibition, *Nature* (*Lond.*) **240**:51.

Hill, R. G., Simmonds, M. A., and Straughan, D. W., 1973, Amino acid antagonists and the depression of cuneate neurones by γ-aminobutyric acid (GABA) and glycine, *Brit. J. Pharmacol.* **47**:642P.

Hösli, L., and Tebēcis, A. K., 1970, Actions of amino acids and convulsants on bulbar reticular neurones, *Exptl. Brain Res.* **11**:111.

Huffman, R. D., and McFadin, L. S., 1972, Effects of bicuculline on central inhibition, *Neuropharmacology* **11**:789.

Inubushi, Y., Kikuchi, T., Isuka, T., Tanaka, K., Saji, I., and Tokane, K., 1972, Total synthesis of the alkaloid (±)-dendrobine, *J. Chem. Soc. Chem. Commun.* **22**:1252.

Iwaskai, S., and Florey, E., 1969, Inhibitory miniature potentials in the stretch receptor neurone of crayfish, *J. Gen. Physiol.* **53**:666.

Jarboe, C. H., and Porter, L. A., 1965, The preparative column chromatographic separation of picrotoxin, *J. Chromatog.* **19**:427.

Jarboe, C. H., Porter, L. A., and Buckler, R. T., 1968, Structural aspects of picrotoxinin action, *J. Med. Chem.* **11**:729.

Jöel, E., and Arndts, F., 1925, Beiträge zur Pharmakologie der Körperstellung und der Labyrinthreflexe, *Pflüger's Arch.* **210**:280.

Johnson, E. S., Roberts, M. H. T., and Straughan, D. W., 1970, Amino-acid induced depression of cortical neurones, *Brit. J. Pharmacol.* **38**:659.

Johnston, G. A. R., and Mitchell, J. F., 1971, The effect of bicuculline, metrazol, picrotoxin and strychnine on the release of [^{3}H] GABA from rat brain slices, *J. Neurochem.* **18**:2441.

Johnston, G. A. R., Beart, P. M., Curtis, D. R., Game, C. J. A., McCulloch, R. M., and Maclachlan, R. M., 1972, Bicuculline methochloride as a GABA antagonist, *Nature New Biol.* **240**:219.

Kajimoto, Y., Fujimori, H., and Hirota, K., 1955*a*, Study on the toxic components of "Shikimi." I. Chemical study, *Tokushima J. Exptl. Med.* **2**:104.

Kajimoto, Y., Oto, T., Fujimori, H., Harada, K., and Hirota, K., 1955*b*, Study on Akimehishiba. II. General pharmacological property, *Tokushima J. Exptl. Med.* **2**:111.

Kametani, T., 1969, *The Chemistry of the Isoquinoline Alkaloids*, Hirokawa, Tokyo.

Kano, M., and Ishikawa, K., 1972, Effect of tetanus toxin on the inhibitory neuromuscular junction of crayfish muscle, *Exptl. Neurol.* **37**:550.

Kao, L. I., and Crill, W. E., 1972*a*, Penicillin-induced segmental myoclonus: I. Motor responses and intracellular recording from motoneurons, *Arch. Neurol.* **26**:156.

Kao, L. I., and Crill, W. E., 1972*b*, Penicillin-induced segmental myoclonus: II. Membrane properties of cat spinal motoneurons, *Arch. Neurol.* **26**:162.

Kawaguchi, S., and Ono, T., 1973, Bicuculline and picrotoxin sensitive inhibition in interpositus neurones of cat, *Brain Res.* **58**:260.

Kawamura, H., and Provini, L., 1970, Depression of cerebellar Purkinje cells by microiontophoretic application of GABA and related amino acids, *Brain Res.* **24**:293.

Kellerth, J.-O., 1968, Aspects on the relative significance of pre- and postsynaptic inhibition in the spinal cord, in: *Structure and Function of Inhibitory Neuronal Mechanisms* (C. von Euler, S. Skoglund, and U. Söderberg, eds.) pp. 197–212, Pergamon Press, Oxford.

Kellerth, J.-O., and Szumski, A. J., 1966, Post-synaptic inhibitions from muscular afferents differentiated by strychnine and picrotoxin, in: *Muscular Afferents and Motor Control* (R. Granit, ed.) pp. 385–396, Almqvist and Wiksell, Stockholm.

Kelly, J. S., and Renaud, L. P., 1973*a*, On the pharmacology of the γ-aminobutyric acid receptors on the cuneo-thalamic relay cells of the cat, *Brit. J. Pharmacol.* **48**:369.

Kelly, J. S., and Renaud, L. P., 1973*b*, On the pharmacology of the glycine receptors on the cuneo-thalamic relay cells in the cat, *Brit. J. Pharmacol.* **48**:387.

Kelly, J. S., and Renaud, L. P., 1973*c*, On the pharmacology of ascending, descending and recurrent postsynaptic inhibition of the cuneo-thalamic relay cells in the cat, *Brit. J. Pharmacol.* **48**:396.

Kier, L. B., and George, J. M., 1973, Molecular orbital studies on the conformation of bicuculline and β-hydroxy GABA, *Experientia* **29**:501.

Klee, M. R., Faber, D. S., and Heiss, W.-D., 1973, Strychnine- and pentylenetetrazol-induced changes of excitability in aplysia neurons, *Science* **179**:1133.

Kreuger, H. M., 1955, Narcotics and analgesics, in: *The Alkaloids*, Vol. 5 (R. F. Manske, ed.) pp. 2–78, Academic Press, New York.

Krnjević, K., 1971, Effects of drugs on inhibitory synapses, in: *Advances in Cytopharmacology*, Vol. 1 (F. Clementi and B. Ceccarelli, eds.) pp. 419–426, Raven Press, New York.

Krnjević, K., Randić, M., and Straughan, D. W., 1966, Pharmacology of cortical inhibition, *J. Physiol.* (*Lond.*) **184**:78.

Kruglov, N. A., 1964, Effect of the morphine-group analgesics on the central inhibitory mechanisms, *Internat. J. Neuropharmacol.* **3**:197.

Kuffler, S. W., 1960, Excitation and inhibition in single nerve cells, in: *Harvey Lectures, 1958–59*, pp. 176–218, Academic Press, New York.

Kulka, M., 1954, Bisbenzylisoquinoline alkaloids, in: *The Alkaloids*, Vol. IV (R. H. F. Manske, ed.) pp. 199–247, Academic Press, New York.

Kulka, M., 1960, Bisbenzylisoquinoline alkaloids, in: *The Alkaloids*, Vol. VII (R. H. F. Manske, ed.) pp. 439–474, Academic Press, New York.

Kuno, M., 1957, Effects of strychnine on the intracellular potentials of spinal motoneurons of the toad, *Jap. J. Physiol.* **7**:42.

La Grutta, V., and Desmedt, J. E., 1964, Contrastes entre les actions centrales de la coniine et de la strychnine, *Arch. Int. Pharmacodyn. Therap.* **151**:289.

Laidlaw, P. P., 1911, The action of some isoquinoline derivatives, *Biochem. J.* **5**:243.

Lanari, A., and Luco, J. V., 1939, The depressant action of strychnine on the superior cervical sympathetic ganglion and on skeletal muscle, *Am. J. Physiol.* **126**:277.

Landau, E. M., 1967, The effect of strychnine on the neuromuscular junction of the rat, *Life Sci.* **6**:2515.

Larson, M. D., 1969, An analysis of the action of strychnine on the recurrent IPSP and amino acid induced inhibitions in the cat spinal cord, *Brain Res.* **15**:185.

Levy, R. A., and Anderson, E. G., 1972, The effect of the GABA antagonists bicuculline and picrotoxin on primary afferent terminal excitability, *Brain Res.* **43**:171.

Liddell, E. G. T., and Sherrington, C. S., 1925, Further observations on myotatic reflexes, *Proc. Roy. Soc. Lond. Ser. B* **97**:267.

Longo, V. G., and Chiavarelli, S., 1962, Neuropharmacological analysis of strychnine-like drugs, in: *Pharmacological Analysis of Central Nervous Action* (W. D. M. Paton, ed.) pp. 189–198, Pergamon Press, Oxford.

Lovell, F. M., Pepinsky, R., and Wilson, A. J. C., 1959, X-ray analysis of the structure of gelsemine hydrohalides, *Tetrahedron Letters* **4**:1.

MacKay, M., and Crowfoot Hodgkin, D., 1955, A crystallographic examination of the structure of morphine, *J. Chem. Soc.* **1955**:3261.

Maier, W., and Gröger, D., 1971, Über den Einbau von Glycin in Strychnosalkaloide, *Arch. Pharm.* **304**:351.

Maloney, A. H., 1936, Studies on the pharmacological action of coriamyrtin, *J. Pharmacol. Exptl. Therap.* **57**:361.

Manske, R. H. F., 1932, The alkaloids of fumaraceous plants. II. *Dicentra cucullaria* (L.) Bernh., *Can. J. Res.* **7**:265.

Manske, R. H. F., 1933*a*, The alkaloids of fumaraceous plants. III. A new alkaloid, bicuculline, and its constitution, *Can. J. Res.* **8**:142.

Manske, R. H. F., 1933*b*, The alkaloids of fumaraceous plants. VIII. *Corydalis aurea*, Willd. and the constitution of bicucine, *Can. J. Res.* **9**:436.

Manske, R. H. F., 1936, The alkaloids of fumaraceous plants. XI. Two new alkaloids, corlumine and corlumidine, and their constitutions, *Can. J. Res.* **14B**:325.

Marshall, C. R., 1906, The physiological action of tutin, *J. Physiol.* (*Lond.*) **34**:xxix.

Marshall, C. R., 1909, The action of certain convulsants, *J. Physiol.* (*Lond.*) **38**:lxxxiii.

Marshall, C. R., 1912, The pharmacological action of coriamyrtin, *J. Pharmacol. Exptl. Therap.* **4**:135.

McGuigan, H., and Ross, E. L., 1915, The similarity and synergy of morphine and strychnine action, *J. Pharmacol. Exptl. Therap.* **7**:385.

McKinstry, D. N., and Koelle, G. B., 1967, Effects of drugs on acetylcholine release from the cat superior cervical ganglion by carbachol and by preganglionic stimulation, *J. Pharmacol. Exptl. Therap.* **157**:328.

McLennan, H., 1970, Bicuculline and inhibition of crayfish stretch receptor neurones, *Nature* (*Lond.*) **228**:674.

McLennan, H., 1971, The pharmacology of inhibition of mitral cells in the olfactory bulb, *Brain Res.* **29**:177.

Meldrum, B. S., and Horton, R. W., 1971, Convulsive effects of 4-deoxypyridoxine and of bicuculline in photosensitive baboons (*Papio papio*) and in rhesus monkeys (*Macaca mulatta*), *Brain Res.* **35**:419.

Meldrum, B. S., and Horton, R. W., 1973, Physiology of status epilepticus in primates, *Arch. Neurol.* **28**:1.

Mercier, F., and Delphaut, J., 1935, Sur les convulsions produits par la laudanosine, *Compt. Rend. Seanc. Soc. Biol.* **118**:168.

Meyer, H., and Prince, D., 1973, Convulsant actions of penicillin: Effects on inhibitory mechanisms, *Brain Res.* **53**:477.

Moore, C. W,. 1910, The constitutents of gelsemine, *J. Chem. Soc.* **97**:2223.

Morimoto, T., and Kawamura, Y., 1972, Inhibitory postsynaptic potentials of hypoglossal motoneurons of the cat, *Exptl. Neurol.* **37**:188.

Nakamura, Y., and Wu, C. Y., 1970, Presynaptic inhibition of jaw-opening reflex by high threshold afferents from the masseter muscle of the cat, *Brain Res.* **23**:193.

Neal, M. J., 1967, The effect of convulsant drugs on coaxially stimulated guinea-pig ileum, *Brit. J. Pharmacol.* **31**:132.

Nicoll, R. A., 1971, Pharmacological evidence for GABA as the transmitter in granule cell inhibition in the olfactory bulb, *Brain Res.* **35**:137.

Nicoll, R. A., and Barker, J. L., 1971, The pharmacology of recurrent inhibition in the supraoptic neurosecretory system, *Brain Res.* **35**:501.

Obata, K., and Highstein, S. M., 1970, Blocking by picrotoxin of both vestibular inhibition and GABA action on rabbit oculomotor neurones, *Brain Res.* **18**:538.

Obata, K., Takeda, K., and Shinozaki, H., 1970, Further study on pharmacological properties of the cerebellar-induced inhibition of Deiters' neurones, *Exptl. Brain Res.* **11**:327.

O'Connor, M. J., Herman, C. J., Rosenthal, M., and Jöbsis, F. F., 1972, Intracellular redox changes preceding onset of epileptiform activity in intact cat hippocampus, *J. Neurophysiol.* **35**:471.

Owen, A. G. W., and Sherrington, C. S., 1911, Observations on strychnine reversal, *J. Physiol.* (*Lond.*) **43**:232.

Ozeki, M., Freeman, A. R., and Grundfest, H., 1966, The membrane components of crustacean neuromuscular systems. II. Analysis of interactions among the electrogenic components. *J. Gen. Physiol.* **49**:1335.

Parnas, I., and Atwood, J. L., 1966, Differential effects of strychnine on crustacean slow, fast, and inhibitory neuromuscular systems, *J. Cell. Physiol.* **68**:1.

Peck, E. J., Jr., Schaeffer, J. M., and Clark, J. H., 1973, γ-Aminobutyric acid, bicuculline, and post-synaptic binding sites, *Biochem. Biophys. Res. Commun.* **52**:394.

Peerdeman, A. F., 1956, The absolute configuration of natural strychnine, *Acta Crystallog.* **9**:824.

Phillis, J. W., and Tebēcis, A. K., 1967, The responses of thalamic neurones to iontophoretically applied monoamines, *J. Physiol.* (*Lond.*) **192**:715.

Phillis, J. W., and York, D. H., 1967, Strychnine block of neural and drug-induced inhibition in the cerebral cortex, *Nature* (*Lond.*) **216**:922.

Pinto Corrado, A., and Longo, V. G., 1961, An electrophysiological analysis of the convulsant action of morphine, codeine and thebaine, *Arch. Int. Pharmacodyn. Therap.* **132**:255.

Pixner, D. B., 1973, Bicuculline and frog spinal neurones, *Brit. J. Pharmacol.* **47**:637P.

Pollen, D. A., and Ajmone-Marsan, C., 1965, Cortical inhibitory postsynaptic potentials and strychninization, *J. Neurophysiol.* **28**:342.

Pollen, D. A., and Lux, H. D., 1966, Conductance changes during inhibitory postsynaptic potentials in normal and strychninized cortical neurons, *J. Neurophysiol.* **29**:369.

Pong, S. F., and Graham, L. T., Jr., 1972, *N*-Methyl bicuculline, a convulsant more potent than bicuculline, *Brain Res.* **42**:486.

Pong, S. F., and Graham, L. T., Jr., 1973, A simple preparation of bicuculline methiodide, a water soluble GABA antagonist, *Brain Res.* **58**:266.

Porter, L. L., 1967, Picrotoxinin and related substances, *Chem. Rev.* **67**:441.

Precht, W., Baker, R., and Okada, Y., 1973, Evidence for GABA as the synaptic transmitter of the inhibitory vestibulo-ocular pathway, *Exptl. Brain Res.* **18**:415–428.

Precht, W., and Yoshida, M., 1971, Blockage of caudate-evoked inhibition of neurons in the substantia nigra by picrotoxin, *Brain. Res.* **32**:229.

Prince, D. A., 1969, Microelectrode studies of penicillin foci, in: *Basic Mechanisms of the Epilepsies* (H. H. Jasper, A. A. Ward, Jr., and A. Pope, eds.) pp. 320–328, Little, Brown, Boston.

Prince, D. A., 1972, Topical convulsant drugs and metabolic antagonists, in: *Experimental Models of Epilepsy* (D. P. Purpura, J. K. Penry, D. B. Tower, D. M. Woodbury, and R. D. Walter, eds.) pp. 51–83, Raven Press, New York.

Pritchard, J. W., 1971, The effect of strychnine on the leech Retzius cells, *Neuropharmacology* **10**:771.

Quilliam, J. P., and Stables, R., 1968, The effect of cunaniol, a polyacetylenic alcohol isolated from the plant *Clibadium sylvestre*, on piscine behaviour, *Brit. J. Pharmacol.* **34**:678P.

Quilliam, J. P., and Stables, R., 1969, Convulsant effects of Cunaniol, a polyacetylenic alcohol isolated from the plant *Clibadium sylvestre*, on frogs and mice, *Pharmacol. Res. Commun.* **1**:7.

Raffauf, R. F., 1970, *A Handbook of Alkaloids and Alkaloid-Containing Plants*, Wiley-Interscience, New York.

Ramwell, P. W., and Shaw, J. E., 1963, Some observations on the physical and pharmacological properties of picrotoxin solutions, *J. Pharm. Pharmacol.* **15**:611.

Rees, R., and Smith, H., 1967, Structure and biological activity of some reduction products of strychnine, brucine and their congeners, *J. Med. Chem.* **10**:624.

Riban, M. J., 1864, *Bull. Soc. Chim. France* **1**:87.

Riban, M. J., 1867, *Bull. Soc. Chim. France* **7**:79.

Rice, H. V., 1938, Pharmacological actions of corlumine, *J. Pharmacol. Exptl. Therap.* **63**:329.

Robbins, J., 1959, The excitation and inhibition of crustacean muscle by amino acids, *J. Physiol.* (*Lond.*) **148**:39.

Robbins, J., and Van der Kloot, W. G., 1958, The effect of picrotoxin on peripheral inhibition in the crayfish, *J. Physiol.* (*Lond.*) **143**:541.

Robinson, R., 1952, Molecular structure of strychnine, brucine and vomicine, in: *Progress in Organic Chemistry,* (J. W. Cook, ed.) pp. 1–21, Butterworths, London.

Robinson, T., 1968, *The Biochemistry of Alkaloids*, Springer-Verlag, Berlin.

Safe, S., and Moir, R. Y., 1964, Stereochemical configuration of some phthalideisoquinoline alkaloids, *Can. J. Chem.* **42**:160.

Sampson, S. R., 1966, Mechanism of coniine-blockade of postsynaptic inhibition in the spinal cord of the cat, *Internat. J. Neuropharmacol.* **5**:171.

Sampson, S. R., Esplin, D. W., and Zablocka, B., 1966, Effects of coniine on peripheral and central synaptic transmission, *J. Pharmacol. Exptl. Therap.* **152**:313.

Sandberg, F., and Kristianson, K., 1970, A comparative study of the convulsant effects of strychnos alkaloids, *Acta Pharm. Suecia* **7**:329.

Śantavý, F., 1970, Papaveraceae alkaloids, in: *The Alkaloids*," Vol. XII (R. H. F., Manske, ed.) pp. 333–454, Academic Press, New York.

Sauerland, E. K., and Mizuno, N., 1969, Cortically induced presynaptic inhibition of trigeminal proprioceptive afferents, *Brain. Res.* **13**:556.

Saxton, J. E., 1965, Alkaloids of gelsemium species, in: *The Alkaloids*, Vol. VIII (R. H. F. Manske, ed.) pp. 93–117, Academic Press, New York.

Schmidt, R. F., 1971, Presynaptic inhibition in the vertebrate central nervous system, *Ergeb. Physiol. Biol. Chem. Exptl. Pharmacol.* **63**:20.

Sherrington, C. S., 1905, On reciprocal innervation of antagonistic muscles, *Proc. Roy. Soc. Lond. Ser. B* **76**:269.

Sherrington, C. S., 1907, Strychnine and reflex inhibition of skeletal muscle, *J. Physiol.* (*Lond.*) **36**:185.

Smith, G. F., 1965, *Strychnos* alkaloids, in: *The Alkaloids,* Vol. VIII (R. H. F. Manske, ed.) pp. 591–671, Academic Press, New York.

Snatzke, G., Wollenberg, G., Hrbek, J., Śantavý, F., Bláha, K., Klyne, W., and Swan, R. J., 1969, The optical rotatory dispersion and circular dichroism of the phthalideisoquinoline alkaloids and of their α-hydroxybenzyltetrahydroisoquinoline derivatives, *Tetrahedron* **25**:5059.

Spira, M. E., and Bennett, M. V. L., 1972, Penicillin induced seizure activity in the hatchet fish, *Brain Res.* **43**:235.

Stanek, J., 1967, Phthalideisoquinoline alkaloids, in: *The Alkaloids,* Vol. IX (R. H. F. Manske, ed.) pp. 117–131, Academic Press, New York.

Stanek, J., and Manske, R. H. F., 1954, Phthalideisoquinoline alkaloids, in: *The Alkaloids*, Vol. IV (R. H. F. Manske and H. L. Holmes, eds.) pp. 167–198, Academic Press, New York.

Stefanis, C., and Jasper, H., 1965, Strychnine reversal of inhibitory potentials in pyramidal tract neurones, *Internat. J. Neuropharmacol.* **4**:125.

Stone, W. E., 1972, Systemic chemical convulsants and metabolic derangements, in: *Experimental Models of Epilepsy* (D. P. Purpura, J. K. Penry, D. B. Tower, D. M. Woodbury, and R. D. Walter, eds.) pp. 407–432, Raven Press, New York.

Straughan, D. W., Neal, M. J., Simmonds, M. A., Collins, G. G. S., and Hill, R. G., 1971, Evaluation of bicuculline as a GABA antagonist, *Nature* (*Lond.*) **233**:352.

Swanson, E. E., and Chen, K. K., 1936, The pharmacological action of coriamyrtin, *J. Pharmacol. Exptl. Therap.* **57**:361.

Swanson, P. D., 1972, Penicillin-induced metabolic alterations in isolated cerebral cortex, *Arch. Neurol.* **26**:169.

Takagi, K., and Takayanagi, I., 1966, Effects of strychnine, derivatives of phenyl acetate and catecholamines on contraction and acetylcholine output from the cholinergic nerve ending of guinea pig ileum, *Jap. J. Pharmacol.* **16**:211.

Takeuchi, A., and Onodera, K., 1972, Effect of bicuculline on the GABA receptor of the crayfish neuromuscular junction, *Nature New Biol.* **236**:55.

Takeuchi, A., and Takeuchi, N., 1969, A study of the action of picrotoxin in the inhibitory neuromuscular junction of the crayfish, *J. Physiol.* (*Lond.*) **205**:377.

Tatum, A. L., Seevers, M. H., and Collins, K. H., 1929, Morphine addiction and its physiological interpretation based on experimental evidence, *J. Pharmacol. Exptl. Therap.* **36**:447.

Tebēcis, A. K., 1973, Transmitters and reticulospinal neurones, *Exptl. Neurol.* **40**:297.

Tebēcis, A. K., Hösli, L., and Haas, H. L., 1971, Bicuculline and the depression of medullary reticular neurones by GABA and glycine, *Experientia* **27**:548.

Tebēcis, A, K., and Phillis, J. W., 1969, The use of convulsants in studying possible functions of amino acids in the toad spinal cord, *Comp. Biochem. Physiol.* **28**:1303.

Teitel, S., O'Brien, J., and Brossi, A., 1972, Conversion of (−)-β-hydrastine into (−)-bicuculline and related phthalideisoquinolines, *J. Org. Chem.* **37**:1879.

Tower, D. B., 1969, Neurochemical mechanisms, in: *Basic Mechanisms of the Epilepsies* (H. H. Jasper, A. A. Ward, and A. Pope, eds.) pp. 611–638, Little, Brown, Boston.

Turkanis, S. A., and Esplin, D. W., 1968, Evidence for the release and depletion of the postsynaptic inhibitory transmitter by pilocarpine, *Arch. Int. Pharmacodyn. Therap.* **173**:195.

Uhlemann, E. R., and Neims, A. H., 1972, Anticonvulsant properties of the ketogenic diet in mice, *J. Pharmacol. Exptl. Therap.* **180**:231.

Usherwood, P. N. R., and Grundfest, H., 1965, Peripheral inhibition in skeletal muscle of insects, *J. Neurophysiol.* **28**:497.

Van der Kloot, W. G., 1960, Picrotoxin and the inhibitory system of crayfish muscle, in: *Inhibition in the Nervous System and* γ-Aminobutyric Acid (E. Roberts, ed.) pp. 409–412, Pergamon Press, New York.

Van Duijn, H., Schwartzkroin, P. A., and Prince, D. A., 1973, Action of penicillin on inhibitory processes in the cat's cortex, *Brain Res.* **53**:470.

Walker, R. J., Crossman, A. R., Woodruff, G. N., and Kerkut, G. A., 1971, The effect of bicuculline on the gamma-aminobutyric acid (GABA) receptors of neurones of *Periplaneta americana* and *Helix aspersa*, *Brain Res.* **33**:75.

Wall, P. D., and Horwitz, N. H., 1951, Observations on the physiological action of strychnine, *J. Neurophysiol.* **14**:257.

Wall, P. D., McCulloch, W. S., Lettvin, J. Y., and Pitts, W. H., 1955, Effects of strychnine with special reference to spinal afferent fibres, *Epilepsia* **4**:29.

Walsh, G. O., 1971, Penicillin iontophoresis in neocortex of cat: Effects on the spontaneous and induced activity on single neurons, *Epilepsia* **12**:1.

Warnat, K., 1931, Über drei neue Strychnos-alkaloide, *Helv. Chim. Acta* **14**:997.

Washizu, Y., Bonewell, G. W., and Terzulo, C. A., 1961, Effect of strychnine upon the electrical activity of an isolated nerve cell, *Science* **133**:333.

Welch, A. D., and Henderson, V. E., 1934*a*, A comparative study of hydrastine, bicuculline and adlumine, *J. Pharmacol. Exptl. Therap.* **51**:482.

Welch, A. D., and Henderson, V. E., 1934*b*, A note on bicucine, *J. Pharmacol. Exptl. Therap.* **51**:492.

West, R., 1937, A pharmacological study of derivatives of two specimens of tubo-curare, and an examination of four members of genus *Strychnos* and one rubiaceous plant associated with the curares of British Guiana, *Arch. Int. Pharmacodyn. Therap.* **56**:81.

Wikler, A., 1944, Studies on the action of morphine on the central nervous system of cat, *J. Pharmacol. Exptl. Therap.* **80**:176.

Woodward, D. J., Hoffer, B. J., Siggins, G. R., and Oliver, A. P., 1971, Inhibitition of Purkinje cells in the frog cerebellum. II. Evidence for GABA as the inhibitory transmitter, *Brain Res.* **33**:91.

Woodward, R. B., Cava, M. P., Ollis, W. D., Hunger, A., Daeniker, H. V., and Schenker, K., 1963, The total synthesis of strychnine, *Tetrahedron* **19**:247.

Yunusov, M. S., and Yunusov, S. Yu., 1968, Alkaloids of *Corydalis sewerzowi, Khim. Prir. Soedin.* **4**:54.

Zablocka, B., and Esplin, D. W., 1963, Central excitatory and depressant effects of pilocarpine in rats and mice, *J. Pharmacol. Exptl. Therap.* **140**:162.

Zablocka, B., and Esplin, D. W., 1964, Analysis of the effects of arecoline on the central nervous system, *Pharmacologist* **6**:192.

Chapter 7

Ergot Alkaloids and Related Substances

P. B. Bradley and I. Briggs

Medical Research Council Neuropharmacology Unit
The Medical School
University of Birmingham
Birmingham, England

1. INTRODUCTION

Ergot has been called a treasure-house of drugs; possibly no other source of biological products has so many active constituents with such a wide spectrum of pharmacological properties, which has been further expanded by the production of derivatives with qualitatively new actions. Ergot consists of the sclerotia or resting stage produced by fungi of the genus *Claviceps*, most commonly *C. purpurea*, which is principally parasitic on the rye, *Secale cereale.* Many other varieties of ergot are known; over 50 species of *Claviceps* have been described, infesting over 600 recorded host species of the family Gramineae (grasses and cereals) (Bové, 1970). Although possible allusions to ergot are found in early records (see Bové, 1970), the earliest undisputable reference to ergot itself was made in 1582 by Lonicer, who described its use in midwifery. However, it was not widely accepted by physicians until the nineteenth century. The history and pharmacognosy of ergot have been extensively reviewed by Barger (1931) and by Bové (1970).

II. CHEMISTRY OF ERGOT ALKALOIDS

More than 40 different natural ergot alkaloids have been isolated from *Claviceps* species, which are the main sources of these drugs, and some are also found in a few other fungi (e.g., *Aspergillus* and *Agropyrum* spp.) and in a few species of the *Convolvulaceae* (for references, see Bové, 1970; Der Marderosian, 1967). The alkaloids to be described in this chapter are all derived from the ergolene ring system (Table I). The ergolene skeleton is formed from tryptophan and mevalonic acid; the first compound having the skeleton complete is agroclavine, which is a precursor of all the other natural alkaloids. The detailed biochemistry of this compound has been reviewed by Ramstad (1968), who pointed out that the pathways involved in ergot alkaloid biogenesis form a nearly continuous sequence of oxidative steps and speculated that these substances are the products of "detoxification" pathways. After agroclavine, elymoclavine is formed, and this in turn gives rise to lysergic acid, which has Δ_{9-10} instead of Δ_{8-9} (*cf.* Tables I and II). Subsidiary pathways lead to the formation of other clavine alkaloids, some with pharmacological activity. Synthetic clavine derivatives have recently been prepared which have potent and specific pharmacological properties.

Table I. Clavine Alkaloids

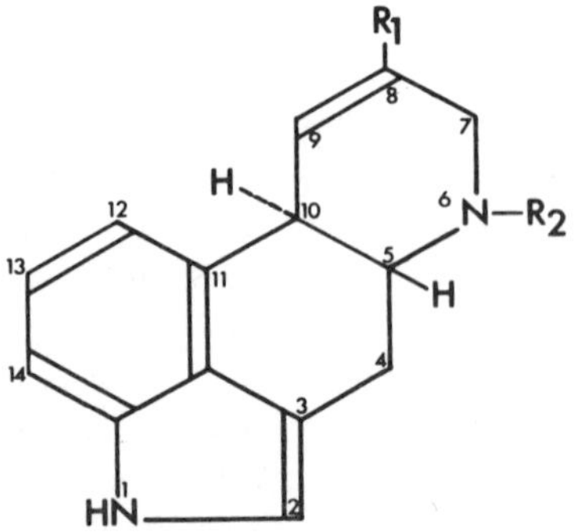

Alkaloid	R_1	R_2
Ergolene	H	H
Agroclavine	CH_3	CH_3
Elymoclavine	CH_2OH	CH_3

Table II. Amine Alkaloids

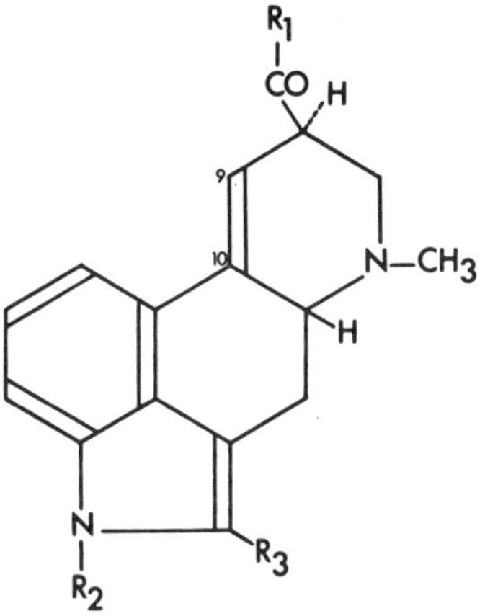

Alkaloid	R_1	R_2	R_3
Lysergic acid	—OH	H	H
LSD-25	$—N(C_2H_5)_2$	H	H
BOL-148	$—N(C_2H_5)_2$	H	Br
Ergometrine	$—NH·CH·(CH_3)·CH_2OH$	H	H
Methylergometrine	$—NH·CH·(CH_2CH_3)·CH_2OH$	H	H
Methysergide	$—NH·CH·(CH_2CH_3)·CH_2OH$	CH_3	H

Lysergic acid is the basis for all of the drugs commonly referred to as ergot alkaloids. These drugs are most easily divided into the two series of optical isomers. Only the *l*-isomers are pharmacologically active; these generally have the suffix *-ine* and are derivatives of *d*-lysergic acid, whereas the inactive *d*-forms have the suffix *-inine*, are derived from *l*-lysergic acid, and are thought to be produced from the natural *l*-isomers during chemical manipulations. This isomerism of lysergic acid is due to an asymmetry at C_8. Another asymmetry at C_5 gives rise to the isolysergic acids, which are pharmacologically inactive derivatives. The pharmacologically active isomers have the R configuration at both C_5 and C_8.

In the natural ergot alkaloids, *d*-lysergic acid is combined with either an amine moiety or an oligopeptide moiety, the two groups of derivatives formed being the "amine" alkaloids (Table II) and the "amino acid" alkaloids of ergot (Table III), respectively. Other active groups of alkaloids are derived semisynthetically from the natural alkaloids; one group is made

Table III. Amino Acid Alkaloids

These derivatives are also based on the structure in Table II. R_1 is an oligopeptide with the general structure

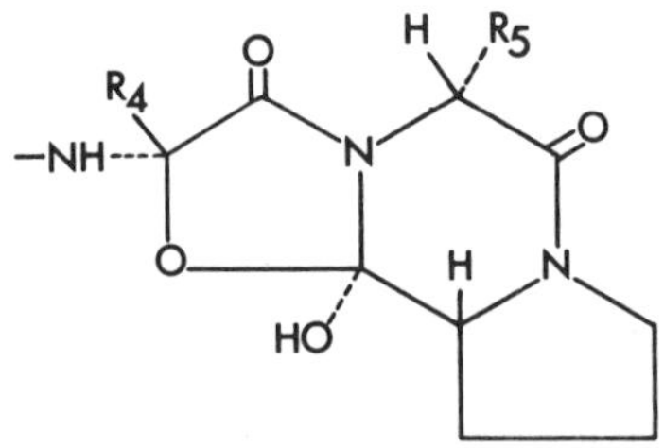

R_2 and R_3 both = H. The different amino acid aklaloids vary in the groups at R_4 and R_5 in the oligopeptide moiety as shown in the table below.

	R_5		
R_4	$—CH_2 \cdot C_6H_5$	$—CH(CH_3)_2$	$—CH_2 \cdot CH(CH_3)_2$
$—CH_3$	Ergotamine	Ergovaline	Ergosine
$—CH_2 \cdot CH_3$	Ergostine	Ergonine	Ergoptine
$—CH \cdot (CH_3)_2$	Ergocristine	Ergocornine	Ergokryptine

by dihydrogenation of the lysergic acid moiety at C_9 and C_{10} to yield a series of analogues of the natural alkaloids. Another group consists of lysergic acid derivatives with synthetic substituents other than natural ones; these include derivatives of all three types of natural alkaloids.

Terminology: In this chapter, the term *ergot alkaloids* will be used to refer to the natural alkaloids (ergometrine and those in Table III); *ergot derivatives* include all the compounds, natural or synthetic, derived from ergot. Compounds other than natural ergot alkaloids will be referred to specifically. *Hydergine* is a mixture of equal amounts of dihydroergocornine, dihydroergocristine, and dihydroergokryptine, as the mesylates.

III. PHARMACOLOGY

Many of the alkaloids derived from ergot have little or no pharmacological activity, but the active alkaloids and derivatives have extremely varied and complex effects, some of them being highly potent. No recent detailed review of the subject is available, but early work has been described by Barger (1931), Rothlin (1947, 1957), Cerletti (1959), and Bové (1970).

Ergot alkaloids can affect the functions of many tissues by virtue of their ability to stimulate directly or to interfere with the actions of monoamines on smooth muscles, nerves, and metabolic processes. At present, it seems unlikely that a unified explanation of all the actions of these drugs can be formulated; the drugs are known to affect mechanisms involving norepinephrine (NorE), dopamine (DA), and 5-hydroxytryptamine (5-HT), and the diversity of the drug actions reflects the diversity of the physiological roles of these monoamines. Possibly other systems are also affected, but the main emphasis of pharmacological research into ergot derivatives has been on their interactions with monoaminergic mechanisms.

The pharmacology of the ergot derivatives is described in this chapter in two main sections, one covering peripheral actions and the other central actions. However, some overlapping is convenient; for example, both centrally and peripherally mediated actions on the cardiovascular system are placed in one section, since the effects of the drugs are frequently the resultant of both central and peripheral actions.

A. Peripheral Actions of Ergot Alkaloids and Their Derivatives

1. *Effects of Ergot Alkaloids and Derivatives on the Uterus*

a. Direct Actions on the Uterus. The abortifacient effects of ergot, the result of its stimulation of strong contractions of the uterus, have long been recognized, and the drug has been used medically for its oxytocic properties for over 400 years. Rothlin (1947, 1957) has described the direct actions of ergot derivatives on the uterus. Ergometrine is the most active; it is absorbed well, so it can be given orally to produce a rapid effect. In contrast, the amino acid alkaloids are ineffective orally and must be given by injection, ergotamine being the most active. Its onset of action is slow, and it is more toxic than ergometrine. Thus ergometrine and its congener methylergometrine are the oxytocics most often used clinically. The dihydrogenated ergot alkaloids have no uterotonic actions in experimental animals. LSD has about two-thirds of the potency of ergometrine on the rabbit uterus, while D-2-bromolysergic acid diethylamide (BOL) has no stimulant actions (Rothlin, 1957). Acetyldihydrolysergamine has been reported to have oxytocic activity comparable or superior to that of ergometrine, while its antiserotonin and antiadrenergic actions and its toxicity are relatively slight (Fregnan and Glässer, 1968). The stimulant actions of ergot derivatives are exerted via α-adrenergic receptors on the uterus, and these effects can be antagonized by α-adrenergic blockers (Konzett, 1960; Brody and Diamond, 1967). The sensitivity of the uterus varies with its state of maturity and during ovarian cycles and gestation; it appears that the numbers and proportions of α- and β-adrenergic receptors on the uterus change in different hormonal states (Miller and Marshall, 1965); in the uterus dominated by estrogen, α-receptors predominate, while in the progesterone-dominated organ, β-receptors predominate (Brody and Diamond, 1967).

b. Interactions of Ergot Derivatives and Catecholamines in the Uterus. The excitatory action of epinephrine on rabbit uterus is antagonized by all of the natural and dihydrogenated alkaloids. Only slight differences in potency are found, with the dihydrogenated alkaloids generally having stronger and longer-lasting effects (Rothlin, 1947). The α-receptor blocking actions of LSD on the uterus are weak (Rothlin, 1957).

The derivatives with predominantly α-blocking actions (e.g., dihydroergotamine) can reverse adrenergic stimulation to relaxation (Miller, 1967). This phenomenon is explained by the selective blockade of the α-adrenergic stimulant receptors, permitting activation of β-receptors to produce relaxation. Dihydroergotamine can block adrenergic inhibition of the rat uterus (Levy and Tozzi, 1963), and there may be some similarity between this action and that on the metabolic receptors involved in lipolysis and in the liver glucogenic response to sympathomimetic agents, which dihydroergotamine also blocks, apparently at a stage subsequent to the formation of cyclic AMP (Hornbrook and Brody, 1963) (cf. Sections IIIA4a and IIIA4b).

c. Interactions of Ergot Derivatives and 5-HT in the Uterus. The dihydrogenated alkaloids and some of the synthetic amide derivatives of lysergic acid are highly potent antagonists of 5-HT-induced contractions of the uterus. Rothlin (1957) and Cerletti and Doepfner (1958) made extensive comparative studies of synthetic lysergic acid derivatives and LSD. Only derivatives of *d*-lysergic acid were active; derivatives of *l*-lysergic acid and of *d*- and *l*-isolysergic acids had less than 1% of the activity of LSD. Methylation or acetylation of LSD in the 1-position or bromination in the 2-position increased anti-5-HT potency, while all other modifications of the LSD structure studied by these authors, including dihydrogenation and alteration of the substituents on the amide group, reduced potency. However, methysergide was later found to be four times as active as LSD (Fanchamps *et al.*, 1960), and methergoline is an extremely potent antagonist of 5-HT in the rat uterus, being 500 times more potent than methysergide (Beretta *et al.*, 1965). Certain clavine alkaloids also antagonize the actions of 5-HT on the rat uterus; the most potent derivative tested, 1-methylelymoclavine, is approximately as potent as methysergide in this respect (Yui and Takeo, 1964). Cerletti and Doepfner (1958) were unable to confirm the reports by Costa (1956) and Delay and Thuillier

(1956) that LSD in low doses appeared to facilitate contractions of the rat uterus due to 5-HT.

d. Effects of Ergot Derivatives on Intestinal Responses to Catecholamines and Serotonin. The actions of both α- and β-adrenergic agonists on the intestine are inhibitory, and ergot alkaloids can block these actions (Rothlin, 1947). The derivatives with polypeptide side-chains (e.g., ergotamine, ergokryptine, dihydroergotamine, and dihydroergocornine) are potent antagonists of epinephrine's inhibitory effects on the rabbit isolated intestine, and are still active in the presence of hexamethonium and atropine, indicating that their actions are exerted directly on receptors on smooth muscle of the tissue, and not via intramural ganglia. The inhibitory action of epinephrine on pendular movements of the intestine is more readily blocked than the action on tonus. Furthermore, the actions of NorE are less readily blocked than are those of epinephrine (Rothlin *et al.*, 1954).

Catecholamines also have inhibitory actions on human isolated taenia coli and isolated jejunum, which, like rabbit intestine, appear to have both α- and β-adrenergic inhibitory receptors. Hydergine blocks the actions of α-adrenergic agonists but not the actions of β-adrenergic agonists on these preparations (Bucknell and Whitney, 1964; Whitney, 1965).

Erspamer (1966) has extensively reviewed the complex interactions of serotonin and lysergic acid derivatives on the intestine. In the limited space available here, this topic cannot be discussed fully; for further details, reference should be made to Erspamer's paper.

2. *Effects of Ergot Derivatives on the Cardiovascular System*

The effects of ergot derivatives on the vascular system are complex, and the net effect of a particular derivative on blood pressure may be the resultant of one or more of the following actions: (1) central effects influencing vascular tone and heart rate, mediated by alterations in tone in adrenergic nerves, by increases in activity in cholinergic sympathetic nerves, or by increases in vagal tone; (2) peripheral effects, including agonistic actions on catecholamine or serotonin receptors and antagonistic actions toward catecholamines or serotonin. In the interests of simplicity, both central and peripheral actions will be described together in this section.

a. Effects on Systemic Blood Pressure. Early work on the vasoactive effects of ergot derivatives has been reviewed by Rothlin (1947, 1957). In intact anesthetized animals, only ergotamine always causes a rise in blood pressure; ergosine in low doses also raises blood pressure, but in high doses causes a fall. The other natural alkaloids, the dihydrogenated alkaloids, LSD, and BOL all reduce blood pressure in intact animals, including cats and dogs. In the spinal cat, the effect of both natural and dihydrogenated alkaloids and of LSD is an increase in blood pressure due to direct constrictor actions on blood vessels, the natural alkaloids being somewhat more active. In man and rats, LSD causes a slight rise in blood pressure (Rothlin, 1957; Salmoiraghi *et al.*, 1957), which in rats is enhanced by pithing or pretreatment with ganglionic blockers; the marked depressor action of BOL in rats is abolished by these treatments.

b. Central Effects of Ergot Derivatives Mediated via Adrenergic Sympathetic Nerves. The hypotensive effects of ergot alkaloids were attributed by Rothlin (1947) to a decreased sympathetic outflow from vasomotor "centers," resulting from either stimulation of inhibitory influences or inhibition of excitatory influences on the "centers." Konzett and Rothlin (1953) showed that the depressor effect of dihydrogenated alkaloids occurs only when at least the medulla oblongata and the spinal cord down to the seventh thoracic segment are intact. Downman (1972) recently reviewed the evidence on central vasomotor control; it appears that both pressor and depressor reflexes are controlled by an extensive system of neurons in the brain stem, diencephalon, and limbic cortex. In the brain stem are a pontomedullary pressor area and a medullary depressor area, each consisting of laterally situated neurons activating more medially placed efferent neurons, but it may be that these areas contain general sympathetic facilitatory and inhibitory mechanisms of which vasomotor components are only a part (Coote *et al.*, 1973). Vasodepression of medullary origin is probably due to inhibitory pathways acting on tonically active spinal segmental pressor reflexes, reducing the excitability of the spinal preganglionic neurons (Downman, 1972). The bulbospinal pathways involved appear to be noradrenergic (Chalmers and Wurtman, 1971; Coote and Macleod, 1972). In man, the central vasodilator actions of ergot derivatives are abolished by sympathectomy and appear to be due to a fall in sympathetic tone originating in the medulla and/or hypothalamus (Bluntschli and Goetz, 1948). There is evidence that stimulation of α-adrenergic receptors in the lower brain stem results in hypotension and bradycardia (Bolme *et al.*, 1972; Share, 1973; Haeusler, 1973), and it thus seems possible that ergot derivatives act by stimulation of adrenergic receptors in this area, increasing the activity of the bulbospinal NorE pathways which inhibit the spinal preganglionic sympathetic neurons. An interaction with serotoninergic mechanisms controlling blood pressure (Ito and Schanberg, 1972) is also a possibility, although the precise location and function of the neurons with these receptors are still uncertain.

Schmitt and Fénard (1970) reported that low doses of dihydroergotamine, dihydroergotoxine, and ergotamine increased electrical activity in the splanchnic nerve, and reduced activity only in high doses. These workers concluded that hypotensive actions could not be related to inhibition of sympathetic tone. However, ergot derivatives appear to have differential effects on tone in different parts of the vasculature. For example, dihydroergocornine, which induces a centrally mediated vasodilatation in most areas, causes a fall in blood flow in the splanchnic area (Bluntschli and Goetz, 1948; Freis *et al.*, 1949), indicating a rise in sympathetic tone, which the results of Schmitt and Fénard also indicate. Thus splanchnic nerve activity may be misleading as an indicator of general sympathetic tone, and data from sympathetic nerves supplying other areas are needed. The differential actions of these drugs on different areas may indicate an action on mechanisms integrating vasomotor control rather than on vasomotor reflexes themselves.

Ergot derivatives can affect vasomotor reflexes evoked by physiological or electrical stimuli; these drugs prevent both depressor responses to stimulation of the aortic (depressor) nerve and pressor responses to bilateral occlusion of the carotids (Rothlin, 1947; Fanchamps *et al.*, 1960). They also reduce the pressor responses to electrical stimulation of the vestibular nuclei and parvocellular reticular nuclei in the medulla (Kovalyov, 1967). The efferent pathway for these reflexes and possibly for the areas activated by Kovalyov (1967) is the bulbospinal NorE pathway (see above), which, when activated, causes a fall in sympathetic tone. The fact that these drugs inhibit both pressor and depressor responses is further evidence that the site of action is not on the reflex pathway itself, but on some mechanism which can affect the responsiveness of the vasomotor reflexes to afferent stimuli.

c. Central Effects of Ergot Derivatives Mediated by Cholinergic Sympathetic Nerves. Mellander and Nordenfelt (1970) found that, among other actions, dihydroergotamine usually dilated resistance vessels (which mainly correspond to arterioles) in skeletal muscle without much affecting vascular resistance in intestine or kidney. In skeletal muscle, NorE constricted resistance vessels, and the authors considered that the dilator responses to dihydroergotamine were related to a central action of the drug leading to a reduction of sympathetic constrictor fiber discharge, since denervation prevented the dilatation. There are two functionally separate central vasodilator mechanisms (Uvnäs, 1960) which are both effected via sympathetic nerves: (1) inhibition of vasoconstrictor tone and (2) initiation of vasodilator activity. The former is not blocked by atropine; it is associated with vasodepressor reflexes in the medulla, which can be affected by ergot derivatives, as has already been discussed. However, more recent evidence has also given support to the second possible explanation of the centrally mediated dilatation. Owen and Stuermer (1971) confirmed the results of Mellander and Nordenfelt (1970) in cats with intact innervation, while in denervated preparations dihydroergotamine was found to cause constriction in the muscle resistance vessels. Chu and Stuermer (1973) reported that in innervated preparations the dilator effect of the drug on skeletal muscle resistance vessels was blocked by atropine but not by phenoxybenzamine, and was potentiated by eserine. After atropine, dihydroergotamine had a constrictor effect on resistance vessels similar to that seen in the denervated preparation. These authors conclude that the dilator effect of dihydroergotamine in cats is mediated centrally via cholinergic innervation of the muscle resistance vessels. It seems that only skeletal muscles receive sympathetic cholinergic vasodilator innervation (Mellander and Johansson, 1968), and it is therefore likely that vasodilator responses in most other organs and tissues are due to reduction of sympathetic constrictor tone.

The sympathetic vasodilator innervation of skeletal muscle can be activated by stimulation of several areas of the brain, including the hypothalamus, where it constitutes part of the mechanism of the coordinated defense reaction; the vasodilatation may be elicited as a relatively isolated response by stimulation of an area dorsal to the cerebral peduncles (Abrahams *et al.*, 1960, 1964). The results of Chu and Stuermer (1973) indicate that dihydroergotamine can activate this mechanism. Horeyseck *et al.* (1972) found that stimulation of the hypothalamic defense area elicited activity in about 10% of the single nerve fibers studied in the cat gastrocnemius soleus sympathetic innervation. These fibers showed no spontaneous activity and were not activated by baroreceptor reflexes. An investigation of the effects of dihydroergotamine on activity in these fibers would be of interest.

d. Centrally Mediated Effects of Ergot Derivatives on Heart Rate. The heart does not seem to be directly affected by ergot derivatives, but there is often a fall in pulse rate which appears to be centrally mediated via the vagal motor nuclei (Rothlin, 1947, 1957). This is supported by observations that intraventricular or intracisternal administration of NorE results in cardiac slowing which can be partly reduced by vagotomy. However, the fact that atropine is not wholly effective and that vagotomy is ineffective in some species indicates that reduction of sympathetic cardioaccelerator tone is an important component of the action (for references, see Bhargava *et al.*, 1972). Similar conclusions were reached in a study of dihydroergocornine in man (Freis *et al.*, 1949).

e. Direct Agonistic Actions on Blood Vessels. The potent vasoconstrictor effects (Rothlin, 1947, 1957) of these drugs are probably due mainly to direct stimulant actions on α-adrenoceptors (Innes, 1962). This is one of the most undesirable effects of the natural alkaloids; they may cause marked constriction of veins and even of arteries as large as the aorta, which may seriously impair circulation. The deleterious consequences of this action will be dealt with in Section IVB.

The dihydrogenated alkaloids, ergometrine, and LSD have direct vasoconstrictor effects weaker than those of the natural alkaloids (Rothlin, 1947, 1957; Ginzel and Kottegoda, 1953; Savini, 1956). The actions of LSD on some vessels are due to stimulation of 5-HT receptors and can be blocked by BOL (Dyer and Gant, 1973), which has no vasoconstrictor actions itself (Savini, 1956).

Mellander and Nordenfelt (1970) found that dihydroergotamine has a strong constrictor action on capacitance vessels (which mainly correspond to veins) in skin and skeletal muscle and on resistance vessels in skin, although centrally mediated dilatation obscures the direct constrictor action on muscle resistance vessels (see Section IIIA2C). Resistance vessels in intestine and kidney and precapillary sphincter vessels in skin, muscle, or intestine are little affected. The constrictor effects are blocked by phenoxybenzamine and are thought to be due mainly or entirely to a direct action on the vascular smooth muscle α-adrenergic receptors (Chu and Stuermer, 1973). Owen and Stuermer (1972) reported the results of similar studies on Hydergine, which differs from ergotamine in that it appears to have little effect on resistance vessels, while it dilates precapillary sphincter vessels, which are not affected by dihydroergotamine (Mellander and Nordenfelt, 1970; Owen and Stuermer, 1971). Dihydroergotamine is about 50 times more potent than Hydergine in constricting capacitance vessels.

Methysergide was found by Fanchamps *et al.* (1960) to have no vasoconstrictor actions in the spinal cat, anesthetized intact dog, or perfused rabbit isolated hind leg. Saxena (1972) observed that both methysergide and ergotamine did have direct vasoconstrictor actions on the external carotid bed in dogs, increasing resistance and decreasing blood flow in doses which did not affect general blood pressure. It seems that these compounds have relatively selective actions on the external carotid circulation.

Aellig and Berde (1969) found that the direct effects of ergot alkaloids on vascular tone in anesthetized dogs were dependent on the preexistent tone; they observed an "inversion-point" phenomenon, in which many derivatives had amphoteric effects, causing vasoconstriction when the existing tone was low and vasodilatation when it was high. Ergotamine, dihydroergotamine, 1-methylergotamine, ergostine, dihydroergostine, and 1-methylergostine all showed this effect. No correlation was found between the degree of existing vasoconstriction represented by the "inversion point" and the potencies of the different alkaloids as vasoconstrictor agents or as α-receptor blockers.

f. Circulatory Actions in Man. Bluntschli and Goetz (1948) studied the circulatory effects of ergot derivatives in man and found that ergotamine and dihydroergotamine have both direct constrictor actions and centrally mediated vasodilator actions. The dilator effects are abolished by sympathectomy, but whether they are due to a fall in adrenergic constrictor outflow or to augmented cholinergic dilator outflow is not known. In fact, it is not yet certain whether cholinergic sympathetic vasodilator fibers exist in man, although Greenfield (1966) reviewed the evidence and considered that these fibers probably do exist in man. Dihydroergocornine has vasodilator actions which are also abolished by sympathectomy, but unlike ergotamine and dihydroergotamine it seems to have no direct constrictor effects (Bluntschli and Goetz, 1948). Freis *et al.* (1949) and Barcroft *et al.* (1951) found that the hypotensive actions of dihydroergocornine and of Hydergine in man seemed to be due to centrally mediated dilatation occurring mainly in the skin, and only slightly in muscle. The effects of dihydroergostine (DE-145) on the human calf have been compared with those of dihydroergotamine by Ulrich and Siggaard-Andersen (1972), using a plethysmographic method. DE-145 gave a significant rise in resting blood flow, possibly indicating a potent dilator effect on resistance vessels, but dihydroergotamine did not raise resting blood flow. A decrease in the limb volume indicated a constriction of capacitance vessels by dihydroergotamine, but DE-145 did not have this effect. It thus seems that in man the effect of DE-145 on muscle blood flow is mainly or wholly centrally mediated, and while dihydroergotamine has little effect on blood flow, it is possible that central vasodilator effects may be counterbalanced by direct constrictor actions.

g. Antagonism of the Actions of Catecholamines by Ergot Derivatives. The abilities of ergot derivatives to antagonize the actions of CAs vary considerably among different species and different test organs. The antagonist activities of the different alkaloids vary with respect to the different CAs.

With the exception of ergometrine, all the natural and dihydrogenated alkaloids cause "reversal" of the action of epinephrine on blood pressure (Rothlin, 1947). The reversal of epinephrine-induced pressor effects to depressor effects is due to blockade of α-adrenergic vasoconstrictor actions, allowing latent β-adrenergic vasodilator actions to predominate (Levy and Ahlquist, 1961). The action of the natural alkaloids is itself of a biphasic nature; the antagonism of epinephrine pressor effects is seen first, and later a sensitization to epinephrine often occurs (Rothlin, 1947). The α-adrenergic blocking actions of LSD and BOL are weak in comparison with those of the natural and dihydrogenated alkaloids (Ginzel and Kottegoda, 1953; Rothlin, 1957; Salmoiraghi *et al.*, 1957; Palmer and Burke, 1971), and LSD can potentiate epinephrine and NorE vasoconstriction in rabbit ear (Gaddum and Hameed, 1954; Savini, 1956) and human veins (Del Bianco *et al.*, 1972). Methysergide has little or no activity on cerebral vasoconstriction induced by NorE in monkeys (White *et al.*, 1971); neither LSD nor methysergide affects NorE-induced venoconstriction in man (Del Bianco *et al.*, 1972). Nicergoline is a potent and highly specific blocker of the effects of epinephrine and of sympathetic nervous stimulation on vascular tone (Arcari *et al.*, 1968).

h. Effects of Ergot Derivatives on the Actions of Serotonin. Vasoconstriction induced by 5-HT in rabbit ear vessels is blocked by LSD, ergotamine, and dihydroergotamine (Gaddum and Hameed, 1954). Savini (1956) found that both 5-HT- and tryptamine-induced constrictions in rabbit ear were antagonized equally by LSD and ergometrine, while the actions of epinephrine and NorE were not affected. BOL had about one-tenth the activity of LSD against the action of 5-HT.

Methysergide prevented 5-HT-induced constriction of dog femoral arteries and the pressor actions of 5-HT in anesthetized dogs (Fanchamps *et al.*, 1960) and pithed rats (Beretta *et al.*, 1965). In rats, LSD and BOL were also effective antagonists of the cardiovascular effects of 5-HT, while their actions in cat and dogs were slight or variable (Salmoiraghi *et al.*, 1957), although LSD does antagonize 5-HT vasoconstriction in the cat's pulmonary circulation; ergotamine and dihydroergotamine were less effective (Gaddum *et al.*, 1953; Ginzel and Kottegoda, 1953). The cerebral vasoconstrictor effects of 5-HT in the monkey were specifically blocked by methysergide (Karlsberg *et al.*, 1963; White *et al.*, 1971). Methysergide, LSD, and methylergometrine had potent and specific actions against 5-HT induced constriction of human veins *in situ* (Del Bianco *et al.*, 1972).

i. Migraine. The therapeutic actions of certain of the ergot derivatives in migraine and in related conditions involving pain of vascular origin, like cluster headache, are probably related to their actions on blood vessels and/or vasomotor control. To explain the actions of the drugs, it is useful to consider briefly the etiology of migraine. The primary cause of migraine is uncertain (Sicuteri, 1967; Sicuteri *et al.*, 1973; Heyck, 1969; Anthony *et al.*, 1969; Dalessio, 1972), but it is generally agreed that in certain people there is an abnormality in the central control of the tone in some vascular beds, which generally includes a hyperreactivity of the reflexes controlling the carotid circulation. When these individuals are subjected to some types of stress, there is a strong vasoconstriction in the carotid beds causing a reduction of blood flow which is associated with the aura preceding a migraine attack. The formation of kinin due to ischemia is thought to initiate release of 5-HT from platelets and mast cells. Both 5-HT and bradykinin are vasoactive and pain-producing; consequently headache develops, due mainly to chemical stimulation of nociceptors. During migraine attacks, there is increased vascular sensitivity to the actions of 5-HT, NorE, and epinephrine; the emetic and vasoconstrictor effects of ergotamine and methysergide and the psychotomimetic actions of LSD and psilocybin are also increased (Sicuteri *et al*., 1973). These last observations appear to indicate a change in central 5-HT functions in migraine.

In the treatment of migraine, methysergide is generally used prophylactically in attempts to prevent or reduce the occurrence of headaches, whereas ergotamine can be used acutely to alleviate developing or existing headaches. The use, side-effects, contraindications, and possible mechanisms of action of these compounds have been reviewed by Dalessio (1972).

The prophylactic value of methysergide in the treatment of migraine has been attributed to several possible actions, and it may be that more than one of these contribute to its effectiveness. One action of methysergide may be to reduce the reactivity of the unstable vasomotor reflexes, preventing the initial vasoconstrictor response to stress, possibly by antagonism of 5-HT in the pons and medulla, where it appears to have a role in cardiovascular control (Ito and Schanberg, 1972). This is one possible explanation of the relative ineffectiveness of this drug as an acute treatment for migraine: once vasoconstriction started, an attack would not be prevented by inhibition of the initial cause. The drug may also reduce the vasodilator actions of 5-HT released from platelets (Anthony *et al*., 1969; Hilton and Cumings, 1972) on arteriovenous anastomoses, although if the vasoconstriction phase is prevented there may be no release of 5-HT. Sicuteri (1967) pointed out that the ability of methysergide to prevent 5-HT-induced sensitization of pain receptors to bradykinin could partly explain why the drug is of little value after an attack starts; if methysergide is given before an experimental.dose of 5-HT, sensitization to bradykinin is inhibited, but if it is given after 5-HT the pain receptors remain sensitized.

Another property of methysergide, which is also shared by ergotamine and methylergotamine, is the ability to prevent the normal aggregation response of platelets to 5-HT (Cumings and Hilton, 1971), which would presumably abolish or reduce the autoregenerative release of 5-HT from these cells.

The effectiveness of ergotamine and the other derivatives used in acute treatment of migraine appears to be due to their ability to cause vasoconstriction (Dalessio, 1972), particularly in the carotid vascular bed (Saxena, 1972), and it may be that in migraine these drugs act on dilated arteriovenous anastomoses in this area, thus restoring capillary circulation and permitting the removal of pain-producing agents from the affected areas.

In view of the evidence of Sicuteri *et al*., (1973) that there is a malfunction in the central control of pain thresholds which may be related to an abnormality in 5-HT functions in the CNS, the possibility must be considered that the drugs act at least partly on the central 5-HT receptors concerned.

3. Effects on the Peripheral Nervous System

a. Effects on the Release of NorE from Sympathetic Nerve Terminals. When the sympathetic nerve supplying an organ is stimulated, the NorE released from the terminals is partly taken back into the terminals and partly lost into the blood or perfusion fluid. The amount of NorE escaping is increased by α-receptor blocking agents. This effect was first explained as an overflow of NorE due to the blockade of postsynaptic receptors, which were thought to act as a "brake" on the diffusion of NorE away from the terminals, and later was ascribed to a blockade of NorE reuptake (for references, see Pacha and Salzmann, 1970).

Ergot derivatives have been and are being used in the study of this mechanism because of their α-receptor blocking properties. The dihydrogenated ergot alkaloids, in particular dihydroergotamine and Hydergine, have been valuable in this respect, but some apparently discordant conclusions have been reached when ergotamine and methylergotamine were used. Salzmann and coworkers (see Pacha and Salzmann, 1970) compared the effects of ergotamine and phenoxybenzamine (PBZ) on release of NorE from cat spleen and on responses of cat nictitating membrane to nerve stimulation and to epinephrine, NorE, tyramine, and 5-HT. High doses of ergotamine caused contractions of the nictitating membrane and spleen by direct stimulation of α-receptors, which PBZ blocked. Low doses of ergotamine potentiated the effects of sympathetic nerve stimulation and of the monoamines on the nictitating membrane and increased stimulation-induced NorE release from the spleen. The authors concluded that the effects of ergotamine were due to inhibition of reuptake of NorE in the absence of α-receptor blockade. Pacha and Salzmann (1970) compared ergotamine, 1-methylergotamine, Hydergine, dihydroergotamine, and PBZ on stimulation-induced release of NorE from isolated cat spleen and found that the first two, which have little α-receptor blocking activity, were roughly as potent as the other drugs with strong α-blocking actions. The authors suggested that these results indicate that the increased NorE release was due to block of NorE reuptake, and not to block of feedback inhibition of release. Ergotamine does have some NorE-uptake blocking activity in cat spleen (Dengler *et al.*, 1961), but Starke and coworkers (see Starke, 1972) found that PBZ and dihydroergotamine enhanced stimulation-evoked release of NorE from rabbit heart in concentrations which did not affect NorE reuptake. The method of Pacha and Salzmann does not specifically determine uptake-blocking activities, and although the two preparations, (i.e., cat spleen and rabbit heart) may not be comparable, it seems that blockade of NorE reuptake is at most only a minor component of the action of the α-blocking drugs on NorE release.

More recent studies have supported an alternative hypothesis: rather than interfering with the reuptake of transmitter, the α-blockers are now thought to increase the stimulation-induced release of NorE from sympathetic terminals by blocking an α-receptor-mediated feedback inhibition of the release (Farnebo and Hamberger, 1971). The precise mechanism is still uncertain. Three possibilities have been proposed:

1. The release of NorE could be regulated by the state of activity of the effector cells; during high activity of the effectors, NorE release would be low, and vice versa. Häggendal (see Stjärne, 1973) compared the effects on NorE release of doses of ergotamine and of PBZ which produced similar degrees of sympathetic blockade in cat skeletal muscle. The release of NorE in the presence of ergotamine was much lower than in the presence of PBZ, and the difference in output was attributed by Häggendal to the stimulating action of ergotamine on the effector cells. He therefore favored the hypothesis of transsynaptic feedback inhibition of release, but apparently did not consider the possibility of stimulation of presynaptic α-receptors by ergotamine, which in the light of later results seems to be as likely an explanation as postsynaptic stimulation. Furthermore, there are several examples of drug actions which do not support this hypothesis (Starke, 1972; McCulloch *et al.*, 1972): certain α-receptor stimulants can reduce NorE release at concentrations lower than those affecting the effector cells, and α-blockers can increase NorE release at concentrations which do not cause postsynaptic blockade.
2. It is possible that the release of prostaglandins E_1 and E_2 (PGE_1 and PGE_2) during sympathetic nerve activity results in local feedback inhibition of NorE release (see Stjärne, 1973; Bergström *et al.*, 1973). The release of NorE from cat spleen is reduced by exogenous PGEs, and PBZ blocks the output of PGE_2 from dog spleen, at the same time increasing the output of NorE (Davies *et al.*, 1968). It is not yet known whether the PGEs are liberated in response to NorE action on postsynaptic receptors or originate presynaptically in the sympathetic terminals.
3. The α-receptors mediating the local feedback inhibition may be situated on the sympathetic terminals (see Stjärne, 1973; McCulloch *et al.*, 1972). Thus the NorE released during sympathetic nerve stimulation activates the α-receptors on the terminals,

causing an autoinhibition of further release, which is disrupted by α-blocking agents.

Stärne (1973) studied the possibility that the prostaglandin-mediated and the α-adrenoceptor mechanisms might be coupled, postulating that locally formed PGE might be the chemical mediator of the control system triggered by α-receptors. He found that inhibition of prostaglandin synthesis did not prevent the enhancement by phentolamine of stimulation-induced release of tritiated NorE or its depression by the α-receptor stimulant methoxamine. The fact that substances acting on α-receptors were still effective during severe depression of PG synthesis makes it unlikely that the α-receptor feedback mechanism requires the mediation of PGE.

A similar type of feedback inhibition mediated by adrenergic receptors seems to operate on release of acetylcholine from postganglionic parasympathetic terminals in the heart (Starke, 1972) and from preganglionic sympathetic terminals (Nishi, 1970).

b. Actions on Autonomic Ganglia. De Groat and Volle (1966*a,b*) found that epinephrine or NorE injected intraarterially in the cat superior cervical ganglion had inhibitory actions on ganglionic transmission, which dihydroergotamine blocked, unmasking a facilitation which was also seen with isoprenaline alone. The facilitation could be blocked by β-adrenergic antagonists. Facilitation of ganglionic transmission was associated with ganglionic depolarization, and inhibition with hyperpolarization.

However, there seems to be no evidence that adrenergic blocking agents can affect ganglionic transmission, and it appears that catecholamines do not have a physiological modulatory role in ganglionic transmission, at least in the superior cervical ganglion of the cat. For a more detailed review of the topics in this section, see Willems (1972).

4. *Metabolic Effects of Ergot Derivatives*

a. Antagonism of Catecholamine-Induced Hyperglycemia. A striking and somewhat paradoxical effect of some ergot derivatives is their ability to inhibit epinephrine-induced hyperglycemia. The paradox is in the fact that although the drugs in question are considered to be mainly α-adrenergic receptor blockers, their action on this response is shared by β-blocking agents such as dichloroisoprenaline (Northrop and Parks, 1964), while other α-blockers have only weak inhibitory effects (Harvey *et al.*, 1951). Harvey *et al.* reported a lack of correlation between the antihyperglycemic actions of ergot derivatives and their abilities to inhibit pressor responses to epinephrine. The mechanism of the effects was elucidated to some extent when it was found that ergotamine blocked the epinephrine-induced formation of cyclic AMP in liver homogenates (Murad *et al.*, 1962) and the activation of liver phosphorylase by epinephrine (Hornbrook and Brody, 1963). Dihydroergotamine is also said to block the hyperglycemic action of cyclic AMP (Northrop and Parks, 1964), but this finding has been disputed (Gothelf and Ellis, 1972).

Chan and Ellis (1969) found that at low doses of dihydroergotamine the blockade of the epinephrine-induced increase in glucose output from liver slices seemed to be competitive, and cyclic AMP effects were not blocked. At the higher concentration needed to block both epinephrine and cyclic AMP effects, the blockade was noncompetitive. It thus seems that the drugs can act in two ways on the hyperglycemic response to epinephrine; with ergotamine and with low doses of dihydroergotamine a competitive block of adrenergic receptors prevents the activation of cyclic AMP, and higher doses of dihydroergotamine exert a noncompetitive action subsequent to the formation of cyclic AMP which prevents the activation of liver phosphorylase.

A large fraction of the hyperglycemic response to epinephrine in intact animals is due to the activation of a central mechanism influencing blood glucose levels, apparently mediated by neurons in the medulla oblongata which are sensitive to epinephrine (Rosenberg and DiStefano, 1962; Ezdinli *et al.*, 1968). Some of the *in vivo* actions of ergot derivatives may thus be due to interference with this mechanism. Those derivatives which have centrally mediated sympathomimetic effects induce hyperglycemia as part of the syndrome (Cerletti, 1959), and it seems possible that the derivatives which reduce central sympathetic tone (e.g., dihydroergotamine; *cf.* Section IIIA2b) may have an opposite effect.

b. Actions of Ergot Derivatives on Lipid Metabolism. The first reports of the ability of catecholamines to induce lipolysis in adipose tissue were closely followed by attempts to block this action, using ergot alkaloids, particularly ergotamine and dihydroergotamine, and other α- and β-blocking agents, in order to define the receptors involved. Most of the work has been carried out on rats or dogs.

In rats, ergotamine can reduce the physiological mobilization of fat caused by fasting, but only if the adrenals are removed, possibly because in intact animals the lipolytic action of corticosteroids can overcome the blocking action of ergotamine. Dihydroergotamine is able to inhibit the release of free fatty acids (FFA) from adipose tissue caused by catecholamines and also by other agents including ACTH, theophylline, and dibutyryl cyclic AMP. Dihydroergotamine in low doses also has a lipolytic action of its own, causing increased accumulation of cyclic AMP, and its effect is potentiated in the presence of growth hormone and dexamethasone or of theophylline. In low doses, it can also potentiate the effect of dibutyryl cyclic AMP (for references, see Himms-Hagen, 1970; Fain, 1973).

In dogs, ergotamine reduces the resting plasma levels of FFA and inhibits the epinephrine-induced rise in FFA, but not that caused by fasting (see Himms-Hagen, 1970). The lipolytic action of dihydroergotamine is greater than in rats. However, in isolated perfused dog adipose tissue, dihydroergotamine and phentolamine have no lipomobilizing effects of their own, but potentiated the release of FFA and glycerol following stimulation of the sympathetic innervation of the tissue. They reduce the latency of the onset of release and increase the output of FFA and glycerol, the effect being more marked at higher stimulation rates (Fredholm and Rosell, 1968). It thus appears that the lipolytic effect of low doses of dihydroergotamine may be due to blockade of an α-adrenergic inhibitory influence on the lipolytic mechanism; this could be mediated by inhibitory α-receptors either on the fat cells themselves (Himms-Hagen, 1970) or on the sympathetic terminals—if feedback inhibition of transmitter release were blocked, the increased release of NorE would cause increased lipolysis. A third possible explanation of the effects of dihydroergotamine on lipolysis is derived from its actions on adenyl cyclase and phosphodiesterase. Catecholamine-induced stimulation of adenyl cyclase is blocked by the drug, thus preventing the catecholamine-induced lipolysis mediated by increased cyclic AMP formation. The lipolytic action of dihydroergotamine and its potentiation of the lipolytic actions of other drugs are ascribed to inhibition of phosphodiesterase, thus decreasing the catabolism of cyclic AMP and elevating its levels (Fain, 1973; Iwangoff and Enz, 1972).

High doses of dihydroergotamine cause a "nonspecific" reduction of lipolysis induced by several agents, indicating an action subsequent to the formation of cyclic AMP (*cf.* its action on hyperglycemia responses). It has been suggested that the drug may act by inhibiting the lipase activated by cyclic AMP (Nakano *et al.*, 1969).

Obviously, the effects of ergot alkaloids on lipid metabolism are complex, and more detailed study is needed to establish which of the possible modes of action are involved.

B. Central Effects of Ergot Derivatives

1. *Introduction*

In the CNS, as in the periphery, ergot derivatives have a multiplicity of actions. Different alkaloids can have opposite actions, and some have different actions at different doses. Although it is probable that most or all of the effects are due to interactions with monoaminergic neuron systems, the variety of possible interactions has generally made it much more difficult in the CNS than in the periphery to ascribe effects to a particular mode of action. Receptors for NorE, 5-HT, and DA have been reported to be either stimulated or blocked by ergot derivatives, and since often two or more neuron systems containing different monoamines innervate areas in which the drugs appear to act, the interpretation of experimental findings can be difficult.

Among the central actions of these compounds are effects on behavior, including psychotomimetic, excitatory, and sedative actions; on central autonomic control; on respiration; on thermoregulation; and on neuroendocrine control of prolactin and gonadotropin secretion. Many of the drugs have emetic actions exerted via the CNS.

The psychotomimetic effect of some of the lysergic acid derivatives is one their most prominent central actions; however, many derivatives are inactive in this respect, and often sedative effects are seen (Yui and Takeo, 1958; Isbell *et al.*, 1959; Isbell and Gorodetsky, 1965). The psychotomimetic effects of lysergic acid derivatives, and in particular of LSD, the most potent, have been the subject of many reviews (Evarts, 1957; Purpura, 1957; Rothlin, 1957; Cerletti, 1959; Eiduson *et al.*, 1964; Cohen, 1967; Hoffer and Osmond, 1967; Freedman, 1963, 1969; Brawley and Duffield, 1972; Aghajanian, 1972*a*). Only a relatively brief discussion is possible here, and further details of less recent studies may be found via these reviews.

The psychotomimetic actions of LSD and related agents are characterized in man by excitation, mood changes, perceptual disturbances, hallucinations (particularly visual ones), depersonalization, and behavior which has some similarities to "psychotic" behavior.

2. *Biochemical Effects of Psychotomimetic Lysergic Acid Derivatives*

The psychotomimetic properties of LSD can be related to certain of its biochemical effects. The principal change appears to be in the metabolism of 5-HT in the brain. Although high doses of LSD have usually been used in order to produce detectable changes, it has recently been shown that changes in 5-HT levels occur after doses as low as 25 μg/kg (King *et al.*, 1972). After LSD, the turnover rate of 5-HT is reduced (Lin *et al.*, 1969; Freedman *et al.*, 1970), and 5-HT synthesis from tryptophan is reduced, although total 5-HT synthesis is not changed (Shields and Eccleston, 1973). The fall in 5-HT synthesis is probably a consequence of reduced synthesis of 5-HTP from tryptophan (Carlsson and Lindqvist, 1972). The fraction of 5-HT affected by LSD is thought to represent a small functional pool which can be released by nerve impulses (Shields and Eccleston, 1973).

Katz and Kopin (1969) also found that LSD selectively inhibited the release of 5-HT induced by electrical stimulation of rat brain slices. Since the slices were from brain areas without 5-HT-containing cell bodies, this effect was probably due to an action on the 5-HT terminals. However, only high concentrations of LSD were effective.

In contrast with 5-HT, levels of NorE fall and NorE turnover is increased (Freedman, 1963). The rise in 5-HT levels occurs mainly in the pons and medulla, and the fall in NorE is most marked in the cerebral hemispheres (I. L. Martin, personal communication).

Using the fluorescence histochemical technique, Andén *et al.* (1968) found that in high doses LSD reduces the turnover of 5-HT and increases that of NorE in terminals containing the amines: the disappearance of 5-HT from terminals after inhibition of tryptophan hydroxylase is markedly retarded by LSD, while the disappearance of NorE after inhibition of tyrosine hydroxylase is accelerated.

3. Behavioral and Central Physiological Effects of Ergot Derivatives

Many attempts have been made to identify relationships between the hallucinogenic effects of LSD and related drugs and other behavioral and physiological effects which are more susceptible to analysis.

a. Effects on Arousal and Sleep. Cerletti (1959) showed that the psychotomimetic effects of different lysergic acid derivatives vary in parallel with a variety of sympathomimetic effects, including piloerection, tachycardia, hyperglycemia, and hyperthermia, and he considered that this pattern of central sympathetic stimulation is one of the major factors determining psychotomimetic properties. The active compounds also cause increased behavioral and reflex responses to sensory stimuli. Sensory thresholds are reduced, although primary sensory responses in specific cortical areas are not increased, and may be reduced. The EEG shows arousal patterns, and sleep is reduced. Habituation to repetitive stimuli is abolished; the control of attention by the filtering and integration of sensory input is impaired, and the functioning of all the senses is disturbed.

The increases in arousal levels and responsiveness to stimuli after LSD appear to be due to an action in the reticular formation of the lower brain stem, facilitating the input to this area from sensory collaterals (see Key, 1965*a,b*; Brawley and Duffield, 1972). The action does not appear to be on the sensory collaterals themselves, but on the processes regulating the level of significance of the information; these processes appear to be involved in sensory habituation, and when they are disrupted the filtering out of irrelevant stimuli fails, reducing sensory and arousal thresholds. The particular neurons which control these functions are not yet known with certainty, but it seems probable that the serotonin-containing cells of the raphe at least impinge on the process. Treatment of animals with *p*-chlorophenylalanine (PCPA), which inhibits 5-HT synthesis, or surgical destruction of raphe neurons has some effects similar to those of LSD, including reduction of sleep (both slow-wave and REM), induction of continuous pontogeniculooccipital (PGO) spiking, inhibition of habituation, and increased irritability (for review, see Jouvet, 1972).

Studies of the interactions of LSD with drugs or treatments which alter brain monoamine levels have also provided evidence that the effects of LSD involve monoaminergic neurons. Pretreatment of rats or mice with reserpine or tetrabenazine, which deplete both 5-HT and catecholamines, or with PCPA, which depletes 5-HT relatively selectively, enhanced the sensitivity of the animals to LSD (Appel and Freedman, 1964; Appel *et al*., 1970*a*; Gessner, 1970). Lesions in the midbrain raphe which selectively reduced brain 5-HT concentrations also enhanced the sensitivity of rats to subthreshold doses of LSD (Appel *et al*., 1970*b*). Furthermore, treatment with 5-HTP has been found to reduce the tremorogenic effect of LSD in mice (Gessner, 1970). Although a single dose of α-methyl-*p*-tyrosine (AMPT) apparently did not affect the action of LSD in rats (Appel *et al*., 1970*a*), pretreatment with AMPT for 24 hr did attenuate the behavioral actions but not the hyperthermic actions of LSD in rabbits (Horita and Hamilton, 1973). It is possible that in the experiments of Appel *et al*. (1970*a*) the brain catecholamines were not effectively depleted. The administration of L-DOPA to AMPT-treated rabbits restored the behavioral actions of LSD (Horita and Hamilton, 1973). It thus appears that the actions of LSD are exerted in some way counter to the physiological functions of 5-HT, and possibly in synergism with those of NorE or DA.

It seems probable that many of the effects of LSD are due to impairment of the functional roles of the 5-HT-containing raphe neurons. Aghajanian and coworkers have shown that LSD administered intravenously or directly to raphe neurons by microiontophoresis causes a marked inhibition of the activity of these cells, which are also inhibited by iontophoretically applied 5-HT (Haigler and Aghajanian, 1972; Aghajanian *et al*., 1972). This finding offers an explanation of the biochemical and histochemical observations described earlier that LSD reduces 5-HT turnover in the brain. The inhibition of the release of 5-HT from terminals in brain slices has already been described in Section IIIB2. Also, the postsynaptic actions of 5-HT released from the terminals of raphe and other 5-HT-containing neurons might be blocked by LSD. Evidence for a block of the excitatory actions of 5-HT by LSD has been obtained by Roberts and Straughan (1967), Boakes *et al*. (1970), and Couch (1970). Couch found that LSD simultaneously blocked the excitations evoked synaptically by stimulation of a region which contains 5-HT cell bodies and the excitations evoked by iontophoretically applied 5-HT. Certain methylated tryptamine derivatives with LSD-like behavioral effects also selectively antagonized 5-HT excitations of neurons in the reticular formation of the pons and medulla (Bradley and Briggs, 1974). It thus seems that hallucinogens can reduce the activity of raphe neurons by a direct action, can reduce the release of 5-HT from neurons, and also can antagonize the postsynaptic excitatory actions of 5-HT. All these actions would lead to a reduction of the influence of raphe cells on other systems.

The reduction of both slow-wave sleep (SWS) and rapid eye movement (REM) sleep by LSD and by methysergide (Stern *et al.*, 1972; Tabushi and Himwich, 1971) is probably also closely related to these actions. The mechanisms of induction and maintenance of sleep are controlled at least partly by 5-HT- and NorE containing neurons; 5-HT seems to be associated primarily with the control of SWS and the "priming" of REM sleep, whereas the catecholamines appear to be involved in tonic mechanisms concerned with arousal and REM sleep (for review, see Jouvet, 1972).

SWS appears to be induced by an inhibitory influence of structures in the lower pons and medulla on more rostal activating areas. The inhibitory mechanisms seem to be situated in the caudal pontine and medullary reticular formation, the nucleus tractus solitarius (NTS), and the area postrema. The area postrema appears to act as a "gain control" regulating the NTS. It has been suggested (Koella, 1969; Bronzino, 1972; Bronzino *et al.*, 1972) that 5-HT, acting via the area postrema, can facilitate the excitability of the NTS; the most significant projections of the NTS are to the medullary reticular formation (Morest, 1967), which exerts a strong inhibitory influence on the EEG-desynchronizing mechanisms (Jouvet, 1972; Bolme *et al.*, 1972). The extensive projections of the raphe neurons to the midbrain and forebrain, including the locus coeruleus, hypothalamus, and hippocampus, also appear to be important in the control of sleep and arousal (Jouvet, 1972; Morgane and Stern, 1972; Mabry and Campbell, 1973).

Mechanisms in the pons and medulla are also involved in the regulation of REM sleep. The pontine raphe nuclei appear to have a "REM-sleep-priming"role, acting on the NorE-containing neurons of the locus coeruleus which maintain the state of REM sleep (Jouvet, 1972).

Clearly, these systems could be affected by LSD and methysergide at several points; the antagonism of 5-HT excitations of single neurons in the medulla and pons (Boakes *et al.*, 1970) and pontine raphe (Couch, 1970) and the direct inhibitory action of LSD on midbrain raphe neurons (Aghajanian *et al*., 1972) have already been described, while the area postrema, the NTS, and the locus coeruleus might also be involved in the effects of these drugs on sleep.

Another aspect of sleep which is affected by LSD and methysergide is the phenomenon of PGO spiking. These waves can be recorded from the pons, lateral geniculate nucleus, and occipital cortex and from certain other areas; they normally occur mainly in association with REM sleep episodes and are strongly correlated with the eye movements of this state. The PGO waves appear to be under the control of a noradrenergic "pacemaker" in the dorsolateral pontine tegmentum, probably the medial part of the locus coeruleus (Jovet, 1972). The PGO pacemaker appears to be subject to an inhibitory serotoninergic influence, since administration of PCPA, or lesions of the raphe, can induce PGO waves outside REM sleep which are suppressed by 5-HTP (Jouvet, 1972). LSD also induces PGO spikes outside REM sleep; this action is not shared by methysergide or BOL (Stern *et al*., 1972; Monachon *et al*., 1972). Reserpine induces PGO spiking during SWS and waking, and, somewhat paradoxically, LSD and methysergide counteract this effect of reserpine (Jouvet, 1972; Monachon *et al*., 1972).

A reduction of the serotoninergic inhibitory influence on the pacemaker by LSD would account for its facilitatory action on PGO spiking, and this effect could be achieved by the mechanisms already discussed in relation to the sleep states. The contrasting effect of LSD in reducing PGO spikes in reserpinized animals is difficult to explain in the same terms. Possibly the mechanism depends on a balance of opposing influences which may be altered by LSD in opposite directions in reserpine-treated and nontreated animals.

Other actions of LSD and related compounds have been suggested to be related to their psychotomimetic properties. These include suggestions of stimulation of 5-HT receptors (Aghajanian, 1972*a,b,c*; Andén *et al*., 1968; Berridge and Prince, 1973), stimulation of NorE receptors or potentiation of the actions of NorE (Costa and Zetler, 1959), and inhibition of the release of an unknown transmitter (Tebēcis and Di Maria, 1972: see Section IIIB3b; Ambache *et al*., 1973). The first of these receives most support as an alternative to the hypothesis described above, that LSD antagonizes the functions of serotoninergic neurons. In some mammalian peripheral organs and in some invertebrate test organs, LSD can stimulate 5-HT receptors. Andén *et al*. (1968) suggested that a stimulant action on 5-HT receptors could explain the facilitatory action of LSD on spinal extensor reflexes in acutely spinal rats. This effect was like that following combined nialamide and 5-HTP treatment, which presumably was due to increased 5-HT levels in the spinal cord. At the same time, LSD reduced the turnover of 5-HT in terminals. This was attributed to a hypothetical inhibitory feedback loop activated by direct stimulation of 5-HT receptors, which reduces the activity of the 5-HT-containing neurons. Further evidence for this has been described by Aghajanian (1972*c*), who also attributes the LSD-induced reduction of firing of raphe neurons to an inhibitory feedback circuit, although he has also shown a direct inhibitory action of LSD on raphe neurons (Aghajanian *et al.*, 1972; Haigler and Aghajanian, 1972). A possible link in a feedback loop is the nonfluorescing neuron group in the anterior pole of the median raphe nucleus and the linearis caudalis nucleus. Neurons in this group receive 5-HT-containing terminals from the raphe, and following intravenous administration of LSD the firing of these is accelerated. This action is suggested to be due to the mimicking of an excitatory action of 5-HT on postsynaptic receptors on these neurons, which leads to compensatory inhibition of the raphe neurons (Aghajanian, 1972*c*). However, a reciprocal innervation of the raphe neurons by the neurons of the linearis caudalis nucleus has not yet been identified. Furthermore, the action of 5-HT on the latter neurons is not known, but no neurons in other areas studied appear to be excited by both 5-HT and LSD. Even if LSD does mimic 5-HT excitations of these neurons, the results of a study of four methylated derivatives of tryptamine, which have some 5-HT-mimicking actions (Bradley and Briggs, 1974), indicate that their LSD-like psychotomimetic properties are not related to their potencies in mimicking 5-HT excitations. Without more evidence, it is not possible to decide whether the feedback hypothesis is correct. At present, one reasonable alternative explanation is that the increased firing of linearis caudalis neurons after intravenous LSD is a consequence of the direct inhibition of raphe neurons by the drug.

b. Actions of Ergot Derivatives in the Lateral Geniculate Nucleus. Because of the prominence of visual disturbances and hallucinations among the subjective effects of psychotomimetics in man, there have been a large number of studies of the actions of these drugs in the visual system. The earlier studies on this problem have been reviewed by Brawley and Duffield (1972) and Tebēcis and Di Maria (1972). LSD given by intracarotid injection depresses the transmission of optic nerve impulses through the lateral geniculate nucleus (LGN). At present, the transmitter released from optic nerve terminals is unidentified, and the mechanism of action of LSD is unexplained. Tebēcis and Di Maria (1972) reinvestigated the effects of iontophoretically applied monoamines and LSD on spontaneous and evoked activity in the LGN of the cat. With low ejecting currents, 5-HT depressed spontaneous activity and orthodromic activation of LGN neurons by light or optic nerve stimulation, but affected firing evoked by ACh, glutamate, or aspartate, or by antidromic activation, only when higher ejecting currents were used. The actions of LSD were similar to those of 5-HT but of longer duration. The authors supported the hypothesis that 5-HT and LSD either blocked the release of the optic nerve transmitter or prevented its access to receptors on the LGN neurons. Higher concentrations of both agents had direct depressant actions on the LGN neurons, which were suggested to be mediated by 5-HT receptors. Horn and McKay (1973) studied the effects of intravenous LSD (25–300 μg per cat) on LGN neurons and found that spontaneous activity was generally depressed, although some cells were excited, particularly by the lower doses tested; responses to photic stimuli delivered to the center and surround regions of the receptive fields were also depressed. The size and shape of receptive fields did not change. BOL did not have effects like those of LSD. The changes in spontaneous activity caused by LSD were not correlated with changes in the responses to stimuli, and it seems that at the doses used LSD had no direct uniform depressant effect on the neurons. An indirect depressant action mediated via the reticular formation was considered possible.

Although the significance of these effects for the psychotomimetic actions of LSD is uncertain, they offer a possible explanation of the decreased photosensitivity of the baboon *Papio papio* observed after administration of LSD and other lysergic acid derivatives, including nonpsychotomimetic ones (Walter *et al.*, 1971; Meldrum and Naquet, 1971; Vuillon-Cacciuttolo and Balzano, 1972). The reduction of photically evoked epileptic responses in these animals appeared to be related to a depression of evoked responses in the LGN and visual cortex. The effects were not related to the psychotomimetic potencies of the drugs.

c. Actions on the Nigrostriatal DA System. Stone (1973) found that 1–2 mg/kg agroclavine in rats caused sedation and stereotyped sniffing and gnawing, while higher doses (5–10 mg/kg) induced transient sedation followed by hypermotility, excitation, and aggression. He considered that the stereotyped movements were similar to those observed with drugs such as apomorphine which are thought to stimulate DA receptors in the basal ganglia, and suggested that agroclavine had a similar mode of action. Support for this idea was provided by Corrodi *et al.*, (1973), who compared ergocornine and 2-bromo-α-ergokryptine (CB-154) with apomorphine in rats with unilateral lesions induced by 6-hydroxydopamine in the substantia nigra. All three drugs caused stereotyped sniffing and gnawing and rotation of the animals toward the unlesioned side. Pimozide, which blocks DA receptors, blocked these effects, and Corrodi *et al.* (1973) proposed that the drugs all act by stimulation of DA receptors. However, it seems difficult to reconcile a direct action of the ergot alkaloids on DA receptors with the observation of Corrodi *et al.* (1973) that after pretreatment with reserpine and AMPT the effects of the two derivatives were greatly reduced, unlike those of apomorphine, which were increased by this pretreatment. The effects of the ergot alkaloids thus seem to be mediated at least partly by the release of DA from DA-containing neurons, or by a potentiation of the effect of DA. The action of DA on receptors has been suggested to be due to the activation of adenyl cyclase, leading to increased cyclic AMP formation (Kebabian and Greengard, 1971). The enzyme which catabolizes cyclic AMP, phosphodiesterase, has been found by Iwangoff and Enz (1972) to be strongly inhibited by dihydrogenated ergot alkaloids in homogenates of cat brain gray matter. This enzyme appears to be localized predominantly in dendrites, immediately adjacent to subsynaptic membranes, possibly indicating a role related to the action of transmitters (Florendo *et al.*, 1971). If the two derivatives used by Corrodi *et al.* (1973) also inhibit phosphodiesterase, then the retardation of the catabolism of cyclic AMP would potentiate the effects of stimulation of adenyl cyclase by DA. Corrodi *et al.* (1973) also found that NorE levels were reduced and 5-HT levels increased by the two derivatives, as with LSD (Andén *et al.*, 1968), and attributed these effects to block of NorE receptors and stimulation of 5-HT receptors, respectively. In view of the results of Corrodi *et al.* (1973), it is possible that some of the effects of lysergic acid derivatives on arousal (see Section IIIB3a) might be mediated by the nigrostriatal DA neurons, which may have a role in the control of behavioral arousal (Jouvet, 1972).

d. Actions on Spinal Reflexes. The facilitatory action of LSD on spinal extensor reflexes (Andén, *et al.*, 1968) has been described in Section IIIB3a. Andén *et al.* considered it to be due to stimulation of 5-HT receptors by LSD. Methysergide and BOL did not have effects like those of LSD.

The effects of LSD, methysergide, and BOL on the bulbospinal influences on spinal reflexes have been discussed in a review by Anderson (1972). Administration of 5-HTP, tryptophan, or monoamine oxidase inhibitors to acutely spinalized rats causes a slowly developing but marked increase in monosynaptic spike size, a decrease in latency of the reflex, and spontaneous ventral root discharges, indicating increased excitability of α-motoneurons. At the same time, the reflex response recorded from an adjacent dorsal root is depressed. LSD, methysergide, and BOL, and other structurally unrelated 5-HT antagonists, can rapidly reverse the facilitatory effect of 5-HTP but not the depression of the dorsal root reflex. The effects of 5-HTP are thought to be exerted via 5-HT-containing nerve terminals which appear to increase motoneuron excitability. This idea receives support from work of Barasi and Roberts (1973), who found that stimulation of the rat hindbrain in the region of the raphe facilitated the monosynaptic reflex and that the facilitation was potentiated by intravenous injection of tryptophan. Both the facilitation and its potentiation by tryptophan were blocked by intravenous LSD or cinanserin. In other experiments, negative field potentials elicited in the motoneuron pool by dorsal root stimulation were increased in amplitude by iontophoretic application of 5-HT, and by hindbrain stimulation; iontophoretic application of methysergide or cinanserin prevented the effect of hindbrain stimulation on the size of the potential. The hindbrain stimulation was associated with depolarization of spinal motoneurons, and these workers proposed the existence of an excitatory 5-HT synapse in the ventral horn, possibly on the motoneurons. However, Anderson and coworkers (see Anderson, 1972) found that stimulation of the raphe region of the pons and medulla could cause either potentiation or inhibition of the monosynaptic reflex; only the depressant effects were reduced by LSD, methysergide, and BOL. This discrepancy may be due to species or dosage differences.

e. Effects in the Cerebral Cortex. The desynchronizing effects of certain ergot derivatives on the activity of the cerebral cortex are now generally thought to be caused indirectly by actions in other areas, especially the lower brain stem (see Evarts, 1957; Purpura, 1957; Brawley and Duffield, 1972; and Sections IIIB3a and IIIB3c of this chapter). However, direct actions of these drugs on the cortex have been described. Krnjević and Phillis (1963) found that LSD, ergometrine, methylergometrine, methysergide, and 12-hydroxyergometrine could all affect cortical single-unit activity when applied iontophoretically, but the specificity of the effects is uncertain. Roberts and Straughan (1967) found that lysergic acid derivatives (LSD, methysergide, and BOL) depressed neuronal firing rates and spike amplitudes, and also preferentially antagonized 5-HT excitatory effects on single neurons. LSD was the most potent of the three in this respect. Davidson *et al.* (1969) found that somatosensory evoked potentials in the cortex were reduced by NorE topically applied to the same cortical area. This inhibitory effect of NorE was antagonized by LSD and by agroclavine, also applied topically. Somatosensory evoked potentials in the cortex were found by Samanin *et al.* (1972) to be inhibited by stimulation of the midbrain raphe area in rats. LSD potentiated the inhibitory effect of raphe stimulation. This finding seems to support the hypothesis that LSD can either potentiate the actions of 5-HT released from raphe neuron terminals or activate 5-HT receptors directly.

f. Emetic Actions of Ergot Derivatives. Many of the ergot derivatives have emetic activity. Wang and coworkers (see Wang, 1965) found that the site of action of dihydroergotoxine was in a "chemoreceptive emetic trigger zone" situated in the area postrema. A mode of action involving blockade of α-adrenergic receptors was suggested. Fuxe and Owman (1965) considered the monoamine-containing neurons of the area postrema to be important in the emetic reflex, and the projection of the area postrema to the nucleus tractus solitarius (Morest, 1967) has been proposed as another link in the reflex.

g. Effects on Respiration. It was demonstrated very early that ergot derivatives can depress or stimulate respiration (Barger, 1931; Horita and Dille, 1954), but there has been little further study of these actions. However, recent studies on respiratory control may help to explain the effects, although only speculation is possible at present. Bolme and Fuxe (1973) have postulated that there is a central noradrenergic inhibitory influence on respiration and suggested that the locus coeruleus might have a pneumotaxic role mediated via neurons in the nucleus tractus solitarius (NTS). An alternative or additional mechanism has been proposed by Ylitalo *et al.* (1970), who suggested that 5-HT-containing neurons in the area postrema, projecting to the NTS, are also involved in respiratory depression. If the existence of these mechanisms is substantiated, then the ability of ergot derivatives to act on NorE or 5-HT receptors is a possible explanation of their effects on respiration. A study of their interactions with monoamines on the medullary neurons controlling respiration would be of interest.

4. Effects of Ergot Derivatives on Neuroendocrine Functions.

Certain of the ergot derivatives have been known for some time to affect processes regulating reproduction and lactation; recently, these actions have been the subject of a considerable amount of research, and the ergot drugs have proved to be useful tools in the investigation of the regulation of secretion and functions of prolactin, one of the hormones involved in the control of these processes.

a. Control of Prolactin Secretion. Meites and Clemens (1972) and Meites *et al.* (1972) have reviewed recent work on prolactin, including studies of the inhibitory actions of ergot derivatives on the secretion of this hormone, and as only a brief account it is possible here, these reviews should be consulted for further information.

The secretion of prolactin (P) from the anterior pituitary is controlled by the hypothalamus, which in mammals secretes a prolactin-release inhibiting factor (PIF) into the pituitary portal circulation. A prolactin releasing factor (PRF) is also thought to play a role. The secretion of PIF is regulated by hypothalamic monoaminergic neurons, in particular dopamine (DA) containing neurons with cell bodies in the arcuate nuclei projecting to the external layer of the median eminence (see McCann *et al.*, 1972; Porter *et al.*, 1972; Hökfelt and Fuxe, 1972*a,b*; Björklund *et al.*, 1973; Björklund and Nobin, 1973). Increased activity in these DA neurons induces increased

PIF secretion and a fall in pituitary P release. NorE also inhibits P release but is much less potent than DA, where as 5-HT appears to stimulate P release. The DA-containing neurons seem to form part of the feedback mechanism by which plasma P levels influence the rate of release of further P. The activity of the neurons varies during the ovarian cycle; it increases markedly when plasma P levels are high, for example, during lactation or early pregnancy (Hökfelt and Fuxe, 1972*a,b*). The functions of NorE and 5-HT in this system are less well understood, but they may include the maintenance of basal release of P and the control of diurnal variations in its secretion. The mechanisms inducing release of P are not at present understood; there is preliminary evidence in some species that thyrotropin releasing factor (TRF) has high P releasing activity and may serve to regulate release of both thyrotropin and prolactin.

The results of iontophoretic studies of the actions of monoamines on hypothalamic neurons are so far difficult to relate to this system.

b. Inhibitory Effects of Ergot Derivatives on Prolactin Secretion. The derivatives which cause reductions in secretion of P have diverse structures; compounds with variations in both the ring system and the side-chain are active, but slight alterations in structure can cause marked differences in potency. Among the active compounds are ergokryptine, ergocornine, their dihydrogenated derivatives, 2-bromo-α-ergokryptine, ergometrine, ergotamine, LSD, agroclavine, elymoclavine, and other synthetic ergoline derivatives; inactive compounds include lysergic acid, ergocorninine, and compounds with substituents on N_1. Variations in the peptide side-chain of the compounds can cause differences in potency, so it appears that this part of the molecule influences the activity, but an elaborate side-chain is not essential, since agroclavine, for example, is active with only a methyl group in the corresponding position (for references, see Meites and Clemens, 1972).

The inhibitory action of these drugs on P release seems to be exerted in two ways: they act on the hypothalamus to increase synthesis and release of PIF, which then affects pituitary P release, and they also act directly on the pituitary, apparently blocking the P release mechanism without affecting P synthesis, since the number of P granules in the pituitary cells increases. The mechanisms of action underlying these effects are not clear, but it seems likely that the hypothalamic actions involve a stimulation of the DA receptors which increase PIF secretion (Hökfelt and Fuxe, 1972*a*) (*cf.* Section IIIB3c).

The direct actions on pituitary release of P are at present difficult to explain. It has not been possible to demonstrate the presence of monoamines in the hypophyseal portal blood, and infusions of monoamines into the anterior pituitary via the portal vessels have no effect on the secretion of P or of LH or FSH (for references, see McCann *et al.*, 1972); it thus seems that monoamines in portal blood do not affect hypophyseal cells, but the presence of monoamines in many cells of the adenohypophysis (Björklund and Falck, 1969) leads to the suggestion that the effects of ergot derivatives may be related in some way to these cells.

c. Effects of Ergot Derivatives Mediated by Inhibition of Prolactin Secretion. Since the demonstration that ergot derivatives inhibit P release, they have been used in the study of the processes in which P has regulatory functions.

Certain ergot derivatives prevent the rapid increase in P secretion during proestrus, estrus, and metestrus and inhibit the involution of corpora lutea during the ovarian cycle; corpora lutea therefore accumulate in the ovaries. On the other hand, when given to rats in early pregnancy, the drugs prevent the rise in prolactin secretion which normally occurs at this time; the corpora lutea then undergo involution, thus terminating the secretion of progesterone by the ovaries and preventing normal implantation of the ova. The animals then return to the estrous state, and ovulation recurs, usually followed by pseudopregnancy. These drug effects in early pregnancy resemble those produced by surgical removal of active corpora lutea and can be counteracted by administration of progesterone or P. These effects indicate that P has a dual function with respect to rat corpora lutea: it is important for maintenance of active corpora and secretion of progesterone in early pregnancy, but in cyclic rats luteolysis is dependent on the action of P. Although the ergot derivatives suppress the normal changes in P secretion, the estrus cycle itself is not altered and ovulation is not blocked (Wuttke *et al.*, 1971); it thus seems that P is of slight importance in this respect.

Daily administration of ergot derivatives to rats during the second half of pregnancy does not terminate pregnancy, although the animals do lose weight, a significant part of this being a fall in mammary gland weight. After parturition, lactation is significantly impaired, as judged by the rate of weight gain of the pups (Shaar and Clemens, 1972). In women, 2-bromo-α-ergokryptine (CB-154) is highly effective in preventing puerperal lactation and breast engorgement, by suppressing the increase in P levels in the postpartum period. The drug also stops nonpuerperal galactorrhea in patients with high serum P levels (Del Pozo *et al.*, 1972) and galactorrhea induced by psychotropic drugs (see Daughaday and Jacobs, 1972).

It has been suggested (Flückiger and Wagner, 1968) that the inhibitory actions of ergot derivatives on fertility and lactation are achieved by actions on more than one mechanism, since ergocornine and 2-bromo-α-ergokryptine have differential actions on the two processes; the latter drug is significantly more selective in preventing pregnancy.

In rodents, some ergot derivatives cause an inhibition of the growth of mammary and pituitary tumors, which is probably mediated by their effect on P secretion. It has been suggested that this action may be clinically valuable in the treatment of mammary tumors in women, but in a trial of 2-bromo-α-ergokryptine in 19 women with advanced tumors no objective remissions were observed (European Breast Cancer Group, 1972). However, Stoll (1972) did find regression of mammary tumors in several patients treated with a combination of L-DOPA and estrogen, which is also supposed to act by inhibition of P secretion. Further work in this field is obviously desirable; treatment at an earlier stage might prove more effective.

In nonmammalian vertebrates, P is the most important hormone in osmoregulation, but until recently there was little evidence of such a function in mammals. Richardson (1973) found that chronic administration of 2-bromo-α-ergokryptine to rats reduced the incidence of spontaneous nephrosis, decreased urinary Ca^{2+} and specific gravity, and increased the daily volume of urine as well as its pH and its Na^+ and K^+ content. He suggests that these findings support a possible role of P in the control of electrolyte and water balance in rats.

d. Effects of Ergot Derivatives on Gonadotropin Secretion. Relatively high doses of the derivatives which inhibit the release of P can also alter the secretion of LH and FSH (Meites *et al.*, 1972). The release of these hormones is regulated by a releasing hormone (one hormone appears to control both FSH and LH; Schally *et al.*, 1973), which is itself controlled by monoaminergic neurons in the median eminence. The work of some groups indicates that DA neurons in this area have a facilitatory role in FRF/LRF release, whereas others suggest that their role is inhibitory. Serotonin appears to have an inhibitory effect on gonadotropin release (for references, see McCann *et al.*, 1972; Hökfelt and Fuxe, 1972*a,b*).

Ergot derivatives do not affect spontaneous ovulation in adult rodents, but it has been found that ovulation induced in immature mice or rats by pregnant mare serum (PMS) gonadotropin is facilitated by 5-HT and inhibited by LSD, methysergide, ergocornine, and 2-bromo-α-ergokryptine (see Brown, 1968; Hökfelt and Fuxe, 1972*a*). PMS-induced ovulation has been suggested as a model for the study of the neuroendocrine mechanisms controlling LH release during the critical period for ovulation. The actions of the ergot derivatives in this system are of uncertain mechanism, but it has been suggested that the effects are at least partly mediated indirectly by the increased activity of the tuberoinfundibular DA neurons resulting from the inhibition of P secretion. On the other hand, the inhibition of 5-HT synthesis by PCPA also inhibits PMS-induced ovulation, so the effects of the drugs may thus be due to an antagonism of 5-HT or to reduced activity in a serotoninergic input to the hypothalamus.

Although the secretion of at least some other hypothalamic regulating hormones is also thought to be affected by the DA neurons in the median eminence, ergot derivatives do not seem to affect the production of other pituitary hormones, so far as is known. It thus seems that their main effect is on P secretion, and the effects on gonadotropins of high doses of the drugs are possibly due to feedback mechanisms influenced by P levels.

5. *Effects of Ergot Derivatives on Thermoregulation*

The effects of ergot derivatives on the regulation of body temperature depend on the type of alkaloid, the dose, the species, and especially in small animals, the ambient temperature. Shemano and Nickerson (1958) first established the importance of this factor and found that an inversion of the effect of drugs on body temperature usually occurred around a particular ambient temperature for each drug. Above this temperature hyperthermia occurred, and below it hypothermia. The inversion temperature for Hydergine, ergotamine, and LSD was 30°C, which is in the range of thermal neutrality for the rat. In this range, constant body temperature is maintained with minimal physiological control, and the observation that these drugs have an inversion temperature around 30°C suggests that in the rat the drugs induce poikilothermia by inhibition of the processes of thermoregulation in the CNS. In other species (cat, dog, and rabbit), LSD causes marked hyperthermia (Horita and Dille, 1954). Rothlin (1947, 1957) pointed out a parallelism between the hyperthermic responses to ergot derivatives and other central effects, including nausea, vomiting, and general excitation. This observation was extended by Cerletti (1959), who reported a parallelism between the pyretogenic effects of lysergic acid derivatives and the "central excitatory syndrome" (see Section IIIB3a), which itself paralleled the psychotogenic properties of the drugs in man. There is thus a relationship between the hyperthermic effects of the drugs in animals and their psychotomimetic effects in man, although a dissociation of the two effects is seen in, for example, BOL and 1-methylated derivatives of lysergic acid. Horita and Hamilton (1973) produced a pharmacological dissociation between the behavioral excitatory effects and the hyperthermic effects of LSD in rabbits by pretreating the animals with α-methyl-p-tyrosine. This abolished the behavioral but not the hyperthermic effects of low doses of LSD. The latter effect thus did not appear to depend on catecholaminergic mechanisms.

The mechanisms controlling thermoregulation are at present poorly understood. Both heat production and heat loss can be varied to accomplish body temperature changes; the control mechanisms have been suggested to be influenced by 5-HT, NorE, DA, ACh, and prostaglandins (for reviews, see Borison and Clark, 1967; Avery, 1972; Fuxe and Sjöqvist, 1972; Hellon, 1972; Lomax and Schönbaum, 1973).

In view of the known interactions of ergot derivatives with 5-HT, NorE, and DA neuron systems, it is not surprising that thermoregulation is disrupted by these drugs. As the roles of the monoamines in thermoregulation are still uncertain, it is not possible at present to identify the modes of actions of the drugs. Only LSD has been studied in any detail; it inhibits the 5-HT-containing neurons in the raphe which are activated when body temperature rises (Corrodi *et al.*, 1967; Simmonds, 1970; Weiss and Aghajanian, 1971), but so far the physiological role, if any, of the raphe neurons in thermoregulation is not known, and no conclusions can be drawn until both thermoregulatory control and the central actions of the drugs are better understood.

IV. POISONING

Ergot alkaloids and their derivatives are highly toxic, and may cause acute or chronic poisoning. Acute poisonings by the ergot derivatives fall into two main types; one type results from attempts to procure abortion, another from the nonmedical abuse of LSD and related psychotomimetic ergot derivatives taken for their mental effects. Chronic poisoning by ergot alkaloids was formerly not uncommon; widespread epidemics occurred frequently during the Middle Ages (Barger, 1931; Bové 1970), due usually to ingestion of bread contaminated with ergot. This type of chronic poisoning is now rare, thanks to better quality control of grain and flour, but chronic poisoning by the pure alkaloids from ergot is not rare, as a result of the use of the drugs in migraine and obstetrics. Toxic effects may result either from repeated or prolonged ingestion of excessive doses of ergot derivatives or from normally therapeutic doses, apparently due to hypersensitivity to the drugs.

A. Acute Poisoning

1. Nonpsychotomimetic Derivatives

The symptoms of acute poisoning by ergot or ergot alkaloids include tingling, itching, and coldness of the skin, thirst, vomiting, diarrhea, confusion, and coma. Hemorrhage from the uterus and abortion may occur in pregnant women, but fatal poisoning may ensue in these cases without abortion taking place. The natural alkaloids are much more toxic than their dihydrogenated analogues (Rothlin, 1947).

2. *Psychotomimetic Derivatives*

The use of LSD and related agents as psychedelics has continued in spite of strong governmental measures against their illicit use. The complications of LSD use have been classified by Cohen (for reference, see Connell, 1972) into psychotic disorders, nonpsychotic disorders, and neurological reactions. The "psychotic" side-effects of LSD consist of schizophrenic-type reactions indistinguishable from paranoid, schizoaffective, or catatonic types of schizophrenia; paranoia; delusions; prolonged or recurrent LSD-like states; and psychotic depressions. "Nonpsychotic" reactions include chronic anxiety and acute panic. Neurological side-effects include epileptiform convulsions and EEG abnormalities. Some workers have suggested that LSD can precipitate psychosis in people without previous apparent disorder (Smart and Bateman, 1967), but other evidence suggests that persistent adverse reactions to LSD occur in predisposed individuals (Hollister, 1972). Díaz and Huttunen (1971) found that in rats given low doses of LSD daily for 1 month brain serotonin levels and turnover were increased, in contrast to the reduced turnover after acute doses of LSD. This change was considered to be persistent since the animals were not killed until 18 hr after the last dose of LSD, and the authors suggested that behavioral alterations among chronic users of the drug might be associated with similar persistent metabolic effects of LSD.

In 1967, it was suggested that there was a higher incidence of congenital abnormalities in the offspring of LSD users, and it has been found that, *in vitro,* LSD causes chromosome breakages in cultured cells. The possibility of genetic damage by LSD has been the subject of several reviews. Jacobson and Berlin (1972) considered that their findings did indicate that LSD taking was associated with teratogenic effects, although the ingestion of other illicit drugs, the presence of diseases, and marginal maternal nutrition precluded any definite conclusion with regard to the effect of LSD itself. Similar conclusions were reached by Dishotsky *et al.* (1971), Nichols (1972), and Long (1972), who considered that pure LSD in moderate amounts does not damage chromosomes *in vivo,* does not cause detectable genetic damage, and is not teratogenic or carcinogenic in man. When chromosome damage was found, it appeared to be related to extraneous factors associated with drug abuse, such as hepatitis, virus infections, and malnutrition, and not to LSD alone. A distinction was drawn between pure and illicit LSD: use of the latter did seem to be associated with increased incidence of malformations and spontaneous abortions.

Another effect of LSD which may be significant for its use in humans was recently reported by Voss *et al.* (1973). *In vitro,* LSD appears to interfere with immunoglobulin synthesis by preventing tryptophan incorporation into protein molecules, either by terminating the peptide chain or by taking the place of tryptophan in the chain. It was therefore suggested that LSD could significantly interfere with antibody production. Lysergic acid also has this effect.

B. Chronic Poisoning

The symptoms of chronic ergotism have been described graphically in the historical monograph by Barger (1931). Chronic ergot poisoning, whether a consequence of overdosage or of hypersensitivity, appears in two forms; the more common is characterized principally by circulatory changes, the other by nervous symptoms including convulsions.

1. Gangrenous Ergotism

In gangrenous ergotism, intense vasoconstriction of arteries and veins and probably of lymph vessels occurs; the pulse often disappears in affected limbs; and the feet, legs, and sometimes the hands become cold, pale, and numb. Painful muscle cramps occur, and in severe cases gangrene and amputation of the limbs may result from the lack of circulation. Besides the vasoconstriction, hypercoagulability of the blood appears to develop (Cranley *et al.,* 1963), and thrombosis results in complete occlusion of the smaller arteries. Internal organs, as well as the limbs, can be affected: angina is aggravated by coronary vasoconstriction, gangrene of the bowel may follow constriction of the arterial supply, and renal failure may result from spasm of the renal arteries. The constriction of the renal arteries (Fedotin and Hartmann, 1970) has been suggested by Lewis and Lee (1972) to be a possible triggering factor in the postpartum renal failure sometimes associated with ergometrine. The fall in blood pressure in the kidney due to renal arterial constriction is suggested to cause excessive renin secretion from the juxtaglomerular apparatus, resulting in renal failure.

Vascular sensitivity to the ergot alkaloids is greatly increased in fever, infections, liver disease, and diseases in which vascular disorders already exist.

2. *Convulsive Ergotism*

Convulsive ergotism is said to occur mainly in people with vitamin A deficiency (Barger, 1931), which has been suggested to cause an increased sensitivity of the CNS to the ergot alkaloids. The symptoms usually start with twitching and numbness in the hands and feet, drowsiness, dizziness, weakness, formication and itching of the skin, and diarrhea. The clonic and tonic convulsions which follow in severe cases are extremely painful, and fatalities were formerly common. Convulsions have also been observed after LSD (see Connell, 1972).

3. *Fibrotic Effects*

As a result of the long-term use of methysergide in the prophylaxis of migraine, another serious side-effect, inflammatory fibrosis, has been observed (Graham, 1967; Graham *et al.*, 1967). The fibrosis may develop in the retroperitoneal space, causing compression of arteries, veins, and lymphatic vessels, leading to ischemic and obstructive lesions; in the connective tissue of cardiac valves, causing heart murmurs; and in the pleura and lungs, causing chest pain and respiratory difficulties due to pleural thickening and friction. The etiology of these fibrotic processes has been discussed by Graham *et al.*, (1967), who drew attention to the similarity of these effects to those found in various forms of vascular disease, including ergotism. It is possible that the inflammatory and fibrotic lesions are secondary to vascular changes caused by methysergide, which can have many effects similar to those seen in ergotism (Curran *et al.*, 1967).

C. Treatment of Poisoning

In general, the main methods of treatment involve withdrawal of the offending drug, if the drug is still being taken, and symptomatic measures to counteract the effects.

1. *Poisoning with Nonpsychotomimetic Ergot Alkaloids*

In cases where the main toxic effect is excessive vasoconstriction, the treatment is designed to maintain adequate circulation in affected areas. Vasodilator agents, α-receptor blocking agents, heparin, and low molecular weight dextran are all considered useful. Ganglionic blockade and epidural anesthesia have also been used to reduce any nervous component of the vasoconstriction, but since the constrictor action of the ergot alkaloids is directly on the vessels (see Section IIIA2e), the value of these treatments is questionable.

2. *Psychotomimetic Agents*

In the treatment of LSD intoxication, sedation and symptomatic relief are the primary objectives: oral or intravenously administered phenothiazines, benzodiazepines, or short-acting barbiturates are effective (Isbell and Logan, 1957; Taylor *et al.*, 1970; Hasse *et al.*, 1971). In cases of illicit drug use, the situation is complicated by the possibility that the drug taken by the patient might not be LSD, or might be contaminated by other agents. In particular, the effects of anticholinergic agents are aggravated by phenothiazines, so since the psychotoxic symptoms of poisoning with anticholinergics can be difficult to distinguish from those of LSD, benzodiazepines or barbiturates are preferred to the phenothiazines by some practitioners for treatment of hallucinogen abuse (Taylor *et al.*, 1970).

V. CONCLUSIONS

Although the present state of knowledge of the pharmacology of the ergot alkaloids and their derivatives is wide and complex, the field is by no means exhausted. The spectrum of effects is still being extended by discoveries of new properties, and the more detailed study of well-known actions is leading to a better understanding of their mechanisms. However, many aspects of the subject are controversial, and further research is needed to clarify the apparently conflicting findings. In view of the established importance and possible future value of these compounds both in clinical practice and in research, a more complete understanding of their actions is of great importance.

VI. REFERENCES

Abrahams, V. C., Hilton, S. M., and Zbrożyna, A. W., 1960, Active muscle vasodilation produced by stimulation of the brain stem: Its significance in the defence reaction, *J. Physiol.* (*Lond.*) **154**:491.

Abrahams, V. C., Hilton, S. M., and Zbrożyna, A. W., 1964, The role of active muscle vasodilation in the altering stage of the defence reaction, *J. Physiol.* (*Lond.*) **171**:189.

Aellig, W. H., and Berde, B., 1969, Studies of the effect of natural and synthetic polypeptide type ergot compounds on a peripheral vascular bed, *Brit. J. Pharmacol.* **36**:561.

Aghajanian, G. K., 1972*a*, LSD and CNS transmission, *Ann. Rev. Pharmacol.* **12**:157.

Aghajanian, G. K., 1972*b*, Influence of drugs on the firing of serotonin-containing neurons in brain, *Fed. Proc.* **31**:91.

Aghajanian, G. K., 1972*c*, Chemical feedback regulation of serotonin-containing neurons in brain, *Ann. N.Y. Acad. Sci.* **193**:86.

Aghajanian, G. K., Haigler, H. J., and Bloom, F. E., 1972, Lysergic acid diethylamide and serotonin: Direct actions on serotonin-containing neurons in rat brain, *Life Sci.* **11**:615 (Part I).

Ambache, N., Dunk, L. P., Verney, J., and Aboo Zar, M., 1973, An inhibition of postganglionic motor transmission in the mammalian vas deferens by D-lysergic acid diethylamide, *J. Physiol.* (*Lond.*) **231**:251.

Andén, N.-E., Corrodi, H., Fuxe, K., and Hökfelt, T., 1968, Evidence for a central 5-hydroxytryptamine receptor stimulation by lysergic acid diethylamide, *Brit. J. Pharmacol.* **34**:1.

Anderson, E. G., 1972, Bulbospinal serotonin-containing neurons and motor control, *Fed. Proc.* **31**:107.

Anthony, M., Hinterberger, H., and Lance, J. W., 1969, The possible relationship of serotonin to the migraine syndrome, *Res. Clin. Stud. Headache* **2**:29.

Appel, J. B., and Freedman, D. X., 1964, Chemically-induced alterations in the behavioral effects of LSD-25, *Biochem. Pharmacol.* **13**:861.

Appel, J. B., Lovell, R. A., and Freedman, D. X., 1970*a*, Alterations in the behavioral effects of LSD by pretreatment with *p*-chlorophenylalanine and α-methyl-*p*-tyrosine, *Psychopharmacologia* (*Berl.*) **18**:387.

Appel, J. B., Sheard, M. H., and Freedman, D. X., 1970*b*, Alterations in the behavioral effects of LSD by midbrain raphe lesions, *Commun. Behav. Biol.* **5**:237.

Arcari, G., Dorigotti, L., Fregnan, G. B., and Glässer, A. H., 1968, Vasodilating and alpha-receptor blocking activity of a new ergoline derivative, *Brit. J. Pharmacol.* **34**:700P.

Avery, D. D., 1972, Thermoregulatory effects of intrahypothalamic injections of adrenergic and cholinergic substances at different environmental temperatures, *J. Physiol.* (*Lond.*) **220**:257.

Barasi, S., and Roberts, M. H. T., 1973, The action of 5-hydroxytryptamine antagonists and precursors on bulbospinal facilitation of spinal reflexes, *Brain Res.* **52**:385.

Barcroft, H., Konzett, H., and Swan, H. J. C., 1951, Observations on the action of the hydrogenated alkaloids of the ergotoxine group on the circulation in man, *J. Physiol.* (*Lond.*) **112**:273.

Barger, G., 1931, *Ergot and Ergotism*, Gurney and Jackson, London.

Beretta, C., Ferrini, R., and Glässer, A. H., 1965, 1-Methyl-8β-carbobenzyloxy-aminomethyl-10α-ergoline, a potent and long-lasting 5-hydroxytryptamine antagonist, *Nature* (*Lond.*) **207**:421.

Bergström, S., Farnebo, L.-O., and Fuxe, K., 1973, Effect of prostaglandin E_2 on central and peripheral catecholamine neurons, *Europ. J. Pharmacol.* **21**:362.

Berridge, M. J., and Prince W. T., 1973, Mode of action of hallucinogenic molecules, *Nature New Biol.* **243**:283.

Bhargava, K. P., Mishra, N., and Tangri, K. K., 1972, An analysis of central adrenoceptors for control of cardiovascular function, *Brit. J. Pharmacol.* **45**:596.

Björklund, A., and Falck, B., 1969, Histochemical characterization of a tryptamine-like substance stored in cells of the mammalian adenohypophysis, *Acta Physiol. Scand.* **77**:475.

Björklund, A., and Nobin, A., 1973, Fluorescence histochemical and microspectrofluorometric mapping of dopamine and noradrenaline cell groups in the rat diencephalon, *Brain Res.* **51**:193.

Björklund, A., Moore, R. Y., Nobin, A., and Stenevi, U., 1973, The organisation of tubero-hypophyseal and reticulo-infundibular catecholamine neuron systems in the rat brain, *Brain Res.* **51**:171.

Bluntschli, H. J., and Goetz, R. H., 1948, The effect of ergot derivatives on the circulation in man with special reference to two new hydrogenated compounds (dihydroergotamine and dihydroergocornine), *Am. Heart J.* **35**:873.

Boakes, R. J., Bradley, P. B., Briggs, I., and Dray, A., 1970, Antagonism of 5-hydroxytryptamine by LSD 25 in the central nervous system: A possible neuronal basis for the actions of LSD 25, *Brit. J. Pharmacol.* **40**:202.

Bolme, P., and Fuxe, K., 1973, Pharmacological studies on a possible role of central noradrenaline neurons in respiratory control, *J. Pharm. Pharmacol.* **25**:351.

Bolme, P., Fuxe, K., and Lidbrink, P., 1972, On the function of central catecholamine neurons—Their role in cardiovascular and arousal mechanisms, *Res. Commun. Chem. Pathol. Pharmacol.* **4**:657.

Borison, H. L., and Clark, W. G., 1967, Drug actions on thermoregulatory mechanisms, *Advan. Pharmacol.* **5**:129.

Bové, F. J., 1970, *The Story of Ergot*, Karger, Basel.

Bradley, P. B., and Briggs, I., 1974, Further studies on the mode of action of psychotomimetic drugs: Antagonism of the excitatory actions of serotonin by methylated derivatives of tryptamine, *Brit. J. Pharmacol.* **50**:345–354.

Brawley, P., and Duffield, J. C., 1972, The pharmacology of hallucinogens, *Pharmol. Rev.* **24**:31.

Brody, T. M., and Diamond, J., 1967, Blockade of the biochemical correlates of contraction and relaxation in uterine and intestinal smooth muscle, *Ann. N.Y. Acad. Sci.* **139**:772.

Bronzino, J. D., 1972, Evoked response study of postulated neural circuit associated with sleep–waking process, *Life Sci.* **11**:419 (Part I).

Bronzino, J. D., Morgane, P. J., and Stern, W. C., 1972, EEG synchronization following application of serotonin to area postrema, *Am. J. Physiol.* **223**:376.

Brown, P. S., 1968, The effect of drugs on induced ovulation, *J. Reprod. Fertil. Suppl.* **4**:61.

Bucknell, A., and Whitney, B., 1964, A preliminary investigation of the pharmacology of the human isolated taenia coli preparation, *Brit. J. Pharmacol.* **23**:164.

Carlsson, A., and Lindqvist, M., 1972, The effect of L-tryptophan and some psychotropic drugs on the formation of 5-hydroxytryptophan in the mouse brain *in vivo, J. Neural Trans.* **33**:23.

Cerletti, A., 1959, in: *Neuropsychopharmacology,* Proceedings of the First International Congress of Neuropsychopharmacology (P. B. Bradley, P. Deniker, and C. Radouco-Thomas, eds.) pp. 117–123, Elsevier, Amsterdam.

Cerletti, A., and Doepfner, W., 1958, Comparative study on the serotonin antagonism of amide derivatives of lysergic acid and of ergot alkaloids, *J. Pharmacol. Exptl. Therap.* **122**:124.

Chalmers, J. P., and Wurtman, R. J., 1971, Participation of central noradrenergic neurons in arterial baroreceptor reflexes in the rabbit, *Circ. Res.* **28**:480.

Chan, P. S., and Ellis, S., 1969, Dihydroergotamine antagonism of glucose release by rabbit liver slices induced by catecholamines, glucagon and 3′,5′-AMP, *Fed. Proc.* **28**:742.

Chu, D., and Stuermer, E., 1973, Studies on the mechanism of action of dihydroergotamine (DHE) on the vascular bed of cat skeletal muscle, *Brit. J. Pharmacol.* **48**:331P.

Cohen, S., 1967, Psychotomimetic agents, *Ann. Rev. Pharmacol.* **7**:301.

Connell, P. H., 1972, Hallucinogens, in: *Side Effects of Drugs*, Vol. VII (L. Meyler and A. Herxheimer, eds.) pp. 38–50, Excerpta Medica, Amsterdam.

Coote, J. H., and Macleod, V.H., 1972, The possibility that noradrenaline is a sympathoinhibitory transmitter in the spinal cord, *J. Physiol.* (*Lond.*) **225**:44P.

Coote, J. H., Hilton, S. M., and Zbrożyna, A. W., 1973, The pontomedullary area integrating the defence reaction in the cat and its influence on muscle blood flow, *J. Physiol.* (*Lond.*) **229**:257.

Corrodi, H., Fuxe, K., and Hökfelt, T., 1967, A possible role played by central monoamine neurons in thermo-regulation, *Acta Physiol. Scand.* **71**:224.

Corrodi, H., Fuke, K., Hökfelt, T., Lidbrink, P., and Ungerstedt, U., 1973, Effect of ergot drugs on central catecholamine neurons: Evidence for a stimulation of central dopamine neurons, *J. Pharm. Pharmacol.* **25**:409.

Costa, E., 1956, Effects of hallucinogenic and tranquilizing drugs on serotonin evoked uterine contractions, *Proc. Soc. Exptl. Biol. Med* **91**:39.

Costa, E., and Zetler, G., 1959, Interactions between epinephrine and some psychotomimetic drugs, *J. Pharmacol. Exptl. Therap.* **125**:230.

Couch, J. R., 1970, Responses of neurons in the raphe nuclei to serotonin, norepinephrine and acetylcholine and their correlation with an excitatory synaptic input, *Brain Res.* **19**:137.

Cranley, J. J., Krause, R. J., Strasser, E. S., and Hafner, C. D., 1963, Impending gangrene of four extremities secondary to ergotism, *New Engl. J. Med.* **269**:727.

Cumings, J. N., and Hilton, B. P., 1971, Effects of methysergide on platelets incubated with reserpine, *Brit. J. Pharmacol.* **42**:611.

Curran, D. A., Hinterberger, H., and Lance, J. W., 1967, Methysergide, *Res. Clin. Stud. Headache* **1**:74.

Dalessio, D. J., 1972, *Wolff's Headache and Other Head Pain*, 3rd ed., Oxford University Press, New York.

Daughaday, W. H., and Jacobs, L. S., 1972, Human prolactin, *Ergeb. Physiol.* **67**:169.

Davidson, N., Edwardson, J. A., and Schwab, D. I., 1969, Agroclavine antagonises depression induced by noradrenaline in the cerebral cortex of the rat, *Nature* (*Lond.*) **223**:1166.

Davies, B. N., Horton, E. W., and Withrington, P. G., 1968, The occurrence of prostaglandin E_2 in splenic venous blood of the dog following splenic nerve stimulation, *Brit. J. Pharmacol.* **32**:127.

de Groat, W. C., and Volle, R. L., 1966*a*, The actions of the catecholamines on transmission in the superior cervical ganglion of the cat, *J. Pharmacol. Exptl. Therap.* **154**:1.

de Groat, W. C., and Volle, R. L., 1966*b*, Interactions between the catecholamines and ganglionic stimulating agents in sympathetic ganglia, *J. Pharmacol. Exptl. Therap.* **154**:200.

Delay, J., and Thuillier, J., 1956, Dualité d'action du diéthylamide de l'acid lysergique sur la contraction utérine provoquée par la 5-hydroxytryptamine (sérotonine), *Compt. Rend. Soc. Biol.* **150**:1335.

Del Bianco, P. L., Franchi, G., Fanciullacci, M., and Sicuteri, F., 1972, Clinical pharmacology of 5-hydroxytryptamine and catecholamines venomotor receptors, *Arch. Int. Pharmacodyn. Therap.* **196**: Suppl. 113.

Del Pozo, E., Brun del Re, R., Varga, L., and Friesen, H., 1972, The inhibition of prolactin secretion in man by CB154 (2-bromo-alpha-ergocryptine), *J. Clin. Endocrinol. Metab.* **35**:768.

Dengler, H. J., Spiegel, H. E., and Titus, E. O., 1961, Effects of drugs on uptake of isotopic norepinephrine by cat tissues, *Nature* (*Lond.*) **191**:816.

Der Marderosian, A., 1967, Hallucinogenic indole compounds from higher plants, *Lloydia* **30**:23.

Díaz, J.-L., and Huttunen, M. O., 1971, Persistent increase in brain serotonin turnover after chronic administration of LSD in the rat, *Science* **174**:62.

Dishotsky, N. I., Loughman, W. D., Mogar, R. E., and Lipscomb, W. R., 1971, LSD and genetic damage, *Science* **172**:431.

Downman, C. B. B., 1972, The vasomotor centre, in: *Modern Trends in Physiology* (C. B. B. Downman, ed.) pp. 292–308, Butterworth, London.

Dyer, D. C., and Gant, D. W., 1973, Vasoconstriction produced by hallucinogens on isolated human and sheep umbilical vasculature, *J. Pharmacol. Exptl. Therap.* **184**:366.

Eiduson, S., Geller, E., Yuwiler, A., and Eiduson, B. T., 1964, *Biochemistry and Behavior*, Van Nostrand, Princeton, N.J.

Erspamer, V., 1966, Peripheral physiological and pharmacological actions of indolealkylamines, *Handbook Exptl. Pharmacol.* **19**:245.

European Breast Cancer Group, 1972, Clinical trial of 2-Br-α-ergocryptine (CB 154) in advanced breast cancer, *Europ. J. Cancer* **8**:155.

Evarts, E. V., 1957, A review of the neurophysiological effects of lysergic acid diethylamide (LSD) and other psychotomimetic agents, *Ann. N.Y. Acad. Sci.* **66**:479.

Ezdinli, E. Z., Rouliah, J., Owens, G., and Sokal, J. E., 1968, Effect of high spinal cord section on epinephrine hyperglycemia, *Am. J. Physiol.* **214**:1019.

Fain, J. N., 1973, Biochemical aspects of drug and hormone action on adipose tissue, *Pharmacol. Rev.* **25**:67.

Fanchamps, A., Doepfner, W., Weidmann, H., and Cerletti, A., 1960, Pharmakologische Charakterisierung von Deseril, einem Serotonin-Antagonisten, *Schweiz. Med. Wschr.* **90**:1040.

Farnebo, L.-O., and Hamberger, B., 1971, Drug-induced changes in the release of [^{3}H]-noradrenaline from field stimulated rat iris, *Brit. J. Pharmacol.* **43**:97.

Fedotin, M. S., and Hartmann, C., 1970, Ergotamine poisoning producing renal arterial spasm, *New Engl. J. Med.* **283**:518.

Florendo, N. T., Barrnett, R. J., and Greengard, P., 1971, Cyclic 3′,5′-nucleotide phosphodiesterase: Cytochemical localization in cerebral cortex, *Science* **173**:745.

Flückiger, E., and Wagner, H. R., 1968, 2-Br-α-ergokryptin: Beeinflussung von Fertilität und Laktation bei der Ratte, *Experientia* **24**:1130.

Fredholm, B., and Rosell, S., 1968, Effects of adrenergic blocking agents on lipid mobilization from canine subcutaneous adipose tissue after sympathetic nerve stimulation, *J. Pharmacol. Exptl. Therap.* **159**:1.

Freedman, D. X., 1963, Psychotomimetic drugs and brain biogenic amines, *Am. J. Psychiat.* **119**:843.

Freedman, D. X., 1969, The psychopharmacology of hallucinogenic agents, *Ann. Rev. Med.* **20**:409.

Freedman, D. X., Gottlieb, R., and Lovell, R. A., 1970, Psychotomimetic drugs and brain 5-hydroxytryptamine metabolism, *Biochem. Pharmacol.* **19**:1181.

Fregnan, G. B., and Glässer, A. H., 1968, Structure–activity relationship of various acyl derivatives of 6-methyl-8β-aminomethyl-10α-ergoline (dihydrolysergamine), *Experientia* **24**:150.

Freis, E. D., Stanton, J. R., Litter, J., Culbertson, J. W., Halperin, M. H., Moister, F. C., and Wilkins, R. W., 1949, The hemodynamic effects of hypotensive drugs in man. II. Dihydroergocornine, *J. Clin. Invest.* **28**:1387.

Fuxe, K., and Owman, C., 1965, Cellular localization of monoamines in the area postrema of certain mammals, *J. Comp. Neurol.* **125**:337.

Fuxe, K., and Sjöqvist, F., 1972, Hypothermic effect of apomorphine in the mouse, *J. Pharm. Pharmacol.* **24**:702.

Gaddum, J. H., and Hameed, K. A., 1954, Drugs which antagonize 5-hydroxytryptamine. *Brit. J. Pharmacol.* **9**:240.

Gaddum, J. H., Hebb, C. O., Silver, A., and Swan, A. A. B., 1953, 5-Hydroxytryptamine: Pharmacological action and destruction in perfused lungs, *Quart. J. Exptl. Physiol.* **38**:255.

Gessner, P. K., 1970, Pharmacological studies of 5-methoxy-*N,N*-dimethyltryptamine, LSD and other hallucinogens, in: *Psychotomimetic Drugs* (D. H. Efron, ed.) pp. 105–118, Raven Press, New York.

Ginzel, K. H., and Kottegoda, S. R., 1953, A study of the vascular actions of 5-hydroxytryptamine, tryptamine, adrenaline and noradrenaline, *Quart. J. Exptl. Physiol.* **38**:225.

Gothelf, B., and Ellis, S., 1972, Effect of dihydroergotamine (DHE) on liver glycogenolysis and hyperglycemia induced by epinephrine, glucagon and cyclic AMP (cAMP) in the rat, in: *Fifth International Congress of Pharmacology,* San Francisco, p. 86 (abst.).

Graham, J. R., 1967, Methysergide, *Practitioner* **198**:302.

Graham, J. R., Suby, H. I., Le Compte, P. M., and Sadowsky, N. L., 1967, Inflammatory fibrosis associated with methysergide therapy, *Res. Clin. Stud. Headache* **1**:123.

Greenfield, A. D. M., 1966, Survey of the evidence for active neurogenic vasodilatation in man, *Fed. Proc.* **25**:1607.

Haefely, W. E., 1969, Effects of catecholamines in the cat superior cervical ganglion and their postulated rôle as physiological modulators of ganglionic transmission, *Prog. Brain Res.* **31**:61.

Haeusler, G., 1973, Activation of the central pathway of the baroreceptor reflex, a possible mechanism of the hypotensive action of Clonidine, *Naunyn-Schmiedeberg's Arch. Pharmakol.* **278**:231.

Haigler, H. J., and Aghajanian, G. K., 1972, Mescaline and LSD: Direct and indirect effects on serotonin-containing neurons in brain, *Europ. J. Pharmacol.* **21**:53.

Harvey, S. C., Wang, C.-Y., and Nickerson, M., 1951, Blockade of epinephrine-induced hyperglycemia, *J. Pharmacol. Exptl. Therap.* **104**:363.

Hasse, H. E., Scheifgen, W., and Schönhöfer, P. S., 1971, Notfallsituationen bei jugendlichen Drogenkonsumenten, *Deutsch. Med. Wschr.* **96**:449.

Hellon, R., 1972, Central transmitters and thermoregulation, in: *Essays on Temperature Regulation* (J. Bligh and R. E. Moore, eds.) pp. 71–85, North-Holland, Amsterdam.

Heyck, H., 1969, Pathogenesis of migraine, *Res. Clin. Stud. Headache* **2**:1.

Hilton, B. P., and Cumings, J. N., 1972, 5-Hydroxytryptamine levels and platelet aggregation responses in subjects with acute migraine headache, *J. Neurol. Neurosurg. Psychiat.* **35**:505.

Himms-Hagen, J., 1970, Adrenergic receptors for metabolic responses in adipose tissue, *Fed. Proc.* **29**:1388.

Hoffer, A., and Osmond, H., 1967, *The Hallucinogens,* Academic Press, New York.

Hökfelt, T., and Fuxe, K., 1972*a*, On the morphology and the neuroendocrine role of the hypothalamic catecholamine neurons, in: *Brain–Endocrine Interaction. Median Eminence: Structure and Function* (K. M. Knigge, D. E. Scott, and A. Weindl, eds.) pp. 181–223, Karger, Basel.

Hökfelt, T., and Fuxe, K., 1972*b*, Effects of prolactin and ergot alkaloids on the tuberoinfundibular dopamine (DA) neurons, *Neuroendocrinology* **9**:100.

Hollister, L. E., 1972, Psychiatric syndromes due to drugs, in: *Drug-Induced Diseases*, Vol. 4 (L. Meyler and H. M. Peck, eds.) pp. 561–570, Excerpta Medica, Amsterdam.

Horeyseck, G., Jänig, W., Kirchner, F., and Thämer, V., 1972, Electrophysiological studies on the hindlimb vasodilators on anesthesized cats, *Pflügers Arch.* **332**: Suppl. R64.

Horita, A., and Dille, J. M., 1954, Pyretogenic effect of lysergic acid diethylamide, *Science* **120**:1100.

Horita, A., and Hamilton, A. E., 1973, The effects of DL-α-methyltyrosine and L-DOPA on the hyperthermic and behavioral actions of LSD in rabbits, *Neuropharmacology,* **12**:471.

Horn, G., and McKay, J. M., 1973, Effects of lysergic acid diethylamide on the spontaneous activity and visual receptive fields of cells in the lateral geniculate nucleus of the cat, *Exptl. Brain. Res.* **17**:271.

Hornbrook, K. R., 1970, Adrenergic receptors for metabolic responses in the liver, *Fed. Proc.* **29**:1381.

Hornbrook, K. R., and Brody, T. M., 1963, Phosphorylase activity in rat liver and skeletal muscle after catecholamines, *Biochem. Pharmacol.* **12**:1407.

Innes, I. R., 1962, Identification of the smooth muscle excitatory receptors for ergot alkaloids, *Brit. J. Pharmacol.* **19**:120.

Isbell, H., and Gorodetsky, C. W., 1966, Effect of alkaloids of ololiuqui in man, *Psychopharmacologia* (*Berl.*) **8**:331.

Isbell, H., and Logan, C. R., 1957, Studies on the diethylamide of lysergic acid. II. Effects of chlorpromazine, azacyclonol and reserpine on the intensity of the LSD-reaction, *A.M.A. Arch. Neurol. Psychiat.* **77**:350.

Isbell, H., Miner, E. J., and Logan, C. R., 1959, Relationships of psychotomimetic to antiserotonin potencies of congeners of lysergic acid diethylamide (LSD-25), *Psychopharmacologia* (*Berl.*) **1**:20.

Ito, A., and Schanberg, S. M., 1972, Central nervous system mechanisms responsible for blood pressure elevation induced by *p*-chlorphenylalanine, *J. Pharmacol. Exptl. Therap.* **181**:65.

Iwangoff, P., and Enz, A., 1972, The influence of various dihydroergotamine analogues on cyclic adenosine-3′,5′-monophosphate phosphodiesterase in the grey matter of cat brain *in vitro*, *Agents and Actions* **2**:223.

Jacobson, C. B., and Berlin, C. M., 1972, Possible reproductive detriment in LSD users, *J.A.M.A.* **222**:1367.

Jouvet, M., 1972, The role of monoamines and acetylcholine-containing neurons in the regulation of the sleep-waking cycle, *Ergeb. Physiol.* **64**:166.

Karlsberg, P., Elliott, H. W., and Adams, J. E., 1963, Effect of various pharmacologic agents on cerebral arteries, *Neurology* **13**:772.

Katz, R. I., and Kopin, I. J., 1969, Effect of D-LSD and related compounds on release of norepinephrine-H^3 and serotonin-H^3 evoked from brain slices by electrical stimulation, *Pharmacol. Res. Commun.* **1**:54.

Kebabian, J. W., and Greengard, P., 1971, Dopamine-sensitive adenyl cyclase: Possible role in synaptic transmission, *Science* **174**:1346.

Key, B. J., 1965*a*, Effect of lysergic acid diethylamide on potentials evoked in the specific sensory pathways, *Brit. Med. Bull.* **21**:30.

Key, B. J., 1965*b*, The effects of drugs in relation to the afferent collateral system of the brain stem, *Electroenceph. Clin. Neurophysiol.* **18**:670.

King, A. R., Seymour, K. A., and Martin, I. L., 1972, Reversal learning enhanced by LSD 25: Correlation with levels of brain amines, *Psychopharmacologia* (*Ber.*) **26**: Suppl. 121.

Koella, W. P., 1969, Neurohumoral aspects of sleep control, *Biol. Psychiat.* **1**:161.

Konzett, H., 1960, Specific antagonism of dibenamine to ergometrine, in: *Adrenergic Mechanisms*, CIBA Foundation Symposium (J. R. Vane, G. E. W. Wolstenholme, and M. O'Connor, eds.) pp. 463–465, J. & A. Churchill, London.

Konzett, H., and Rothlin, E., 1953, Investigations on the hypotensive effect of the hydrogenated ergot alkaloids, *Brit. J. Pharmacol.* **8**:201.

Kovalyov, G. V., 1967, Localization and characteristics of the influence of some neurotropic drugs on the bulbar vasomotor centre, *Prog. Brain Res.* **20**:187.

Krnjević, K., and Phillis, J. W., 1963, Actions of certain amines on cerebral cortical neurones, *Brit. J. Pharmacol.* **20**:471.

Levy, B., and Ahlquist, R. P., 1961, An analysis of adrenergic blocking activity, *J. Pharmacol. Exptl. Therap.* **133**:202.

Levy, B., and Tozzi, S., 1963, The adrenergic receptive mechanism of the rat uterus, *J. Pharmacol. Exptl. Therap.* **142**:178.

Lewis, P. J., and Lee, M. R., 1972, Renin release in the rabbit produced by ergometrine infusion, *Brit. J. Exptl. Pathol.* **53**:150.

Libet, B., 1970, Generation of slow inhibitory and excitatory postsynaptic potentials, *Fed. Proc.* **29**:1945.

Lin, R. C., Ngai, S. H., and Costa, E., 1969, Lysergic acid diethylamide: Role in conversion of plasma tryptophan to brain serotonin (5-hydroxytryptamine), *Science* **166**:237.

Lomax, P., and Schönbaum, E. (eds.), 1973, *The Pharmacology of Thermoregulation*, Karger, Basel.

Long, S. Y., 1972, Does LSD induce chromosomal damage and malformations? A review of the literature, *Teratology* **6**:75.

Mabry, P. O., and Campbell, B. A., 1973, Serotonergic inhibition of catecholamine-induced behavioral arousal, *Brain Res.* **49**:381.

McCann, S. M., Kalra, P. S., Donoso, A. O., Bishop, W., Schneider, H. P. G., Fawcett, C. P., and Krulich, L., 1972, The role of monoamines in the control of gonado-tropin and prolactin secretion, in: *Brain-Endocrine Interaction. Median Eminence: Structure and Function* (K. M. Knigge, D. E. Scott, and A. Weindl, eds.) pp. 224–235, Karger, Basel.

McCulloch, M. W., Rand, M. J., and Story, D. F., 1972, Inhibition of ^{3}H-noradrenaline release from sympathetic nerves of guinea-pig atria by a presynaptic α-adrenoceptor mechanism, *Brit. J. Pharmacol.* **46**:523.

Meites, J., and Clemens, J. A., 1972, Hypothalamic control of prolactin secretion, *Vitam. Horm.* **30**:165.

Meites, J., Lu, K. H,. Wuttke, W., Welsch, C. W., Nagasawa, H., and Quadri, S. K., 1972, Recent studies on functions and control of prolactin secretion in rats, *Rec. Prog. Horm. Res.* **28**:471.

Meldrum, B. S., and Naquet, R., 1971, Effects of psilocybin, dimethyltryptamine, mescaline and various lysergic acid derivatives on the EEG and on photically induced epilepsy in the baboon (*Papio papio*), *Electroenceph. Clin. Neurophysiol.* **31**:563.

Mellander, S., and Johansson, B., 1968, Control of resistance, exchange and capacitance functions in the peripheral circulation, *Pharmacol. Rev.* **20**:117.

Mellander, S., and Nordenfelt, I., 1970, Comparative effects of dihydroergotamine and noradrenaline on resistance, exchange and capacitance functions in the peripheral circulation, *Clin. Sci.* **39**:183.

Miller, J. W., 1967, Adrenergic receptors in the myometrium, *Ann. N.Y. Acad. Sci.* **139**:788.

Miller, M. D., and Marshall, J. M., 1965, Uterine response to nerve stimulation; relation to hormonal status and catecholamines, *Am. J. Physiol.* **209**:859.

Monachon, M.-A., Burkard, W. P., Jalfre, M., and Haefely, W., 1972, Blockade of central 5-hydroxytryptamine receptors by methiothepin, *Naunyn-Schmiedeberg's Arch. Pharmakol.* **274**:192.

Morest, D. K., 1967, Experimental study of the projections of the nucleus of the tractus solitarius and the area postrema of the cat, *J. Comp. Neurol.* **130**:277.

Morgane, P. J., and Stern, W. C., 1972, Relationship of sleep to neuroanatomical circuits, biochemistry and behavior, *Ann. N.Y. Acad. Sci.* **193**:95.

Murad, F., Chi, Y.-M., Rall, T. W., and Sutherland, E. W., 1962, Adenyl cyclase III: The effect of catecholamines and choline esters on the formation of adenosine 3′,5′-phosphate by preparations from cardiac muscle and liver, *J. Biol. Chem.* **237**:1233.

Nakano, J., Ishii, T., Oliver, R. D., and Gin, A. C., 1969, Effect of dihydroergotamine and propranolol on dibutyryl cyclic 3′,5′-AMP–induced lipolysis in isolated rat fat cells, *Proc. Soc. Exptl. Biol. Med.* **132**:150.

Nichols, W. W., 1972, The relationship of chromosome aberrations to drugs, in: *Drug-Induced Diseases*, Vol. 4 (L. Meyler and H. M. Peck, eds.) pp. 60–80, Excerpta Medica, Amsterdam.

Nishi, S,. 1970, Cholinergic and adrenergic receptors at sympathetic preganglionic nerve terminals, *Fed. Proc.* **29**:1957.

Northrop, G., and Parks, R. E., Jr., 1964, The effects of adrenergic blocking agents and theophylline on 3′,5′-AMP–induced hyperglycemia, *J. Pharmacol. Exptl. Therap.* **145**:87.

Owen, D. A. A., and Stuermer, E., 1971, Effect of dihydroergotamine (DHG) on the capacitance, resistance and precapillary sphincter vessels of denervated cat skeletal muscle, *Brit. J. Pharmacol.* **42**:655.

Owen, D. A. A., and Stuermer, E., 1972, The effects of Hydergine on acutely denervated cat skeletal muscle vasculature, *Nauyn-Schmiedeberg's Arch. Pharmakol.* **272**:395.

Pacha, W., and Salzmann, R., 1970, Inhibition of the re-uptake of neuronally liberated noradrenaline and α-receptor blocking action of some ergot alkaloids, *Brit. J. Pharmacol.* **38**:439.

Palmer, G. C., and Burks, T. F., 1971, Central and peripheral adrenergic blocking actions of LSD and BOL, *Europ. J. Pharmacol.* **16**:113.

Porter, J. C., Kamberi, I. A., and Ondo, J. G., 1972, Role of biogenic amines and cerebrospinal fluid in the neurovascular transmittal of hypophysiotrophic substances, in: *Brain–Endocrine Interaction. Median Eminence: Structure and Function* (K. M. Knigge, D. E. Scott, and A. Weindl, eds.) pp. 245–253, Karger, Basel.

Purpura, D. P., 1957, Experimental analysis of the inhibitory action of lysergic acid diethylamide on cortical dendritic activity, *Ann. N.Y. Acad. Sci.* **66**:515.

Ramstad, E., 1968, Chemistry of alkaloid formation in ergot, *Lloydia* **31**:327.

Richardson, B. P., 1973, Evidence for a physiological role of prolactin in osmoregulation in the rat after its inhibition by 2-bromo-α-ergokryptine, *Brit. J. Pharmacol.* **47**:623.

Roberts, M. H. T., and Straughan, D. W., 1967, Excitation and depression of cortical neurones by 5-hydroxytryptamine, *J. Physiol.* (*Lond.*) **193**:269.

Rosenberg, F. J., and DiStefano, V., 1962, A central nervous system component of epinephrine hyperglycemia, *Am. J. Physiol.* **203**:782.

Rothlin, E., 1947, The pharmacology of the natural and dihydrogenated alkaloids of ergot, *Bull. Schweiz. Akad. Med. Wiss.* **2**:249.

Rothlin, E., 1957, Pharmacology of lysergic acid diethylamide and some of its related compounds, *J. Pharm. Pharmacol.* **9**:569.

Rothlin, E., Konzett, H., and Cerletti, A., 1954, The antagonism of ergot alkaloids towards the inhibitory response of the isolated rabbit intestine to epinephrine and norepinephrine, *J. Pharmacol. Exptl. Therap.* **112**:185.

Salmoiraghi, G. C., McCubbin, J. W., and Page, I. H., 1957, Effects of *d*-lysergic acid diethylamide and its brom derivative on cardiovascular responses to serotonin and on arterial pressure, *J. Pharmacol. Exptl. Therap.* **119**:240.

Samanin, R., Valzelli, L., and Gumulka, W., 1972, Inhibitory effect of midbrain raphe stimulation on cortical evoked potentials in rats, *Psychopharmacologia* (*Berl.*) **24**:373.

Savini, E. C., 1956, The antagonism between 5-hydroxytryptamine and certain derivatives of lysergic acid, *Brit. J. Pharmacol.* **11**:313.

Saxena, P. R., 1972, The effects of antimigraine drugs on the vascular responses by 5-hydroxytryptamine and related biogenic substances on the external carotid bed of dogs: Possible pharmacological implications to their antimigraine action, *Headache* **12**:44.

Schally, A. V., Arimura, A., and Kastin, A. J., 1973, Hypothalamic regulatory hormones, *Science* **179**:341.

Schmitt, H., and Fénard, S., 1970, Effects des alcaloïdes de l'ergot de seigle sur les centres vasomoteurs et leur inhibition par la clonidine, *Compt. Rend. Soc. Biol.* **164**:1006.

Shaar, C. J., and Clemens, J. A., 1972, Inhibition of lactation and prolactin secretion in rats by ergot alkaloids, *Endocrinology* **90**:285.

Share, N. N., 1973, "Alpha" and "beta" adrenergic receptors in the medullary vasomotor center of the cat, *Arch. Int. Pharmacodyn. Therap.* **202**:362.

Shemano, I., and Nickerson, M., 1958, Effect of ambient temperature on thermal responses to drugs, *Can. J. Biochem. Physiol.* **36**:1243.

Shields, P. J., and Eccleston, D., 1973, Evidence for the synthesis and storage of 5-hydroxytryptamine in two separate pools in the brain, *J. Neurochem.* **20**:881.

Sicuteri, F., 1967, Vasoneuractive substances and their implication in vascular pain, *Res. Clin. Stud. Headache* **1**:6.

Sicuteri, F., Buffoni, F., Anselmi, B., and Del Bianco, P. L., 1972, An enzyme (MAO) defect on the platelets in migraine, *Res. Clin. Stud. Headache* **3**:245.

Sicuteri, F., Anselmi, B., and Del Bianco, P. L., 1973, 5-Hydroxytryptamine supersensitivity as a new theory of headache and central pain: A clinical pharmacological approach with *p*-chlorophenylalanine, *Psychopharmacologia* (*Berl.*) **29**:347.

Simmonds, M. A., 1970, Effect of environmental temperature on the turnover of 5-hydroxytryptamine in various areas of rat brain, *J. Physiol.* (*Lond.*) **211**:93.

Smart, R. G., and Bateman, K., 1967, Unfavourable reactions on LSD: A review and analysis of the available case reports, *Can. Med. Ass. J.* **97**:1214.

Starke, K., 1972, Alpha sympathomimetic inhibition of adrenergic and cholinergic transmission in the rabbit heart, *Naunyn-Schmiedeberg's Arch. Pharmakol.* **274**:18.

Stern, W. C., Morgane, P. J., and Bronzino, J. D., 1972, LSD: Effects on sleep patterns and spiking activity in the lateral geniculate nucleus, *Brain Res.* **41**:199.

Stjärne, L., 1973, Alpha-adrenoceptor mediated feedback control of sympathetic neurotransmitter secretion in guinea-pig vas deferens, *Nature New Biol.* **241**:190.

Stoll, B. A., 1972, Brain catecholamines and breast cancer: A hypothesis, *Lancet* **1**:431.

Stone, T. W., 1973, Studies on the central nervous system effects of agroclavine, an ergot alkaloid, *Arch. Int. Pharmacodyn. Therap.* **202**:62.

Tabushi, K., and Himwich, H. E., 1971, Electroencephalographic study of the effects of methysergide on sleep in the rabbit, *Electroenceph. Clin. Neurophysiol.* **31**:491.

Taylor, R. L., Maurer, J. I., and Tinklenberg, J. R., 1970, Management of "bad trips" in an evolving drug scene, *J.A.M.A.* **213**:422.

Tebēcis, A. K., and Di Maria, A., 1972, A re-evaluation of the mode of action of 5-hydroxytryptamine on lateral geniculate neurones: Comparison with catecholamines and LSD, *Exptl. Brain. Res.* **14**:480.

Ulrich, J., and Siggaard-Andersen, J., 1972, Vascular effects of dihydrogenated ergot alkaloids: Comparative effects of dihydroergostine and dihydroergotamine on the blood flow and the capacitance vessels in the human calf studied by plethysmography, *Angiology* **22**:622.

Uvnäs, B., 1960, Central cardiovascular control, in: *Handbook of Physiology*, Section 1: *Neurophysiology*, Vol. II (J. Field, ed.) pp. 1131–1162, American Physiological Society, Washington, D.C.

Voss, E. W., Jr., Babb, J. E., Metzel, P., and Winkelhake, J. L., 1973, *In vitro* effect of *d*-lysergic acid diethylamide on immunoglobulin synthesis, *Biochem. Biophys. Res. Commun.* **50**:950.

Vuillon-Cacciuttolo, G., and Balzano, E., 1972, Action de quatre dérivës de l'ergot sur la photosensibilité de l'E.E.G. du *Papio papio*, *J. Pharmacol.* (*Paris*) **3**:31.

Walter, S., Balzano, E., Vuillon-Cacciuttolo, G., and Naquet, R., 1971, Effets comportementaux et électrographiques du diéthylamide de l'acide D-lysergique (LSD-25) sur le *Papio papio* photosensible, *Electroenceph. Clin. Neurophysiol.* **30**:294.

Wang, S. C., 1965, Emetic and antiemetic drugs, in: *Physiological Pharmacology*, Vol. 2 (W. S. Root and F. G. Hofmann, eds.) pp. 255–328, Academic Press, London.

Weiss, B. L., and Aghajanian, G. K., 1971, Activation of brain serotonin metabolism by heat: Role of midbrain raphe neurons, *Brain Res.* **26**:37.

White, R. P., Heaton, J. A., and Denton, I. C., 1971, Pharmacological comparison of prostaglandin $F_{2\alpha}$, serotonin and norepinephrine on cerebrovascular tone of monkey, *Europ. J. Pharmacol.* **15**:300.

Whitney, B., 1965, A preliminary investigation of the pharmacology of longitudinal muscle strips from human isolated jejunum, *J. Pharm. Pharmacol.* **17**:465.

Willems, J. L., 1972, On the pharmacology of autonomic ganglia, *Arch. Int. Pharmacodyn. Therap.* **196**: Suppl. 244.

Wuttke, W., Cassell, E. and Meites, J., 1971, Effects of ergocornine on serum prolactin and LH, and on hypothalamic contents of PIF and LRF, *Endocrinology*, **88**:737.

Ylitalo, P., Tammisto, T., and Pohto, P., 1970, Effect of anaesthesia on the behaviour of exogenous 5HT in area postrema of rat and mouse brain studied by fluorescence microscopy, *Ann. Med. Exptl. Fenn.* **48**:94.

Yui, T., and Takeo, Y., 1958, Neuropharmacological studies on a new series of ergot alkaloids, *Jap. J. Pharmacol.* **7**:157.

Yui, T., and Takeo, Y., 1964, Increase in anti-5HT activity by 1-methylation of clavine-type ergot alkaloids, *Jap. J. Pharmacol.* **14**:107.

Index